Management of
Cardiothoracic Trauma

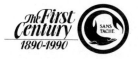

The First Century 1890-1990 SANS TACHE

Management of Cardiothoracic Trauma

Edited by

Stephen Z. Turney, M.D., F.A.C.S.

Chief, Thoracic Surgery
Maryland Institute for Emergency Medical Services Systems
Associate Professor of Surgery
University of Maryland School of Medicine
Baltimore, Maryland

Aurelio Rodriguez, M.D., F.A.C.S.

Attending Traumatologist and Thoracic Surgeon
Maryland Institute for Emergency Medical Services Systems
Assistant Professor of Surgery
University of Maryland School of Medicine
Baltimore, Maryland

R Adams Cowley, M.D., F.A.C.S.

Founder and Director Emeritus
Maryland Institute for Emergency Medical Services Systems
Professor of Thoracic and Cardiovascular Surgery
University of Maryland School of Medicine
Director, Charles McC. Mathias, Jr., National Study Center for Trauma
    and Emergency Medical Systems
Baltimore, Maryland

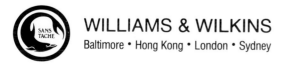

WILLIAMS & WILKINS
Baltimore • Hong Kong • London • Sydney

Editor: Carol-Lynn Brown
Associate Editor: Victoria M. Vaughn
Copy Editor: Peter Binns
Designer: Karen Klinedinst
Illustration Planner: Ray Lowman
Production Coordinator: Barbara J. Felton

Copyright © 1990
Williams & Wilkins
428 East Preston Street
Baltimore, Maryland 21202, USA

Accurate indications, adverse reactions, and dosage schedules for drugs are provided in this book, but it is possible that they may change. The reader is urged to review the package information data of the manufacturers of the medications mentioned.

Printed in the United States of America

Library of Congress Cataloging-in-Publication Data

Management of cardiothoracic trauma / edited by Stephen Z. Turney, Aurelio Rodriguez, R Adams Cowley.
    p.   cm.
   Includes bibliographical references.
   ISBN 0-683-08497-6
   1. Chest—wounds and injuries—Treatment.   2. Heart—wounds and injuries—Treatment.   3. Surgical emergencies.   4. Critical care medicine.   I. Turney, Stephen Z.   II. Rodriguez, Aurelio.   III. Cowley, R Adams.
   [DNLM: 1. Critical Care.   2. Heart Injuries—therapy.   3. Thoracic Injuries—therapy.   WF 985 M266]
   RD536.M258   1990
   617.5'4044—dc20
   DNLM/DLC
   for Library of Congress   90-12013
                                       CIP

90 91 92 93 94
1 2 3 4 5 6 7 8 9 10

To Carolyn, Wendy, Roberta, our children and their families for their support and love

and

To Fiorindo A. Simeone, M.D., surgeon, teacher, and mentor

Foreword

Violence, whether accidental or occasioned by man's inhumanity to fellow man, individually or between organized groups in warfare, has furnished abundant opportunity for observation of the victims and has enabled therapeutic trials and advancement under the stimulus of harsh necessity. Yet, the thorax was the last of the body cavities to become the domain of the surgeon.

From the beginning, the cause of thoracic injuries could generally be attributed to war and violence. Now these injuries are part of the spectrum of trauma associated with our increased tempo of modern living and with technical advances in machines of transport and arms. The trauma surgeon is, by necessity, a generalist, competent in many aspects of surgical and critical care management. While cardiothoracic trauma is a major cause of death and disability, the traumatologist will need to call on the fully trained thoracic surgeon for only relatively severe injuries, those requiring the special expertise acquired in repetitive operations on the heart, great vessels, and major thoracic organs. The trauma surgeon and the emergency room physician should be able to recognize and treat the relatively minor thoracic injuries that constitute the majority of these cases. This book will make the trauma surgeon conversant in the discipline of cardiothoracic trauma and will refresh the thoracic surgeon in the current management of all aspects of the field.

Finally, I wish to express my great pride in and enthusiastic support for the work done by Drs. Turney and Rodriguez in preparing this book.

R Adams Cowley, M.D.

Preface

It has been stated that "injuries are the most serious health problem facing developed societies" (1). Cardiothoracic trauma occurs in about one-third of all acute admissions to a trauma center. From July 1983 through June 1986, 1,704 of the 5,390 acute admissions (32%) to the Maryland Institute for Emergency Medical Services Systems (MIEMSS) Shock Trauma Center in Baltimore had a diagnosis of chest trauma. Seen from this perspective, cardiothoracic trauma is a major health problem fully deserving the attention of the health care system, in particular the trauma care system.

In Maryland, trauma care happens to be embodied in MIEMSS, an agency of state government and a component of the University of Maryland, providing care for the trauma victim from the scene of injury to recovery and rehabilitation, as well as engaging in research and education in trauma-related fields (2). Much of the material presented herein is taken from the experience gained in patient care by the editors and by many others at MIEMSS, but many of the contributors are not MIEMSS faculty or alumni. This is particularly evident in the book's coverage of penetrating injuries, because MIEMSS is not the primary care facility for these cases. The contributors come from many disciplines, emphasizing the multidisciplinary approach required to manage the seriously injured patient successfully. Where possible, we have tried to avoid duplication in the text, although a given procedure or concept may be discussed from the perspective of more than one discipline.

As reflected in the title of this book, the *management* of cardiothoracic trauma will be emphasized. The reader is taken along a fairly orderly route from the scene of injury to initial evaluation and stabilization in the trauma care facility. There are detailed presentations of thoracic imaging techniques and radiographic findings in trauma, anesthesia administration, and critical care considerations. There is also a chapter on the use of heart-assist devices, as applicable to the trauma patient.

Finally, specific cardiothoracic injuries are covered in the last 15 chapters. We have tried to include the full spectrum of cardiothoracic trauma. There are several chapters on penetrating and blunt injuries, each associated with distinct problems in diagnosis and management. Likewise, children and the elderly with chest injuries present uniquely different challenges and are discussed in separate chapters. A special chapter on civilian combat victims is presented apropos of the violence becoming epidemic in our urban centers. These chapters are tailored to the surgeon needing up-to-date information on understanding and managing each injury, with enough background material to refresh the experienced and educate the less experienced clinician. The bibliographies are provided for those needing more substantive detail than space permits in the text.

REFERENCES
1. Baker SP, O'Neill B, Karpf RS. The injury fact book. Lexington: Lexington Books, 1984:1.
2. Cowley RA. A total emergency medical system for the State of Maryland. Md State Med J 1975;24:37–45.

Acknowledgments

The editors wish to acknowledge the following individuals for their invaluable contributions to the preparation of this book: Linda J. Kesselring of the MIEMSS Editorial Staff for her enduring and highly capable assistance in reviewing, editing, and organizing the material from the many contributors and serving as the principal liaison with the publisher; Tom Stevenson, medical illustrator *par excellence*, whose many original contributions provide a unifying visual perspective to the book, helping bridge the variation of literary style among the many contributors; Andy Trohanis, Jim Brown, Jim Faulkner, and the staff of MIEMSS Illustrative Services for their many contributions; Ronda Jennings, medical secretary, for her assistance and patience; and finally the entire staff of MIEMSS, without whom the experience in cardiothoracic trauma reflected in this book would never have happened.

S. Z. T.
A. R.
R A. C.

Contributors

Safuh Attar, M.D., Ph.D. (c), F.A.C.S., F.A.C.C.
Professor of Surgery
Division of Thoracic and Cardiovascular
Surgery
University of Maryland School of Medicine
Baltimore, Maryland

James L. Baker, M.D., M.P.H., F.A.C.E.P.
Assistant Professor
Division of Emergency Medicine
The Johns Hopkins University School of
Medicine
Baltimore, Maryland

**Timothy G. Buchman, Ph.D., M.D., F.A.C.S.,
F.C.C.M.**
Assistant Professor of Surgery
Director, Adult Trauma Services
The Johns Hopkins University School of
Medicine
Baltimore, Maryland

Ellis S. Caplan, M.D., F.A.C.P.
Associate Professor of Medicine
University of Maryland School of Medicine
Chief, Infectious Diseases
Maryland Institute for Emergency Medical
Services Systems
Baltimore, Maryland

Alfred S. Casale, M.D.
Assistant Professor of Cardiac Surgery
The Johns Hopkins University School of
Medicine
Baltimore, Maryland

Joel D. Cooper, M.D., F.A.C.S.
Professor of Surgery
Chief, Section of Thoracic Surgery
Division of Cardiovascular Surgery
Washington University School of Medicine
St. Louis, Missouri

Martin R. Eichelberger, M.D.
Professor of Surgery and Pediatrics
George Washington University School of
Medicine and Health Sciences
Washington, D.C.

Steven K. Gitterman, M.D., Ph.D.
Adjunct Assistant Professor of Medicine
Department of Infectious Diseases
University of Maryland School of Medicine
Baltimore, Maryland

Wendell A. Goins, M.D.
Attending in General and Trauma Surgery
Attending in Surgical Critical Care
District of Columbia General Hospital
Clinical Assistant Professor of Surgery
Howard University College of Medicine
Washington, D.C.

John R. Hankins, M.D., F.A.C.S.
Professor of Surgery (Retired)
Division of Thoracic and Cardiovascular
Surgery
University of Maryland School of Medicine
Baltimore, Maryland

Rao R. Ivatury, M.D., F.A.C.S.
Associate Professor of Surgery
New York Medical College
Director, SICU & Trauma
Lincoln Medical & Mental Health Center
Bronx, New York

Larry R. Kaiser, M.D.
Assistant Professor of Surgery
Section of Thoracic Surgery
Division of Cardiothoracic Surgery
Washington University School of Medicine
St. Louis, Missouri

DiAnne J. Leonard, M.D.
Clinical Assistant Professor of Surgery
Jefferson Medical College
Philadelphia, Pennsylvania
Associate in Trauma Surgery and Critical Care
Geisinger Medical Center
Danville, Pennsylvania

Stuart E. Mirvis, M.D.
Associate Professor of Radiology
University of Maryland Medical System
Director, Trauma Radiology
Maryland Institute for Emergency Medical
   Services Systems
Baltimore, Maryland

Roy A. M. Myers, M.D., F.A.C.S.
Assistant Professor of Surgery
University of Maryland School of Medicine
Director, Hyperbaric Medicine
Attending Traumatologist
Deputy Director, Montebello Rehabilitation
   Hospital
Maryland Institute for Emergency Medical
   Services Systems
Baltimore, Maryland

Kurt D. Newman, M.D.
Assistant Professor of Surgery and of Pediatrics
George Washington University School of
   Medicine and Health Sciences
Washington, D.C.

Ameen I. Ramzy, M.D., F.A.C.S.
Assistant Professor of Surgery
University of Maryland School of Medicine
State EMS Director
Deputy Director, MIEMSS
Attending Traumatologist
Maryland Institute for Emergency Medical
   Services Systems
Baltimore, Maryland

Aurelio Rodriguez, M.D., F.A.C.S.
Assistant Professor of Surgery
University of Maryland School of Medicine
Attending Traumatologist and Thoracic
   Surgeon
Maryland Institute for Emergency Medical
   Services Systems
Baltimore, Maryland

Michael Rohman, M.D., F.A.C.S.
Professor of Surgery
New York Medical College

Chief, Cardiothoracic Surgery
Lincoln Medical & Mental Health Center
Bronx, New York

Robert M. Shorr, M.D.
Assistant Clinical Professor of Surgery
University of Southern California
Los Angeles, California

Thomas R. Smith, M.D.
Senior Trauma Fellow
EMS Systems Fellow
Maryland Institute for Emergency Medical
   Services Systems
Baltimore, Maryland

John K. Stene, M.D., Ph.D.
Assistant Professor of Anesthesiology
Director, Perioperative Trauma Anesthesia
   Services
Milton S. Hershey Medical Center
Pennsylvania State University College of
   Medicine
Hershey, Pennsylvania

Vincent K. H. Tam, M.D.
Fellow, Cardiac Surgery
The Johns Hopkins University School of
   Medicine
Baltimore, Maryland

Stephen Z. Turney, M.D., F.A.C.S.
Associate Professor of Surgery
University of Maryland School of Medicine
Chief, Thoracic Surgery
Maryland Institute for Emergency Medical
   Services Systems
Baltimore, Maryland

Charles E. Wiles III, M.D., F.A.C.S.
Assistant Professor of Surgery
University of Maryland School of Medicine
Critical Care/Traumatology Attending
Maryland Institute for Emergency Medical
   Services Systems
Baltimore, Maryland

Alex T. Zakharia, M.D., F.A.C.S., F.A.C.C.
Associate Professor of Surgery
Clinical Associate Professor
Division of Thoracic and Cardiovascular
   Surgery
University of Miami School of Medicine
Miami, Florida

Contents

1 Prehospital Care of Thoracic Trauma

Thomas R. Smith, MD
Ameen I. Ramzy, MD

Within the context of the overall care of a patient with thoracic trauma, prehospital care may be the shortest component, but in many ways it is the critical beginning. Throughout the continuum of care—from prehospital to hospital to rehabilitation— nowhere other than in the prehospital phase are so many decisions required so rapidly based upon the most limited information. The prehospital care provider has, at his/her disposal, information gathered during physical assessment combined with medical direction via radio, but obviously does not have the diagnostic armamentarium, such as arterial blood gas data, x-rays, and computed tomography (CT) scanning, that are available to the next level of the health care team. Despite this limitation of diagnostic resources, significant assessment and intervention can and should begin in the prehospital phase of care.

Prehospital care takes place within the context of the entire continuum of emergency response and health care in the geographic region. While traumatologists and emergency physicians are expertly versed in their own disciplines, many are not familiar with emergency medical services (EMS) in their community. It is essential that physicians understand who the prehospital providers are in their community as well as their level of training. Throughout the United States, an Emergency Medical Technician-Ambulance (EMT-A) is recognized as being trained to provide a basic life support standard of care based upon a 110-hr curriculum developed by the National Highway Traffic Safety Administration of the United States Department of Transportation. Likewise, such a curriculum also exists for the Emergency Medical Technician-Paramedic (EMT-P), a provider of advanced life support (ALS), based not on a predetermined set of hours, but on knowledge objectives. In most parts of the country, the EMT-P curriculum is achieved with a minimum of 400–500 hr of training beyond that of EMT-A. The intermediate levels of emergency medical technician vary tremendously throughout the country, with as many as 37 different levels of training and certification. The term "first responder" customarily denotes an individual with 40–50 hr of training who can initiate basic care and who knows the kinds of additional resources to call. Typically, individuals trained as first responders are law enforcement officers, who may be the first at the scene of an accident in some communities.

Prehospital care begins with access to the EMS system. The means of gaining access to that system should be well-known, simple, rapid, and efficient. Although emergency

"911" systems have been available for many years, they are universally available in very few states. An ideal 911 system receives all emergency calls for fire, police, and emergency medical services and dispatches the appropriate resources as needed.

While most discussions of acute intervention in thoracic trauma focus on the "ABCs" of airway, breathing, and circulation, it must be emphasized that, in prehospital care, the provider must first assess and secure the safety of the scene before initiating patient care efforts. For example, a prehospital care provider responding to a vehicular crash must first ascertain if there are significant ongoing hazards, e.g., downed electric power lines, that could pose a risk to the responding personnel. Likewise, in the context of penetrating trauma, the provider must obviously determine if all the shooting or stabbing has stopped and if indeed the patient can be approached safely.

Once the scene is secure, the prehospital provider conducts a rapid primary survey to determine if the patient has a patent airway, is breathing, and has a pulse. Problems identified in the primary survey must be addressed before a secondary survey (more specific evaluation) takes place. The training, skill, and experience of the prehospital EMS provider, in conjunction with effective communications for on-line medical direction, are fundamentals in the process of patient assessment. This process is initiated by information gained from the dispatch operator, is continued as the scene is surveyed, and is further formulated by the prehospital providers' on-scene assessment of the patient. As assessment and intervention continue, the patient is assigned a priority level (priority 1, emergent; priority 2, urgent; priority 3, requiring medical care but not emergently or urgently) (1). Prehospital care is much more than the utilization of motor skills, such as airway management, administration of medication, splinting, and bandaging. It comprises the entire assessment and management of the patient from the time the system is accessed until the patient is transported to a medical facility. The goal of prehospital care is to deliver a viable patient to definitive care (2).

ASSESSMENT

Evidence of thoracic trauma ranges from the subtle to the obvious. If subtle signs or symptoms are not recognized, their implications will likely not be appreciated, and the patient may be under-triaged. Assessment of the scene and the patient will enable the trained provider to make timely and appropriate decisions on both prehospital treatment and triage. Evidence of forceful deceleration, steering wheel deformity, vehicle displacement and intrusion, distance of falls, estimated volume of external blood loss, the location of assault instruments, and similar information are all factors that must be considered. Patient assessment begins, as always, with the ABCs but includes subtleties such as hoarseness, abnormal thoracic motion, tracheal deviation, and distended neck veins. Recognition of abnormalities is far more important than establishing the etiology. For example, a patient with a thoracic injury may appear confused because of hypoxia, head injury, or shock; however, determining the exact cause is not of paramount importance in prehospital care. A knowledge of anatomic landmarks is similarly important: penetrating wounds of the chest between the left anterior axillary line and the right midclavicular line are considered as cardiac wounds until proven otherwise.

TREATMENT

A rapid and accurate assessment is the foundation of effective initial treatment. Prehospital treatment should follow protocols developed by the medical authorities of the system. This is essential to ensure uniformity of acceptable practice within the system. The Maryland Medical Protocols for Cardiac Rescue Technicians and Emergency Medical Technician-Paramedics (prehospital ALS protocols) include patient priority, triage, treatment, communications, and advanced skills (cardioversion, defibrillation/ countershock, and airway management). These protocols are intended to allow the prehospital care provider to initiate care while on-line medical communication is established with the receiving physician via radio.

Treatment of patients with thoracic trauma in the prehospital phase begins with ensuring adequacy of the airway and administering supplemental oxygen as close to 100% as possible. Assisted ventilation is utilized when necessary, and hyperventilation should be utilized if there is evidence of significant concomitant head injury.

Obvious external bleeding should be controlled by direct pressure. Although a national controversy persists as to the administration of intravenous fluids in the field, we do advocate the use of intravenous fluids through a large-bore peripheral line. This will allow fluid administration to continue during transport. The volume and value of crystalloid infusion during transport can be debated. One of the subtle values of establishing an intravenous line in the prehospital phase is that, when the patient reaches a definitive care facility, he or she can be given paralyzing agents if necessary for an immediate intubation.

If the patient's mechanism of injury or neurologic assessment reveals the possibility of a spinal injury, the spine should be immobilized, and the EMS provider should make a final check for neck vein distension prior to completing the collar application. Many cervical collars provide a window at the front for repeated assessment of tracheal position at the suprasternal notch. While the significance of tracheal position may be overemphasized, the collar opening does allow frequent monitoring.

The use of tapes, belts, sand bags, bulky dressings, or straps for rib fractures is questionable. If such measures improve patient comfort and, therefore, ventilation, they cannot be abolished summarily. However, the emphasis should be on oxygenation and ventilation during rapid transport.

Impaling objects are left in place. A bulky dressing is constructed in order to stabilize and protect the object from shifting during patient transport and transfer.

A suspected pneumothorax is treated with supplemental oxygen. If there is no reason to suspect spinal cord or spinal column injury from the mechanism of injury, the patient may be transported in a semi-sitting position for comfort as well as for ventilation/perfusion matching. Careful assessment for the development of a possible tension pneumothorax is necessary.

An open pneumothorax ("sucking chest wound") is treated with a three-sided dressing. This prevents further contamination of the wound and, if placed properly, greatly lessens the chance for development of a tension pneumothorax. A totally occlusive dressing presents the risk of converting an open pneumothorax into a tension pneumothorax and therefore should not be utilized.

The treatment of a suspected tension pneumothorax in the field depends tremendously on local conditions, including transport times and medical direction. To our knowledge, the accuracy of the diagnosis of tension pneumothorax in the field has not been critically evaluated, but various treatments have been described (3–6).

There is no specific treatment in the field for a suspected hemothorax. It is more important that the suspected thoracic injury is recognized and the patient assessed rapidly, triaged correctly, and transported to definitive care.

A cardiac contusion rarely requires additional prehospital intervention. In some circumstances, a dysrhythmia detected en route may be treated with antiarrhythmics in addition to adequate oxygenation. It is more important that major anterior chest trauma is recognized and that pertinent information is relayed to the receiving physician.

There is no specific field treatment for suspected cardiac tamponade, diaphragm rupture, tracheobronchial injuries, laryngeal injuries, or traumatic asphyxia. Again, patient assessment and appropriate triage are the critical elements in prehospital management.

CONTROVERSIES

Certain prehospital interventions remain controversial. For trauma patients, specifically, there seems to be considerable discussion regarding the use of medical antishock trousers (MAST), pleural decompression, and cricothyroidotomy. The use of these interventions in the field must be based on a critical appraisal of several factors: the need for the intervention, as well as the risks, must be weighed in relation to the prehospital care providers' response time to the scene and transport time to definitive care.

While recent literature has questioned the value of MAST in the treatment of traumatic hypotension (7), we interpret these results cautiously. We respect the convictions of these authors, but the final word is not yet in. The Maryland prehospital MAST protocol for trauma indicates the use of this device for a blood pressure less than 80 mm Hg in adults. Contraindications include uncontrolled hemorrhage above the site of MAST application, abdominal evisceration, impaled objects in an area of MAST application, respiratory distress, and third-trimester pregnancy.

The use of pleural decompression in the field remains a topic of discussion and consideration. We resist the technologic imperative that says that if a skill *can* be performed it therefore *should* be performed. In the Maryland EMS system, we find it more prudent to focus on whether there is a need for this skill in the field. A review by the Shock Trauma Center of the Maryland Institute for Emergency Medical Services Systems demonstrated 109 instances of tension pneumothorax among 11,771 trauma patients (an incidence of 0.9%). Further analysis demonstrated that there were only 23 instances in which decompression was performed within the first 10 min after arrival at the receiving facility. An earlier review of death certificates revealed no cases in the state in which tension pneumothorax was determined to be the sole cause of death (2). At this time, the Maryland prehospital ALS protocols do not include pleural decompression for suspected tension pneumothorax, but we continue to monitor this question.

Prehospital cricothyroidotomy continues to be the subject of considerable discussion. Despite this, the literature offers a relative paucity of data in this area. A recent article by Spaite and Joseph retrospectively analyzed their experience with prehospital cricothyroidotomy in the EMS region serving a Level I trauma center in Tucson, Arizona (8). Although the number of patients was small, the authors have appropriately pointed out that, regardless of the perceived feasibility of the procedure, they could not demonstrate any patient benefit in terms of improved outcome. They concluded that carefully controlled scientific studies are needed to further evaluate and elucidate the role, if any, of prehospital cricothyroidotomy.

CONCLUSIONS

The essentials of prehospital care of thoracic trauma include a system that allows for prompt activation of the system and dispatch of trained providers with the ability to assess, oxygenate, triage, and transport the patient to definitive care. Definitive care of the trauma patient should take place at a trauma center (9) within a comprehensive trauma system (10). Prehospital care of thoracic trauma is a critical beginning in the care of the injured patient.

REFERENCES

1. Maryland Institute for Emergency Medical Services Systems. The Maryland medical protocols for cardiac rescue technicians and emergency medical technician-paramedics. Baltimore: MIEMSS, 1989.
2. Ramzy AI. Maryland EMS: where are we? Maryland EMS Newsletter 1989;16:1–3.
3. Butman AM, Paturas JL, McSwain NE Jr, Dineen JP, eds. PHTLS, prehospital trauma life support. Akron, OH: Educational Direction, Inc., 1986.
4. American College of Surgeons, Committee on Trauma. Advanced trauma life support, instructor manual program. Chicago: American College of Surgeons, 1989.
5. Gazzariga AB, Iseri LT, Baren M, eds. Emergency care: principles and practices for the EMT-paramedic. 2nd ed. Englewood Cliffs, NJ: Prentice-Hall, 1982.
6. Campbell JE, ed. Basic trauma life support, advanced prehospital care. Alabama Chapter, American College of Emergency Physicians. Bowie, MD: Brady Communications, 1985.
7. Mattox KL, Bickell W, Pepe PE, Burch J, Feliciano D. Prospective MAST study in 911 patients. J Trauma 1989;29:1104–1112.
8. Spaite DW, Joseph M. Prehospital cricothyroidotomy: an investigation of indications, technique, complications, and patient outcome. Ann Emerg Med 1990;19:279–285.
9. Committee on Trauma, American College of Surgeons. Resources for optimal care of the injured patient. Chicago: American College of Surgeons, 1990.
10. West JG, Williams MJ, Trunkey DD, Wolferth CC Jr. Trauma systems: current status—future challenges. JAMA 1988;259:3597–3600.

2 Initial Patient Evaluation and Indications for Thoracotomy

Aurelio Rodriguez, MD

Well-organized prehospital and intrahospital systems of care for injured patients have contributed greatly to the optimization of patient resuscitation. Despite the efforts and expertise of emergency care providers, more than 80,000 trauma victims in the United States die each year—50,000 from automobile accidents and more than 30,000 from assault with handguns, knives, and other instruments (1).

Approximately 50% of those who die from vehicular accidents sustain chest injuries; chest injury is the primary cause of death in 25% of these fatalities (2). Kemmerer (3) studied 585 deaths due to traffic accidents during a 5-year period and found that 133 were related primarily to thoracic trauma; the injuries most frequently encountered were rib fractures, hemothorax, lung lacerations, and rupture of great vessels.

Nevertheless, according to the American College of Surgeons' Trauma Life Support Program, 85% of patients with thoracic trauma can be managed by simple lifesaving techniques that do not require the initial intervention of a thoracic surgeon.

INITIAL ASSESSMENT AND MANAGEMENT

Ideally, a senior surgeon, as team leader, should direct the initial evaluation and treatment. The evaluation of a patient's thoracic injuries is only a part of the total assessment. Furthermore, because thoracic injuries are severe and potentially lethal, the diagnosis and therapy "go hand in hand."

This initial assessment should encompass a pertinent medical history, including alcohol or drug ingestion; assessment of the level of consciousness; a notation of vehicular crash victims' use or nonuse of seat belts; and a record of the mechanisms of injury. This information can be obtained from the prehospital care providers or from lucid patients.

The physical examination of the chest should be carried out expeditiously yet thoroughly. Complete disrobing of the patient is mandatory. The posterior aspect of the torso should be examined for hidden injuries; "log-rolling" the patient will help to avoid iatrogenesis.

Airway Management and Stabilization of the Respiratory System

The assessment and establishment of an airway take precedence over all other problems. The presence of airway obstruction, paradoxic motion of the chest wall, open pneumothorax, and/or tension pneumothorax should be noted and corrective measures taken. The following specific injuries should also be ruled out immediately: cardiac injury with or without tamponade, great vessel injuries, massive hemothorax, and tracheobronchial injuries.

Several modalities of oxygenation and ventilation have been used, ranging from simple procedures such as inserting nasal or oral airways to those requiring higher skill levels such as initiating nasotracheal or orotracheal intubation with or without an ancillary fiber-optic bronchoscope. If the patient cannot be intubated within 60 sec or with several attempts, a cricothyroidotomy should be performed.

Decreased breath sounds and hyperresonance to percussion plus subcutaneous emphysema suggest a pneumothorax. If the symptoms/signs also include a decrease in the blood pressure and deviation of the trachea to the contralateral side, a tension pneumothorax is clearly present. If the hemodynamic condition of the patient is adequate, an erect chest roentgenogram not only will confirm the diagnosis of tension pneumothorax but also will enable the clinician to evaluate the mediastinum better. Blood gas determinations at this point will help monitor the effectiveness of oxygenation and ventilation.

The definitive treatment is placement of a large (#40) chest tube in the fifth intercostal space at the midaxillary line; it should never be placed below this level. In certain circumstances, when the clinical diagnosis is tension pneumothorax, the patient is hemodynamically compromised, and chest tube equipment is not available quickly, needle decompression at the level of the second intercostal space, midclavicular line, could be a temporary lifesaving maneuver (see Chapter 9).

Assessment and Stabilization of Cardiovascular Function

The second immediate priority is the assessment and treatment of cardiovascular function.

HYPOVOLEMIA

The most common cause of cardiovascular alterations is hypovolemia. Most likely due to blood loss, hypovolemia decreases blood return to the heart and, as a consequence, lowers the blood pressure and cardiac output. Low central venous pressure and low urine output complete the clinical picture. Additional thoracic causes of hypovolemia are massive hemothorax and cardiac tamponade. Hypovolemia can also be associated with intraabdominal injuries. Diagnostic peritoneal lavage, computerized tomography, or sonography (4, 5) is necessary to rule out intraabdominal bleeding. The insertion of large-bore (14-gauge) intravenous catheters into the antecubital fossa, plus a cordis introducer into the great saphenous vein, allows the infusion of 2 liters of crystalloid Ringer's lactate to initiate resuscitation. If the patient's blood pressure is below 100 mm Hg, in our institution, resuscitation starts with 2 liters of colloids followed by type-specific blood (6). On many occasions, the use of autotransfused blood from the thoracic drainage is very helpful (6). Care should be taken to warm all administered fluids appropriately.

ACUTE PERICARDIAL TAMPONADE—HEART WOUND

The accumulation of blood in the pericardial sac with impairment of the diastolic filling of the heart should be suspected in any blunt trauma patient with disproportion between the hemodynamic status and the apparent blood loss. In penetrating trauma,

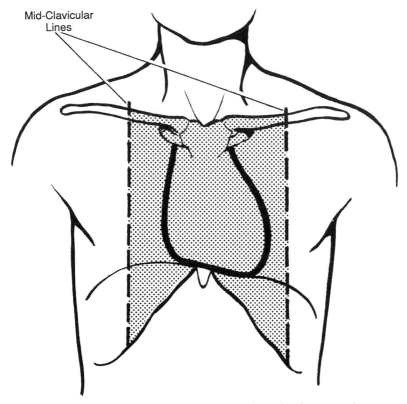

Figure 2.1.   Any penetrating injury between the midclavicular lines is a heart wound until proved otherwise.

the location of the wound is of paramount importance. "Any penetrating wound of the chest between the two midclavicular lines is a heart wound until proved otherwise" (6) (Fig. 2.1). Elevation of central venous pressure in association with an unchanged blood pressure after the administration of fluids may help to confirm the diagnosis (see Chapter 14 for details of other measures such as echocardiogram, pulsus paradoxus, and Swan-Ganz catheter placement). Pericardiocentesis has been advocated as an effective measure to diagnose cardiac tamponade (7, 8). If it is positive, it will also temporarily improve the patient hemodynamically and allow time for the thoracic or trauma surgeon to arrive for the performance of a definitive surgical procedure. It should be remembered that a negative pericardiocentesis does *not* rule out pericardial tamponade. In our view, a more effective and accurate way to diagnose it is by the subxiphoid retrosternal approach (pericardial window) (6, 9, 10).

To create a pericardial window, the anterior chest should be prepared as for anterior thoracotomy. The procedure should be done in the operating room (or in a well-equipped admitting area), with the patient under local or general anesthesia. A head light for the surgeon is ideal. If the hemodynamic status of the patient allows, he or she should be placed in a semi-Fowler's position (see Chapter 14). The xiphoid process should be identified and probably resected for better exposure. The subxiphoid plane should be dissected bluntly and, with good exposure attained with the use of an angled retractor, the surgeon should be able to differentiate the pericardium from the peritoneum. An aid to the surgeon in identifying the pericardium is feeling the heart's pulsation under the finger. After two stay sutures of 2-0 silk have been applied to the pericardium and good hemostasis has been ensured, the sac should be opened with a knife. Free blood in the pericardial sac is diagnostic of hemopericardium (Fig. 2.2). If there is any doubt regarding the procedure or if there is pink fluid egress, the possibility of pericardial rupture should be entertained. Irrigation of the pericardial cavity with warm saline with a soft rubber catheter, demonstrating continued egress of

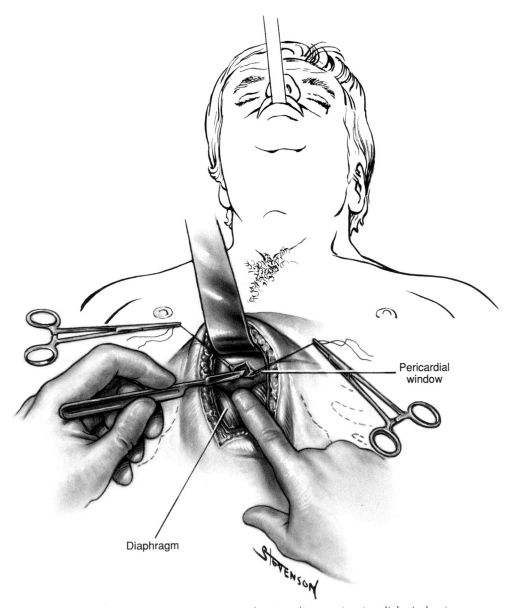

Figure 2.2.   Subxiphoid retrosternal pericardiotomy (pericardial window).

pink/bloody fluid, will help confirm this diagnosis. Interpretation of this finding is subjective and should be based on the surgeon's experience (11, 12).

Finally, the patient may have a myocardial contusion. It is not necessary for patients with this injury to have been in a high-speed vehicular crash or to have external evidence of chest trauma. The diagnosis should be suggested, however, by the mechanism of injury. When myocardial contusion is suspected, a 12-lead electrocardiogram should be obtained and blood should be drawn for assessment of cardiac enzymes (creatine phosphokinase (CPK)), particularly MB bands. If these results are positive (more than 8 IU or more than 5% of total CPK), the diagnosis can be confirmed with a MUGA scan (multigated angiogram) or two-dimensional echocardiogram, which measures the ejection fraction of the ventricles and heart contractility.

Assessment and stabilization of neurologic function are other essential points, but they escape the scope of this book.

SECONDARY ASSESSMENT AND MANAGEMENT

After the main priorities have been assessed and treated properly, a secondary evaluation and management of specific pathologies are initiated.

Identification of Specific Rib Fractures

Fractures of the first and second ribs have been a theme of controversial debate (13–18) because of their potential implication of a major mechanical impact and association with major vascular and visceral injuries. Despite the lack of agreement as to the significance of these injuries, they should be determined.

Flail Chest

Flail chest is not as much a diagnostic problem as it is a treatment problem. Recently, the use of epidural analgesia and other modalities (see Chapter 5) has allowed some patients with flail chest to be treated without mechanical ventilatory support (19, 20). The indications for mechanical ventilatory assistance are shown in Table 2.1.

Chest Tube Drainage
AIR LEAK

Persistent air leak in the chest tube drainage, massive subcutaneous emphysema, or pneumomediastinum with or without hemoptysis should direct attention to the possibility of a ruptured bronchi (21–24). The definite diagnosis can be obtained with fiber-optic bronchoscopy performed by an experienced thoracic surgeon. If more than a third of the bronchial circumference has been transected, surgical repair is indicated (23, 24). However, if there is another associated injury, such as hemoperitoneum, the surgical priorities as to which injury to treat first must be determined (24) in accordance with the hemodynamic and respiratory status of the patient.

BLEEDING

The trend of bleeding is the most important determinant in the decision to perform a thoracotomy. For example, an initial drainage of more than 1,000 ml at chest tube placement or bleeding of 300 ml/hr or more for 3 consecutive hours (100 ml/hr or more for the same period in an elderly person) should be an indication for thoracotomy (see Chapter 9).

Table 2.1.
Indications for Ventilatory Support

Clinical	
Airway obstruction	
Severe brain injury; Glasgow Coma Scale score ≥ 8	
Clinical hypoventilation	
Hypovolemic shock refractory to initial resuscitation	
Respiratory function	
Mechanics	
Respiratory rate	>35/minute
Vital capacity (ml/kg)	<15
Inspiratory force (cm H_2O)	< -25
Oxygenation	
PaO_2 (mm Hg)	<80 (supplemental O_2)
Ventilation	
$PaCO_2$ (mm Hg)	>55

Penetrating Trauma below the Sixth Rib

Patients with penetrating injuries of the lower chest and signs of peritoneal irritation require laparotomy. If those signs are not present, a diagnostic peritoneal lavage should be done; some clinicians use a finding of more than 5,000 red blood cells (RBC)/mm³ as suggestive of intraabdominal injury and others use a threshold of 100,000 RBC (25, 26).

Transmediastinal Injuries

The approach to these injuries depends on the hemodynamic status of the patient. If the patient is stable, the following should be done:

Pericardial window
Bronchoscopy
Esophagoscopy and/or esophagogram
Aortogram of the major vessels

According to our experience, and that of others, use of this set of procedures is the best way to rule out intrathoracic pathology (Fig. 2.3). If the patient is unstable, an immediate thoracotomy should be carried out using the more versatile of the thoracic incisions for trauma, the anterolateral thoracotomy, which can be extended across the midline if necessary (see Chapter 15).

Ruptured Esophagus

This condition is rare in patients with blunt thoracic trauma. It may be suggested by the presence of pneumomediastinum, sustained pain, dysphagia, or fever. A combination of esophagoscopy and esophagogram is indicated for diagnosis (see Chapter 11 for discussion of management).

Scalp Lacerations

Any scalp laceration should be assessed properly. In many cases, it is the only cause of hypovolemia and shock. Unfortunately, such lacerations frequently are missed initially

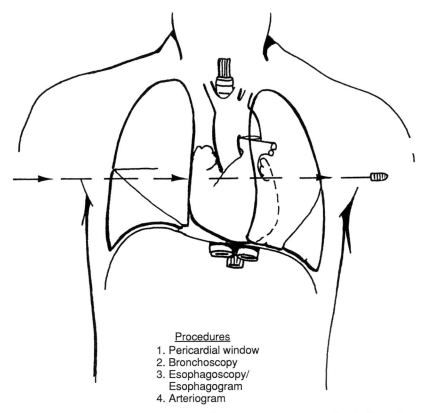

Procedures
1. Pericardial window
2. Bronchoscopy
3. Esophagoscopy/
   Esophagogram
4. Arteriogram

Figure 2.3. Diagnostic procedures for penetrating transmediastinal injuries.

because the bleeding has already subsided at the time of the patient's arrival at the emergency department.

Chest Roentgenogram

In the diagnosis of thoracic trauma, it is very important to obtain a chest roentgenogram with the patient in the upright position to rule out the possibility of wide mediastinum due to a ruptured thoracic aorta. Despite the many signs described (apical cap deviation of the left main stem bronchus, disappearance of the aortopulmonary window, deviation of the nasogastric tube, and increase in size of the paraspinal muscle stripe), in our view, the most important sign indicating the need for an aortogram is the ill-defined visualization of the aortic knob (Figs. 2.4 and 2.5). An aortogram also is indicated if the patient cannot be seated because of a pelvic fracture or spinal injuries. Although the computerized axial tomography scan is not yet an infallible method of diagnosis (see Chapter 4), it helps as a screening procedure in selected cases (27, 28).

EMERGENCY THORACOTOMY

Due to the increasing number of emergency thoracotomies, sound scrutiny of the indications, cost, and final results of the procedure has been advocated in many recent publications. It seems that the mechanism of injury is one area generally agreed as important in determining whether thoracotomy is indicated.

If a patient with penetrating injuries exhibits acute hemodynamic deterioration,

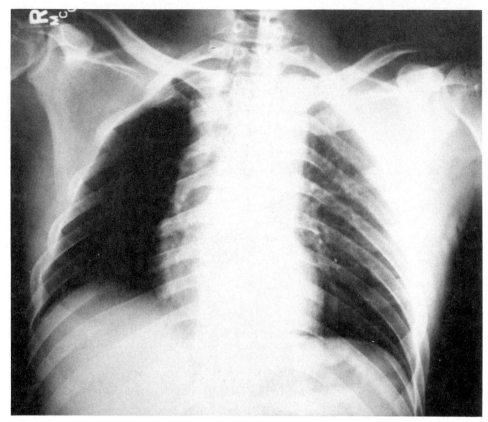

Figure 2.4.   An indistinct aortic knob is an important indicator of the need for an aortogram.

uncontrolled bleeding, or cardiac arrest, a thoracotomy should be performed. Furthermore, if the physician is suspicious of air embolism or of a major vascular injury causing acute hemodynamic deterioration that does not respond to fluid administration, surgical exploration is also warranted (see Chapter 15).

On the other hand, when prehospital care providers report that a blunt-injured patient had vital signs at the scene of injury yet experienced acute deterioration or cardiac arrest in transit to or upon arrival at the hospital, an emergency thoracotomy should be performed.

Technique

Ideally, this procedure should be performed by an experienced trauma surgeon. Many times it is done in conjunction with other resuscitative efforts such as endotracheal intubation and insertion of large-bore intravenous catheters.

The chest is prepared expeditiously with an organic iodine solution.

A left anterolateral thoracotomy is performed at the level of the fifth intercostal space, preferably in the pectoral or mammary crease.

The pectoralis major, serratus anterior, and intercostal muscle are severed with a knife and scissors; no control of the bleeding is necessary at this point.

The chest wall retractor is inserted and opened; cutting the costal cartilages above and below the incision facilitates the exposure.

Initial cardiac massage with the pericardium closed should be followed by immediate opening of the pericardium to obtain better and more effective contraction.

Most times, the pericardium is tense; to open it, it is necessary to apply a traction suture or to cut directly with a scalpel. It is ideal to have a large-bore IV running open before entering the pericardium.

If the heart is in asystole or fibrillation, the initial maneuver is the same: hand compression, preferably using both hands or palms, or compressing the heart against the sternum.

If fibrillation is present or elicited by the compression, direct defibrillation is performed. Usually, no more than 30 W-sec is required.

Epinephrine or calcium may be injected directly into the heart if necessary. Bicarbonate should accordingly be administered intravenously (see Chapter 15).

The best way to evaluate the degree of volemia is by palpating the pulmonary artery and feeling the compliance of the heart.

We recommend prophylactically inserting a chest tube in the right hemithorax to prevent the possibility of a lethal tension pneumothorax (Fig. 2.6).

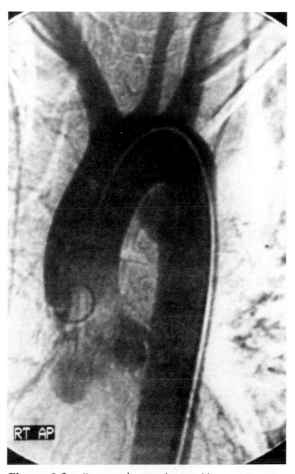

Figure 2.5.   Ruptured aorta depicted by arteriogram.

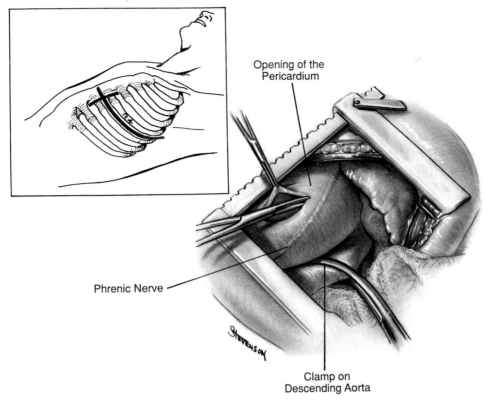

Opening of the
Pericardium

Phrenic Nerve

Clamp on
Descending Aorta

Figure 2.6. Emergency thoracotomy.

Results

Bodai et al. (29) reviewed the published series. They found that the results are different for penetrating and blunt trauma.

PENETRATING TRAUMA

Most patients with noncardiac penetrating chest trauma who arrived at the hospital without vital signs could not be saved (30–32). If the heart is not involved, an emergency department thoracotomy is rarely indicated (33–35). Despite the fact that the number of patients arriving alive at the hospital with penetrating cardiac wounds is small, they benefit the most from emergency thoracotomy, particularly if they have pericardial tamponade. The salvage rate ranges from 34% (in the Steichen series (36)) to 55% (in the Mattox group (37)), survival being directly related to the presence of vital signs. Furthermore, all the series concluded that survivability depends on the presence of signs of life in the field, rapid resuscitative measures, and fast transportation (38–44). Hamar et al. (45) reported a 42% survival rate if there are signs of ventricular activity.

BLUNT TRAUMA

Blunt trauma victims have a very poor chance of survival. Most series (44–46) report a 90–100% mortality. If the patient sustains cardiac arrest at the scene, the prognosis is even poorer. Many possible reasons have been advanced, e.g., associated neurologic injuries, hypoxia, disseminated intravascular coagulation (46).

Complications

The most common complications of this procedure are listed below:

Breast injuries in males or females
Injury of the aorta or esophagus at the time of clamping
Phrenic nerve injury
Heart herniation if the pericardium is closed inadequately
Wound infections
Paraplegia due to prolonged clamping

REFERENCES

1. National Center for Health Statistics. Advance report of final mortality statistics 1980. Monthly Vital Stat Rep 1983;31:22.
2. Trunkey D. Torso trauma. Curr Probl Surg 1987;24:215–265.
3. Kemmerer WT, Eckert WG, Gathright JB, Reemtsma K, Creech O Jr. Patterns of thoracic injuries in fatal traffic accidents. J Trauma 1961;1:595–599.
4. Grüessner R, Mentges B, Düber C, Rückert K, Rothmund M. Sonography versus peritoneal lavage in blunt abdominal trauma. J Trauma 1989;29:242–244.
5. Asher WM, Parvin S, Virgillo RW, Haber K. Echographic evaluation of splenic injury after blunt trauma. Radiology 1976;118:411–415.
6. Cowley RA, Dunham CM. Shock trauma critical care manual. Rockville, MD: Aspen, 1986.
7. Symbas PN, Harlaftis N, Waldo WJ. Penetrating cardiac wounds: a comparison of different therapeutic methods. Ann Surg 1976;183:377–381.
8. Callahan ML. Pericardiocentesis in traumatic and nontraumatic cardiac tamponade. Ann Emerg Med 1984;13:924.
9. Fontenelle LJ, Cuell L, Dooley BN. Subxiphoid pericardial window. Am J Surg 1970;120:679–680.
10. Miller FB, Bond SJ, Shumate CR, Polk HC Jr, Richardson JD. Diagnostic pericardial window: a safe alternative to exploratory thoracotomy for suspected heart injuries. Arch Surg 1987;122:605–609.
11. Fulda G, Rodriguez A, Turney SZ, Cowley RA. Blunt traumatic pericardial rupture: a ten-year experience (1979 to 1989). Presented at the XIX World Congress of the International Society for Cardiovascular Surgery, Toronto, 1989.
12. Fulda G, Brathwaite CEM, Rodriguez A, Turney SZ, Dunham CM, Cowley RA. Blunt traumatic rupture of the heart and pericardium: a ten-year experience (1979-1989), submitted to the Journal of Trauma, 1989.
13. LeGuerrier A, Rosat P, LeBeau G, Dormor D, Kerne J, Rioux C, LoGrais Y. Associated lesions in closed injuries of the thorax: right bronchial rupture, rupture of the right subclavian artery and bilateral fracture of the first rib. J Chir (Paris) 1975;122:561–565.
14. Phillips EH, Rogers WF, Gaspar MR. First rib fractures: incidence of vascular injury and indications for angiography. Surgery 1980;89:42–47.
15. Richardson JD, McEluein RB, Trinkle JK. First rib fracture: a hallmark of severe chest trauma. Ann Surg 1975;181:251–254.
16. Lorentzen JE, Movin M. Fracture of the first rib. Acta Orthop Scand 1976;47:632–634.
17. Galbraith NF, Urschel HC Jr, Wood RF, Razzuk MA, Paulson DL. Fracture of the first rib associated with laceration of subclavian artery. J Thorac Cardiovasc Surg 1973;65:649–652.
18. Pierce GE, Maxwell SA, Boggan MD. Special hazards of first rib fracture. J Trauma 1975;15:264–267.
19. Cullen ML, Staren ED, el-Ganzouri A, Logas WG, Ivankovich AD, Economou SG. Continuous epidural infusion for analgesia after major abdominal operations: a randomized, prospective double-blind study. Surgery 1985;98:718–728.
20. El Baz MMI, Faber LP, Jensik RJ. Continuous epidural infusion of morphine for treatment of pain after thoracic injury: a new technique. Anesth Analg 1984;63:757–764.
21. Hood RM, Sloan HE. Injuries of the trachea and major bronchi. J Thorac Cardiovasc Surg 1959;38:458.
22. Grover FL, Ellestad C, Aromku KV, Root HD, Cruz AB, Trinkle JK. Diagnosis and management of major tracheobronchial injuries. Ann Thorac Surg 1979;28:384–391.

23. Urschel HC, Razzuk MA. Management of acute traumatic injuries of tracheobronchial tree. Surg Gynecol Obstet 1973;136:113–117.

24. Ramzy AI, Rodriguez A, Turney SZ. Management of major tracheobronchial ruptures in patients with multiple system trauma. J Trauma 1988;28:1353–1357.

25. Merlotti GJ, Dillon BC, Lange DA, Robin AP, Barret J. Peritoneal lavage in penetrating thoracoabdominal trauma. J Trauma 1988;28:17–23.

26. Thal ER. Peritoneal lavage reliability of RBC count in patients with stable wounds of the chest. Arch Surg 1984;119:579–584.

27. Mirvis SE, Kostrubiak I, Whitley NO, Goldstein LD, Rodriguez A. Role of CT in excluding major arterial injury after blunt thoracic trauma. AJR 1987;149:601–605.

28. Miller FB, Richardson D, Hollin T. Role of CT in diagnosis of major arterial injury in blunt thoracic trauma. Surgery 1985;106:596–603.

29. Bodai BI, Smith JP, Ward RE, O'Neill MB, Auborg R. Emergency thoracotomy in the management of trauma: a review. JAMA 1983;249:1891–1896.

30. Oparah EE, Mandal AK. Penetrating gunshot wounds of the chest in civilian practice: experience with 250 consecutive cases. Br J Surg 1978;65:45–48.

31. Oparah SS, Mandal AK. Penetrating stab wounds of the chest: experience with 200 consecutive cases. J Trauma 1976;16:868–872.

32. Borja AR, Ransdell HT. Treatment of penetrating gunshot wounds of the chest: experience with 145 cases. Am J Surg 1971;122:81–84.

33. Graham JM, Mattox KL, Beall AC Jr. Penetrating trauma of the lung. J Trauma 1979;19:665–669.

34. Levinsky L, Vidne B, Nudelman I, Salomon J, Kissin L, Levy MJ. Thoracic injuries in the Yom Kippur War: experience in a base hospital. Isr J Med Sci 1975;11:275–280.

35. Trinkle JK, Toon RS, Franz JL, Arom KV, Grover FL. Affairs of the wounded heart: penetrating cardiac wounds. J Trauma 1979;19:467–472.

36. Steichen FM, Dargan EL, Efron G, Pearlman DM, Weil PH. A graded approach to the management of penetrating wounds of the heart. Arch Surg 1971;103:574–580.

37. Mattox KL, Beall AC, Jordan GL, De Bakey ME. Cardiorraphy in the emergency center. J Thorac Cardiovasc Surg 1974;68:886–895.

38. Krome RL, Dalbee DL. Emergency thoracotomy. Emerg Med Clin North Am 1986;4:459–465.

39. Schwab CM, Adcock OT, Max MH. Emergency department thoracotomy (EDT): a 26-month experience using an "agonal" protocol. Am Surg 1986;52:20–29.

40. Roberge RJ, Ivatury RR, Stahl W, Rohman M. Emergency department thoracotomy for penetrating injuries: predictive value of patient classification. Am J Emerg Med 1986;4:129–135.

41. Feliciano DV, Bitondo CG, Cruse PA, Mattox K, Burch JM, Beal AC Jr, Jordan GL Jr. Liberal use of emergency room thoracotomy. Am J Surg 1986;152:654–659.

42. Demetriades D, Rabinowitz B, Sofianos C. Emergency room thoracotomy for stab wounds to the chest and neck. J Trauma 1987;27:483–485.

43. Moore EE. Prognostic factors in emergency department thoracotomy for trauma. Curr Concepts Trauma Care 1982;5:5–9.

44. Cogbill TH, Moore EE, Millikan JS, Cleveland HC. Rationale for selective application of emergency department thoracotomy in trauma. J Trauma 1983;23:453–460.

45. Harnar TJ, Oreskovich MR, Copass MK, Heimbach DM, Herman CM, Carrico CJ. Role of emergency thoracotomy in the resuscitation of moribund trauma victims: 100 consecutive cases. Am J Surg 1981;142:96–99.

46. Bodai BI, Smith JP, Blaisdell FW. The role of emergency thoracotomy in blunt trauma. J Trauma 1982;22:487–491.

3 Management of Thoracic Trauma by the Emergency Physician

James L. Baker, MD, MPH

The initial management of persons suffering significant thoracic trauma is frequently the responsibility of emergency department physicians who are not thoracic surgeons. It is therefore imperative that emergency physicians be able to recognize and stabilize the thoracic injuries that are or will become catastrophic to the patient if not treated properly, as well as those that are more common but less significant (1–6).

In brief, synoptic format, this chapter discusses the thoracic injuries most likely to be encountered in an emergency department practice, as well as certain uncommon injuries that must be identified and managed rapidly to prevent poor outcome. For a more detailed discussion of the initial evaluation, see Chapters 2 and 15.

INJURIES TO THE CHEST WALL
Simple Rib Fractures
DIAGNOSIS

Isolated, uncomplicated rib fractures are usually the result of sports injuries or falls. The patient presents with well-localized rib pain and tenderness, worsened by coughing, deep breathing, or pressure. Frequently, palpation over the painful area will produce a bony "snap." Mild compression of the chest, either anterior-posterior or lateral, will reproduce pain at the fracture site. Nondisplaced rib fractures frequently are not seen on radiographs and, in any event, the clinical diagnosis is reliable. In very young or elderly patients, however, associated injuries may be revealed by chest x-ray studies or special rib views (2) (see Chapter 9).

MANAGEMENT

Relief of pain and preservation of pulmonary function are the primary goals. Patients often request treatments such as rib binders, but such mechanical restrictions predispose the patient to atelectasis or other respiratory problems. A nonnarcotic analgesic will usually suffice, but occasionally an intercostal nerve block will be necessary. The technique of intercostal nerve block is simple, but it is not uncommon for inexperienced personnel to cause a pneumothorax and commit the patient to a chest tube and hospital stay. For this reason, intercostal nerve blocks should be reserved for the patient whose respiratory status may be unduly compromised by pain.

Fracture of the First or Second Rib

DIAGNOSIS

The first and second ribs are anatomically well-protected by clavicles, scapulae, and overlying muscle, and fractures of them are therefore uncommon. Because the force required to fracture these ribs is usually significant, this injury carries the probability of associated thoracic or abdominal injury. Fractures of the first or second rib are usually evident on chest x-ray films.

MANAGEMENT

These fractures by themselves do not require specific therapy. Their principal significance is in serving as a clue to the degree of trauma sustained by the victim. Like fractures of the scapula, their presence should alert the managing physician to possible associated injuries that may not be immediately evident, especially disruption of the great vessels. If these fractures are identified, and there is evidence of aortic dissection, then emergency arteriography must be considered.

Fracture or Dislocation of the Sternum

DIAGNOSIS

Injuries to the sternum most typically result from motor vehicle trauma involving a direct blow to the anterior chest. Contusion may or may not be evident, but localized tenderness and a palpable deformity are frequently present. Lateral chest x-ray films may demonstrate the injury (3) (see Chapter 9).

MANAGEMENT

Sternal fracture is indicative of significant trauma, with a strong possibility of blunt myocardial, pericardial, or pulmonary injury. An electrocardiogram should be obtained, but characteristic electrocardiographic evidence of injury may not be evident initially. Patients with sternal fracture or dislocation should be admitted to a monitored bed for the first 24 hr following injury, with base-line and 12–24-hr myocardial creatine phosphokinase (CPK) enzymes, 12-lead ECG, and ECG monitoring for dysrhythmias (see section on myocardial contusion).

Flail Chest

DIAGNOSIS

Flail chest results from multiple adjacent rib fractures and concomitant loss of normal chest wall integrity. With significant flail, respiration may be compromised and cardiac output reduced. On inspiration, decreased intrathoracic pressure causes the flail segment to collapse paradoxically into the chest; on expiration, the flail segment moves outward. This motion is obvious when the flail segment is large, but muscular splinting or a small segment may make the paradoxical motion subtle. Typically, crepitus is palpable over the fractured area. Radiographically, multiple fractures are usually evident because of displaced fracture margins.

MANAGEMENT

The principal concern with flail chest is preservation of pulmonary function. Upon recognition of significant flail at the prehospital scene, emergency care providers should position the patient on the injured side or stabilize the segment with sand bags to reduce abnormal chest wall motion. At the hospital, hemothorax or pneumothorax should be sought and immediately corrected with tube thoracostomy. If the flail segment is large and respiratory embarrassment is clinically evident, then the patient should be paralyzed and intubated to permit positive pressure ventilation. Intubation decisions must be made on an individualized basis, relying on the total clinical presentation rather than rigid criteria. Most patients with small to moderate flail chest injuries do not require positive pressure ventilatory support immediately. As with all cases of significant blunt thoracic trauma, pulmonary or cardiac contusion should be considered as present, and supportive care should be initiated. On occasion, surgical stabilization of a flail segment becomes necessary; this decision is left to the thoracic surgeon (3, 4).

PULMONARY INJURIES
Pulmonary Contusion
DIAGNOSIS

Pulmonary contusion results from sudden, moderate to severe blunt trauma to the chest. A rapid increase in pulmonic capillary pressure associated with chest compression leads to extravasation into the lung parenchyma and development of localized contusion. Most forms of trauma significant enough to cause multiple rib fractures, sternal fractures, isolated first or second rib fractures, or scapular fractures will also cause pulmonary contusion. No single clinical finding is directly diagnostic of pulmonary contusion, but the radiographic appearance of a hazy infiltrate in an area of blunt trauma is highly characteristic. The radiographic appearance occurs early, usually within several minutes of the traumatic event. Over the ensuing 24 hr, the size and density of the lesion generally increase. Inexperienced clinicians have occasionally interpreted a generalized haziness of an entire single lung field, in the setting of severe blunt trauma, as "pulmonary contusion," when in fact a hemothorax was present and layered out on supine view. This error should be recognized instantly on an erect chest x-ray film (3) (see Chapter 9).

MANAGEMENT

In the emergency setting, there is no specific management which must be employed routinely for pulmonary contusion. The standard efforts of aggressive fluid resuscitation and ventilatory support should be continued. If sufficient lung parenchyma is contused to cause hypoxemia or carbon dioxide retention, or if associated injuries are producing respiratory compromise, then intubation should be performed. For patients without respiratory failure, frequent and aggressive pulmonary toilet is the principal supportive measure. Several "therapeutic" measures have been attempted in the setting of pulmonary contusion, but they have not been shown to be of value. Fluid restriction or diuretic use to keep a patient "dry" will be of no benefit in the treatment of this injury. It is necessary only to avoid overhydration and predisposition to cardiogenic pulmonary edema. Likewise, the use of steroids has not been demonstrated to be effective in altering the course of contusion resolution, and their use may lead to development of secondary pneumonia. Prophylactic antibiotics should not be used for pulmonary contusion because of the possibility of selecting out resistant organisms.

Pneumothorax
DIAGNOSIS

The vast majority of pneumothoraces are clearly evident on chest radiographs, especially on the expiratory view. Smaller pneumothoraces of 5 or 10% are less easily discerned but are equally important to diagnose in the presence of trauma. The pleura should be traced carefully along its course, particularly in the apices. For patients with obvious clinical evidence of tension pneumothorax, such as diminished breath sounds, tympanitic hemithorax, and displacement of the trachea to the contralateral side, delay for a chest x-ray confirmation prior to placement of a chest tube is neither necessary nor desirable.

MANAGEMENT

For pneumothorax following trauma, treatment consists of placement of a chest tube. The midaxillary line at the fifth intercostal space is the preferred site, although some prefer a higher, anterior placement at the midclavicular line. Although a small pneumothorax with minimal symptoms may require only a size 28 French tube, a size 40 French tube should be utilized for traumatically induced pneumothorax. The technique consists of preparation of the site, local infiltration with lidocaine for awake patients, incision along the axis of the ribs, and blunt dissection through the muscular layers and parietal pleura over the superior margin of the rib. Persons inexperienced in chest tube placement frequently make a tentative, too small incision in the skin or too small an opening in the pleura. Particularly in the obese or very muscular patient, it is important to make an adequate skin incision to permit effective blunt dissection of the fatty or muscular layers. The pleura should then be pierced with a hemostat or clamp, which should be opened widely after insertion to create a passage that can be located readily for insertion of the tube. The pleural cavity should be explored with the gloved finger to confirm that the pleural cavity has indeed been entered and that no lung tissue is adherent to the chest wall. After the tube is inserted and placed to suction (Fig. 3.1), it is secured with a no. 2 nylon suture and sealed with petrolatum gauze. A chest x-ray film should be obtained routinely after placement to ensure adequate reexpansion. If a persistent air leak is present and the lung is not reexpanding, a second chest tube at another site of the hemithorax should be placed. Continued air leak or lack of reexpansion after two chest tubes will necessitate urgent consultation by a thoracic surgeon, who most likely will perform a bronchoscopy to rule out tracheobronchial injury (5–7).

Hemothorax
DIAGNOSIS

This clinical entity is also confirmed quickly by chest x-ray study, if more than a few hundred milliliters of blood have accumulated in the chest. On upright chest film, the layer of accumulated blood is easily identified. On supine film, the layering of blood may make smaller amounts of accumulated blood somewhat less evident. In penetrating trauma of the chest, however, hemopneumothorax is essentially universal, and chest x-ray films are generally not necessary prior to tube placement.

MANAGEMENT

As with pneumothorax, treatment consists of placement of a chest tube. Again, a size 40 French tube is preferred, and the lateral approach is used. For the emergency physician who is resuscitating a trauma victim, placement of a chest tube for hemothorax is straightforward, but massive drainage of blood from the chest may present a more significant challenge. Certainly, if autotransfusion is available it should be utilized if there are no contraindications. If more than 1000 to 1500 ml of blood are evacuated on initial placement, or if drainage continues at a rate greater than 300 ml/hr for 3

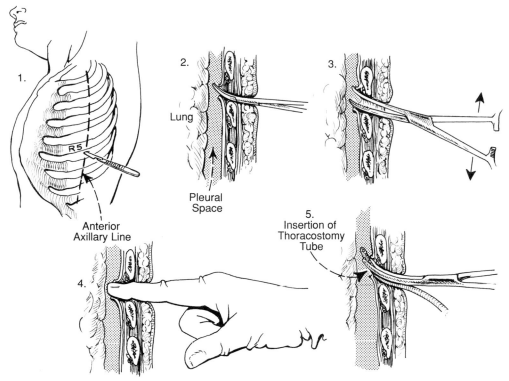

Figure 3.1. Technique for insertion of chest tube. *1,* location of the skin and subcutaneous incision at the level of the fifth intercostal space midaxillary line. *2,* a small hemostat is used to perforate the pleural cavity. No tunneling is necessary. *3,* a larger hemostat is used to expand the intercostal muscles. *4,* a finger should be introduced to ensure that the lung is not adherent to the chest wall. *5,* the chest tube is inserted with the help of a curved hemostat.

consecutive hours, the patient will need emergent exploration by a thoracic surgeon consultant. If the patient deteriorates rapidly after drainage of a massive hemothorax and death is imminent despite maximal fluid resuscitation, then immediate thoracotomy and control of continued hemorrhage must be considered. Obviously, this procedure should be performed by the surgical team if one is available; however, if the patient will clearly die prior to the arrival of the surgeon, then the emergency physician must act accordingly, proceed with thoracotomy, and attempt to gain proximal control by initial finger compression of the bleeding site(s), reserving clamping of the bleeding structure(s) only when clearly safe to do so. Rapid fluid resuscitation will be successful only if major bleeding can be brought under control quickly (1).

Tracheobronchial Injury
DIAGNOSIS
Disruption of the tracheobronchial tree usually occurs within 3 cm of the carina, with a shearing or tearing of the distal bronchi from more fixed proximal structures. Rapid deceleration, such as occurs in motor vehicle trauma or falls from a height, is a common cause. A large amount of subcutaneous air is frequently detected on presentation, and chest radiographs may reveal mediastinal air or pneumothorax. Persisting air leak after

chest tube placement is highly suggestive of disruption. The final diagnosis is made by bronchoscopy performed by an experienced thoracic surgeon.

MANAGEMENT

This injury must be managed by a thoracic surgeon. The role of the emergency physician in this case is rapid recognition of the problem, placement of chest tubes if pneumothorax is present, and continuation of aggressive resuscitative efforts until definitive management can be performed (5, 8, 9).

CARDIAC AND GREAT VESSEL INJURIES
Myocardial Contusion
DIAGNOSIS

Severe blunt chest trauma frequently results in contusion of the myocardium. Steering wheel imprint, fracture of the sternum, flail chest, and other indications of a direct blow to the chest should be considered presumptive evidence of myocardial contusion. In patients who have symptoms of this injury, chest pain and unexplained sinus tachycardia are the most common, followed by atrial fibrillation and extrasystole. The electrocardiogram may show evidence of block or frank ischemia, but in most cases the tracing is normal. The diagnosis is initially made on clinical grounds, based on the mechanism of injury and presence of associated characteristic injuries.

MANAGEMENT

In the patient with a diagnosis of myocardial contusion, prophylactic treatment is usually with a bolus of lidocaine (1 mg/kg) followed by a drip of 1–3 mg/min for at least 24 hr. Alternative agents are bretylium tosylate or procainamide. In all suspected cases, admission to a monitored bed is necessary. Serial CPK isoenzymes should also be monitored. Patients with acidosis or hypoxemia resulting from other injuries are at particular risk of dysrhythmias in the setting of myocardial contusion; these problems should be identified and corrected (3, 10).

Myocardial Rupture
DIAGNOSIS

If blunt chest trauma is severe enough, myocardial rupture may occur. This catastrophic injury is usually rapidly fatal, but if a low-pressure chamber is ruptured, the patient may survive. The presentation will be consistent with pericardial tamponade: distended neck veins, diminished heart tones, and narrowed pulse pressure; however, if the patient is symptomatic from other injuries, these classic signs may not be apparent. Penetrating cardiac injury may also be survivable if only low-pressure chambers are involved (the right ventricle is the most commonly injured chamber in stab wounds to the heart). The presence of central chest injury, when coupled with progressive sinus tachycardia and hypotension, is suggestive of possible myocardial rupture.

MANAGEMENT

The primary concern in the emergency department resuscitation of patients with suspected myocardial rupture is aggressive volume replacement. Multiple peripheral line placement is preferred over central line placement because the thoracic vascular architecture may be distorted by this injury. Salt solutions are used initially, followed by type-specific blood as soon as it is available. A cardiothoracic surgeon should be contacted as soon as this injury is suspected, even if the patient is not immediately decompensating. If pericardial tamponade is suspected and the patient is deteriorating, pericardiocentesis should be performed. Myocardial rupture can be managed definitively only in the operating room. However, if the patient is dying despite volume replacement and standard resuscitative measures, the emergency physician may elect to perform thoracotomy to relieve pericardial tamponade and attempt a temporizing repair of identified myocardial injury (see Chapter 2 for a description of emergency thoracotomy technique).

Ruptured Thoracic Aorta

The diagnosis and management of this lethal injury are discussed extensively in Chapter 13.

REFERENCES

1. Callaham ML. Current therapy in emergency medicine. Toronto: Decker, 1987.
2. Kattan KR. What to look for in rib fractures and how. JAMA 1980;243:262.
3. Kirsch MM, Sloan H. Blunt chest trauma. Boston: Little, Brown, 1977.
4. McSwain NE, Kerstein M. Evaluation and management of trauma. East Norwalk, CT: Appleton-Century-Crofts, 1986.
5. Moore EE. Critical decisions in trauma. St. Louis: Mosby, 1984.
6. Rosen P, Baker FJ, Barkin RM, Braen GR, Dailey RH, Levy RC. Emergency medicine: concepts and clinical practice. St. Louis: Mosby, 1988.
7. Sabiston DC, Spencer FG. Gibbon's surgery of the chest. Philadelphia: Saunders, 1976.
8. Shields TW. General thoracic surgery. Philadelphia: Lea & Febiger, 1989.
9. Trunkey DD, Lewis FR. Chest trauma. Surg Clin North Am 1980;60:1541–1549.
10. Trunkey DD, Lewis FR. Current therapy of trauma-2. Toronto: Decker, 1986.

4 Imaging of Thoracic Trauma

Stuart E. Mirvis, MD

Diagnostic imaging plays a major role in the emergency assessment of the multitrauma victim, particularly the patient with major thoracic trauma. At the Shock Trauma Center of the Maryland Institute for Emergency Medical Services Systems, chest radiography is the primary modality used in such assessment but, depending on the individual circumstances, other modalities may include computed tomography (CT), digital subtraction angiography (DSA), sonography, and magnetic resonance imaging (MRI). This chapter focuses primarily on imaging findings related to thoracic pathology encountered in the acute posttrauma period (less than 24 hr); however, it also addresses some pathologic processes that typically develop after the acute phase of injury as well as iatrogenic complications that can occur during the resuscitation and physiologic monitoring of the patient with thoracic trauma.

DIAGNOSTIC IMAGING IN THE ACUTE SETTING

Chest radiography, the principle diagnostic screening test performed emergently after admission of the multitrauma patient, is often obtained while resuscitation efforts are in progress. Radiographic observations can confirm clinical diagnoses such as tension pneumothorax, hemothorax, or pulmonary contusion and can suggest other injuries, such as mediastinal hemorrhage, diaphragmatic rupture, or bronchial or esophageal laceration, that may be clinically occult.

Technical Considerations

The wide range of tissue density differences in the chest makes it difficult to optimally image the entire chest with a single radiograph. Although a fast-exposure and high-kilovoltage technique (120–140 kV) (1) best displays all the information present on the chest film with limited motion artifacts, it is a difficult technique to achieve with the single-phase, line-operated portable radiographic units commonly used in the acute setting (2). Ideal exposures are best obtained using three-phase radiographic generators and fast-film/screen combinations to acquire rapid exposures. However, at the Shock Trauma Center, a single-phase, high-frequency overhead generator system combines mobility and compactness with improved image quality compared to standard mobile radiographic units (2).

In clinical situations in which blunt thoracic trauma is suspected, my colleagues and I routinely obtain both a supine chest radiograph, exposed to accentuate lung parenchymal detail, and a "true erect" anteroposterior (AP) chest radiograph (see below) with increased exposure to penetrate the mediastinum for assessment of the aortic arch and descending aorta, the tracheobronchial tree, and the retrocardiac lung field. In general, the erect AP chest radiograph allows easier detection of pneumothorax, hemothorax, and basilar lung infiltrates than the supine view (1). In some cases, my colleagues and I utilize contrast-enhanced CT scanning of the thorax in the emergency setting to evaluate the thorax in patients who cannot sit upright (see below); this technique provides increased sensitivity for detecting many pathologic processes.

Mediastinal Hemorrhage/Aortic Rupture

Traumatic rupture of the aorta (TRA) accounts for 16% of the fatalities resulting from motor vehicle accidents. The mortality from TRA prior to reaching a medical facility has been reported at 85–90% but can be expected to improve with increasing use of regional trauma centers and rapid helicopter transportation (3). The danger of rapid exsanguination remains a constant risk in patients who initially survive aortic injury; the study of Parmley et al. (4) emphasized the need for prompt diagnosis and surgical management. Of 35 patients who survived to reach a medical facility but whose aortic injuries were not diagnosed, 30% died within 6 hr, and 40% by 24 hr after admission. Unfortunately, clinical signs and symptoms in patients with TRA have not provided sufficient sensitivity or specificity to dictate the need for thoracic angiography. Overall, suggestive clinical findings are present in less than one-half of patients, and up to one-third have no evidence of external thoracic trauma (3, 5–7).

At the Shock Trauma Center, the decision to proceed to thoracic angiography has been based largely on interpretation of the admission chest radiograph in light of a clinical history of significant decelerating thoracic trauma. Over the past two decades, a wide variety of radiologic signs have been promoted for their value as indicators of mediastinal hemorrhage and potential great vessel injury (Table 4.1). A retrospective analysis of chest radiographs and thoracic aortograms of more than 200 patients, including 42 with arteriographically diagnosed and surgically confirmed great vessel ruptures, was conducted at the Shock Trauma Center to determine the value of these signs (Table 4.2). It must be emphasized that all of the radiologic signs described indicate the presence of mediastinal hemorrhage and are only indicators of *potential* thoracic great vessel rupture.

Radiographic assessment of the mediastinal contour should be based whenever possible on the true erect view of the thorax. Ayella et al. (8) argued that an AP projection with the patient erect and leaning 10–15° beyond the vertical most closely simulated the routine posteroanterior chest radiograph. As illustrated in Figures 4.1 and 4.2, the true erect view provides a more accurate display of the anatomy of the superior mediastinum than either supine or semierect projections. Schwab at al. (9) assessed the effect of patient position on the plain radiographic diagnosis of TRA. In their study, 21 of 55 patients (38%) had apparently widened mediastinums as shown on supine chest radiographs obtained after blunt chest trauma but were considered to have normal chest radiographs in the erect position; all were found to be normal by aortography. However, 4 of 12 patients with widened mediastinal contours on both views had TRA. These authors recommended the erect view to avoid unnecessary aortograms. In a retrospective review of 49 patients in whom both supine and true erect chest radiographs were obtained prior to thoracic aortography, both views were found to be equally sensitive in detecting patients with TRA, but only 20% of patients with negative aortograms were considered to have normal supine chest radiographs, while the true erect view was considered normal in 48% of patients with negative aortograms (10).

RADIOLOGIC SIGNS
Mediastinal Widening

In 1975, Marsh and Sturm (11) concluded that a mediastinum greater than 8 cm in width at the level of the aortic knob on a 100-cm AP chest radiograph constituted a highly sensitive sign of aortic rupture. However, in a later publication (12), Sturm et al. demonstrated significant overlap in the measured mediastinal width of traumatized patients with and without TRA, thus diminishing the value of this sign. In 1981, Seltzer et al. (13) introduced the concept of the mediastinal-width/chest-width ratio (M/C), suggesting that a ratio of 0.25–0.28 on an AP supine chest radiograph was 95% sensitive and 75% specific. Subsequent studies by Marnocha et al. (14) challenged this concept. They found an M/C ratio greater than 0.38 to be only 40% sensitive and 60% specific. In the experience of my colleagues and myself, an M/C ratio greater than 0.25 was 53% sensitive and 59% specific as an indicator of aortic rupture (10).

Progressive widening of the superior mediastinum on serial radiographs due to a gradually expanding hematoma has been suggested as another sign of TRA. Applebaum et al. (15) recommended serial chest radiographs during the first 48 hr after admission to detect delayed mediastinal bleeding. Ayella et al. (8) challenged this concept because, in their extensive clinical experience, no patient with an aortic rupture exhibited a gradually expanding hematoma. They argued that lysis of a mediastinal hematoma initially containing an aortic rupture or rupture of the adventitia would result in a sudden, massive hemorrhage that would not permit time for serial radiographs. They suggested that descriptions of gradually widening mediastinums were either from nonaortic sources of bleeding or lack of concern in reproducing technically equivalent chest radiographs. The experience of my colleagues and myself over the past 6 yr has validated this impression.

Abnormal Aortic Arch/Descending Aorta Contour

Several authors have stressed the importance of abnormalities of the contour or obscuration of the aortic outline as an indicator of TRA (Figs 4.3–4.5). Marsh and Sturm (11) reported this sign in all of their patients with aortic rupture, but also in 45% of those with normal aortas. Marnocha et al. (14) reported this sign to be sensitive (88%) but nonspecific (42%) as an indicator of TRA. They observed that the outline of the aorta may be blurred if the radiograph is underexposed or if there is excessive motion. Adjacent lung infiltrates due to aspiration or pulmonary contusion can obscure the aortic outline as can venous hemorrhage into the mediastinum. Overall, previous series have found a 53–100% sensitivity and 21–53% specificity for this sign as an indicator of TRA. The review by my colleagues and myself similarly found a 72% sensitivity and 47% specificity for this sign (10).

Shift of the Trachea/Nasogastric Tube

By virtue of anatomic proximity, a contained hematoma or pseudoaneurysm of the proximal descending aorta might be expected to affect the course of the adjacent trachea and esophagus. Gerlock et al. (16) reported that, if both the trachea and esophagus were shifted to the right on an AP chest radiograph, then the patient had a 96% probability of TRA (Figs. 4.4, 4.5). In their series of 45 patients, no patient without a shifted nasogastric tube had a ruptured aorta. Wales et al. (17) demonstrated deviation of the nasogastric tube to the right in only five of eight patients with TRA. A study by Dart and Braitman (18) found normal tracheal position in many patients with TRA.

Table 4.1.
Sensitivity and Specificity of Plain Chest Radiologic Findings for Traumatic Rupture of the Aorta in Previous Series[a]

Observations		Marnocha et al. (14) (13/73)[b]	Sturm/ Olson (82) (26/—)	Sefzcek et al. (83) (12/54)	Gundry et al. (84) (25/173)	Barcia et al. (7) (17/113)	Kirsh et al. (6) (43/—)	Marsh/ Sturm (11) (12/47)	Woodring et al. (85) (15/20)	Akins et al. (86) (44/—)
Widened mediastinum	Sensitivity	100%[c]	81%	90%	89%	94%[e]	97%	100%[f]	82–92%[g]	95%
	Specificity	(85)[d] 1[c] (34)[d]				60		50		
Abnormal aortic contour	Sensitivity	88	88	100	82	100[b]	95	100	53	
	Specificity	42				21		55		
Tracheal shift	Sensitivity	45[i]	46	50		12	32	100	53	
	Specificity	89				95		80		
Nasogastric tube shift	Sensitivity	71		40	23	50			71	
	Specificity	94				90				
Left apical cap	Sensitivity	62		20	39	63[j]			53	
	Specificity	75				76				
Left paraspinal stripe thickened	Sensitivity	40			62	83[j]			40[k]	
	Specificity	90				89				
Right paraspinal stripe thickened	Sensitivity			50		29[j]				
	Specificity					94				
Depressed left mainstem bronchus	Sensitivity	41		30[l]	25	7[m]	30	80[m]	40	
	Specificity	90				100		80		

Finding	Measure					
Lung contusion	Sensitivity	38	42	18	80	
	Specificity	77		58	40	
Rib fractures	Sensitivity	27	28	41[n]	80	
	Specificity	76	24[n]	49	0	
Pneumothorax	Sensitivity	15	19	12	20	
	Specificity	93		72	85	
Hemothorax	Sensitivity	19	36	38	60	
	Specificity	79		76	55	7[o]
Aorticopulmonary window opacification	Sensitivity	84	0	80	100	
	Specificity			56	80	40
Right paratracheal wall thickening	Sensitivity					
	Specificity					90
Displaced superior vena cava	Sensitivity		46	46	40	
	Specificity			77	100	
Opacification of medial left lung	Sensitivity	50		100		
	Specificity			95		

[a]From Mirvis SE, Bidwell JK, Buddenmeyer EU, Diaconis JN, Pais OS, Whitley JE. Imaging diagnosis of traumatic aortic rupture: a review and experience at a major trauma center. Invest Radiol 1987;22:187–196.
[b]Ratios in parentheses are ruptures/nonruptures.
[c]Mediastinum/chest > 0.25.
[d]Subjective impression.
[e]Subjective determination.
[f]>8 cm at aortic arch (100 cm anteroposterior supine).
[g]82% for mediastinal width > 8 cm; 92% for mediastinum/chest > 0.25.
[h]Aortic knob not discernible on overpenetrated view.
[i]Left tracheal wall to right of the T4 spinous process.
[j]Without coexisting rib fractures.
[k]Right or left paraspinal stripe.
[l]Left bronchus > 40 degrees below horizontal.
[m]Carinal angle < 40 degrees.
[n]First and second ribs.
[o]Left hemothorax.

Table 4.2.
Sensitivity, Specificity, and Predictive Values of the Signs of Traumatic
Aortic Rupture[a, b]

| Sign | Incidence | | Sensitivity | Specificity | Predictive Values | |
	Positive Diagnosis	Negative Diagnosis			Positive	Negative
Aortic knob outline	113	323	72%	47%	26%	87%
Widened mediastinum[c]	82	249	53	59	25	83
Tracheal shift[d]	31	48	20	92	39	82
Left mainstem bronchus[e]	5	5	3	99	50	80
Left hemothorax	7	16	5	97	30	80
Nasogastric tube displaced to right	14	23	9	96	38	80
Left apical cap						
Fracture	3	31	2	95	9	79
No fracture	14	27	9	96	34	80
Rib fracture first through fourth	24	98	15	84	20	79
Widened left paraspinal stripe [f]						
Fracture	4	24	3	96	14	79
No fracture	18	21	12	97	46	81
Widened right paraspinal stripe[g]						
Fracture	3	4	2	99	43	80
No fracture	3	7	2	99	30	80
Lung contusion	18	88	12	86	17	79
Loss of descending aorta	98	283	63	53	26	85
Loss of aortico-pulmonary window	65	101	42	83	39	85
Opacified medial left lung field	18	32	12	95	36	81
Pneumothorax or pneumo-mediastinum	18	69	12	89	21	80
Displaced superior vena cava to right[g]	11	23	7	96	32	80
Negative	2	84	—	—	—	98

[a]From Mirvis SE, Bidwell JK, Buddemeyer EU, Diaconis JN, Pais SO, Whitley JE, et al. Value of chest radiography in excluding traumatic aortic rupture. Radiology 1987;163:487–493.
[b]Total of all examiners. Based on 156 total positive and 606 total negative studies.
[c]Subjective impression, or >8 cm at the aortic knob, or >0.25 mediastinal width/chest width.
[d]Left tracheal wall to the right of the T4 spinous process.
[e]Subjective or shifted >40 degrees below horizontal.
[f]Greater than 5 mm or greater than one-half the width of descending aorta, or greater than one-half the distance from the spine to the left margin of the descending aorta.
[g]Subjective impression.

Difficulties in utilizing these signs include rotation of the chest, failure to place a nasogastric tube, and the potential of a balancing hematoma in the right mediastinum. In previous series, deviation of the trachea has demonstrated a poor sensitivity (12–53%) but better specificity (80–89%), whereas deviation of a nasogastric tube to the right has a higher sensitivity (40–71%) and specificity (90–94%). In the review by my colleagues and myself, tracheal shift to the right of the spinous process of the T4 vertebra was 20% sensitive and 92% specific, whereas bowing of the nasogastric tube was 9% sensitive and 96% specific (10).

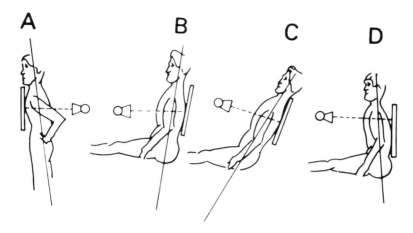

Figure 4.1. The true erect anteroposterior chest radiograph. **A,** position for normal posteroanterior chest radiograph in a standing patient. **B,** usual position for portable AP radiograph. **C,** "cheating" AP chest radiograph with x-ray tube tilted to be perpendicular to the patient. **D,** "true erect" portable AP chest radiograph that most closely mimics the position of the thorax for a posteroanterior radiograph and produces the least distortion of mediastinal contours of all anteroposterior views. (From Ayella RA. Radiologic management of the massively traumatized patient. Baltimore: Williams & Wilkins, 1978:86.)

The Apical Pleural Cap Sign

In 1975, Simeone et al. (19) stressed the value of the extrapleural left apical cap as a sign of an aortic isthmus region tear (Fig. 4.4). Blood from an aortic tear could extend along the left subclavian artery in the potential space between the left parietal pleura and the extrapleural soft tissue, producing an apical soft-tissue density. In their original study, this sign was present in 25 of 27 patients with TRA. However, a subsequent evaluation in 1981 by Simeone et al. (20) noted that the apical cap was usually accompanied by another sign of TRA such as a widened mediastinum or poorly defined aortic arch; they believed that aortography was not indicated if an apical cap was the only positive radiologic sign. Other series indicate a sensitivity of 20–63% and a specificity of 75–76% for this sign (Table 4.1)

The false-positive rate of the apical pleural cap sign is increased by the similar radiologic appearance produced by hematoma arising from adjacent rib or clavicle fractures or by an ectatic subclavian artery. My colleagues and I have observed this sign in only 9% of our patients with TRA; however, half of the patients with this sign but without associated fractures, had aortic rupture diagnosed (10). In agreement with Simeone et al. (19, 20), I have observed no patient in whom an apical pleural cap has been the only sign of a ruptured aorta.

Widened Paraspinal Lines

Bleeding within the mediastinum can distend the paraspinal stripes. Barcia and Livoni (7) reported a displaced left paraspinal line, defined as greater than one-half the distance from the spine to the left margin of the descending aorta, in 83% of patients with aortic rupture (Fig. 4.5). This sign was also 83% specific without concomitant spine or sternal fractures. Other series have determined a somewhat lower sensitivity of

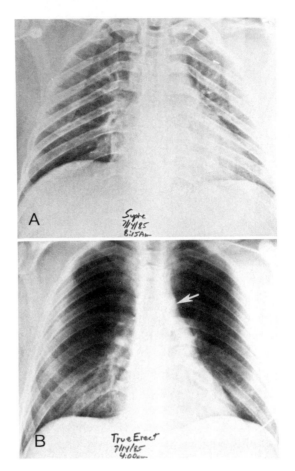

Figure 4.2. Comparison of mediastinal contour in supine and erect view of same patient. **A,** supine projection tends to widen mediastinum and distorts normal contours. **B,** erect view with increased exposure clearly reveals a normal mediastinal width and sharply defined aortic arch contour *(arrow)*. (From Mirvis SE. Traumatic disruption of the thoracic aorta: imaging diagnosis. Trauma Q 1988;4:49–60.)

40–62% (Table 4.1). Barcia and Livoni (7) found displacement of the right paraspinal line to be less sensitive (seen in only 4 of 14 patients with TRA) but 94% specific without spine or sternal fractures. Peters and Gamsu (21) found this sign in 8 of 14 patients with TRA and in none without this injury.

Sensitivity of the paraspinal stripe sign is likely to be compromised by failure to visualize even widened paraspinal lines on underexposed chest radiographs and specificity is decreased by hematomas arising from concomitant spine fractures. Widening of the right and left paraspinal stripes without associated thoracic fracture occurred in only 2 and 12%, respectively, of my patients with TRA (10).

Depression of the Left Mainstem Bronchus

Hematoma or pseudoaneurysm arising from the aortic isthmus may depress the left mainstem bronchus and narrow the carinal angle (Fig. 4.4). Barcia and Livoni (7)

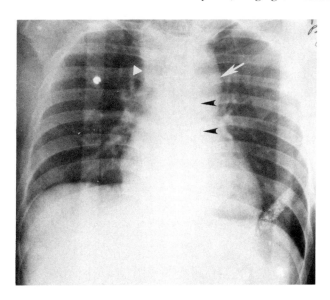

Figure 4.3. Mediastinal hemorrhage (radiography). An AP chest radiograph demonstrates abnormal mediastinal contours with distortion of aortic arch outline *(white arrow)* and widened right paratracheal soft-tissue stripe *(white arrowhead)*. Left paraspinal stripe *(black arrowheads)* is slightly widened as well. The aorta was ruptured at arteriography.

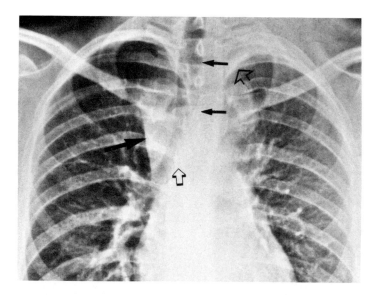

Figure 4.4. Mediastinal hemorrhage (radiography). An AP chest radiograph after blunt chest trauma reveals a tracheal shift to the right *(small black arrows)*, a widened right paratracheal stripe *(solid black arrow)*, and a left apical pleural "cap" of extrapleural fluid *(open arrow.)* The carinal angle appears narrowed *(closed white arrow)*. The aorta was ruptured at arteriography. (From Mirvis SE. Traumatic disruption of the thoracic aorta: imaging diagnosis. Trauma Q 1988;4:49–60).

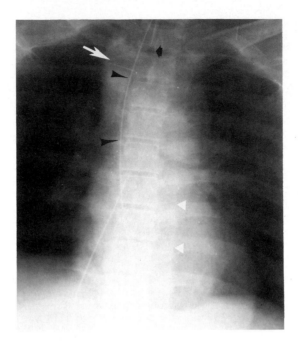

Figure 4.5.   Mediastinal hemorrhage (radiography). An AP chest radiograph after blunt thoracic trauma reveals a tracheal shift to the right of the T4 spinous process *(black arrow)*, bowing of the nasogastric tube to the right *(black arrowheads)*, widening of the right paratracheal soft tissues *(white arrow)*, and widening of the left paraspinal stripe *(white arrowheads)*. The patient had a ruptured thoracic aorta at angiography.

measured the carinal angle in 113 patients with blunt chest trauma. In 17 patients with aortic injury, the carinal angle varied from 56 to 92° (mean, 75°) and, in patients without vascular injury, the range was 49–108° (mean, 71°). They believed this measurement had no predictive value. Other series using various criteria to measure left mainstem bronchus depression have shown a low sensitivity (4–41%) but high specificity (80–100%) for this sign (Table 4.1). Decreased sensitivity may be related in part to difficulty in accurately visualizing the mainstem bronchi on underexposed portable chest radiographs. This sign was present in only 3% of patients seen at this institution with TRA, but 50% of patients with this sign had TRA diagnosed angiographically (10).

Injury to Ribs, Lungs, and Pleura
Other signs (pulmonary contusion, rib fractures, pneumothorax, and hemothorax) present on chest radiographs following blunt chest trauma have been assessed for potential association with TRA. In general, these signs have not shown sufficient sensitivity or specificity to be of diagnostic value in dictating the need for thoracic angiography.

Combining Radiologic Signs: Diagnostic Values
Analysis of the study at this institution, as well as that of previous studies, demonstrates that no single plain chest radiographic sign is either completely sensitive or specific in diagnosing TRA (Tables 4.1 and 4.2). Thus, some authors have suggested that any patient

with a history of blunt decelerating chest trauma should have diagnostic angiography despite the appearance of the chest radiograph. My colleagues and I believe that this procedure would result in an excessive number of normal aortograms that might delay diagnoses and treatment of other life-threatening craniocerebral or abdominal injuries. Mirvis et al. (10) have noted that the simultaneous absence of certain combinations of radiologic signs has a high negative predictive value (Table 4.3). For instance, a normal aortic arch, normal descending aorta, and clear aorticopulmonary window had a 91% negative predictive value on both supine and erect radiographs of the chest. A normal aortic arch and normal descending aorta had an 87% negative predictive value on the erect view and a 91% negative predictive value on the supine study. A normal chest radiograph had a 98% negative predictive value (Table 4.2).

It must be recalled, however, that these statistics are derived from a population of patients whose radiographs were already "suspicious" enough to warrant aortography. At the Shock Trauma Center, a substantial majority of patients with blunt chest trauma are excluded from arteriography after consideration of their clinical presentation,

Table 4.3.
Effect of Combining Signs on Diagnosis of Traumatic Aortic Rupture[a]

Signs Present (or Conditions)	Sensitivity		False Positive Rate		Positive Predictive Value	
	Supine	Erect	Supine	Erect	Supine	Erect
Widened mediastinum or abnormal aortic arch	88%	72%	76%	55%	21%	34%
Abnormal aortic knob or loss of descending aorta contour	90	76	75	45	22	34
Abnormal aortic arch, or loss of aortico-pulmonary window	88	86	70	55	22	33
Widened mediastinum, abnormal aortic arch, loss of descending aorta, loss of aortico-pulmonary window	93	89	84	58	20	32

Signs Present (or Conditions)	Sensitivity		False Negative Rate		Negative Predictive Value	
	Supine	Erect	Supine	Erect	Supine	Erect
Normal aortic arch and descending aorta	25%	49%	11%	23%	91%	87%
Normal aortic arch, descending aortic, and aortico-pulmonary window	22	45	9	14	91	91
Normal aortic arch, aortico-pulmonary window, and left paraspinal stripe	27	56	12	22	91	89
Normal aortic arch, aortico-pulmonary window, and tracheal position	20	44	8	13	91	92

[a]From Mirvis SE, Bidwell JK, Buddemeyer EU, Diaconis JN, Pais SO, Whitley JE, et al. Value of chest radiography in excluding traumatic aortic rupture. Radiology 1987;163:487–493.

mechanism of injury, and screening admission chest radiographs, which demonstrate normal mediastinal contours, i.e. a normal aortic arch, normal descending aorta, clear aorticopulmonary window, lack of tracheal or esophageal shift, and a normal left paraspinal stripe. To my knowledge, and based on analysis of the admission chest radiograph, my colleagues and I have not missed an aortic injury that was later clinically manifest and have, at the same time, avoided aortography on a large percentage of patients admitted with blunt chest trauma.

COMPUTED TOMOGRAPHY

The potential role of dynamic contrast-enhanced computed tomography (DCECT) in assessing the mediastinum for hemorrhage or its potential to directly visualize great vessel injury is controversial. In a small series of 10 patients, Heiberg et al. (22) demonstrated the ability of CT to demonstrate direct evidence of aortic injury in four patients and to identify normal aortas in six. However, other studies have cited a lack of both sensitivity and specificity for CT in diagnosing TRA and emphasize problems with motion and volume averaging in identifying intimal injuries (23, 24).

In a previous study, Mirvis et al. (25) evaluated the results of DCECT in 20 patients who were suspected of having mediastinal hemorrhage and in whom angiography was also performed. All patients were studied using DCECT scanning methods with CT table incrementation at 1-cm intervals. Contrast boluses of 50 ml were delivered through a large peripheral intravenous line, starting just above the aortic arch and again at the level of the carina. CT scans demonstrated direct aortic injury or mediastinal hematomas in all four patients ultimately confirmed to have TRA (Figs. 4.6 and 4.7). Although six patients with mediastinal hematomas but no aortic injury were also identified, 10 patients without evidence of mediastinal hematoma or direct aortic injury by CT were confirmed as normal by angiography. Larger prospective studies are needed to assess the role of DCECT in the diagnosis of mediastinal hematomas and thoracic great vessel injury.

In my opinion, any patient with radiologic evidence of mediastinal hemorrhage following an appropriate history of blunt decelerating thoracic injury, particularly when based upon interpretation of the true erect chest radiograph, should undergo immediate aortography. In patients for whom there is limited indication for aortography based on the reported mechanism of injury or for whom the chest radiographs are equivocal or of suboptimal quality, DCECT may function as an ancillary screening study in selecting patients for aortography. Demonstration of mediastinal hemorrhage by DCECT even without direct demonstration of great vessel injury should lead to performance of aortography. DCECT is particularly appropriate for patients for whom CT is already required to evaluate other injuries such as craniofacial or abdominal trauma.

AORTOGRAPHY: DIGITAL SUBTRACTION TECHNIQUE

Ultimately, the diagnosis of great vessel injury requires confirmation by arteriography prior to thoracotomy. Aortography should be performed as soon as possible. During the past 4 yr, my colleagues and I have exclusively used intraarterial digital subtraction angiography (IADSA) to evaluate the great thoracic vessels (Fig. 4.8). Initially, 61 patients, including 10 with TRA (26) were studied by IADSA. Conventional cut-film aortograms were also performed in the first 10 patients evaluated. IADSA was about 50%

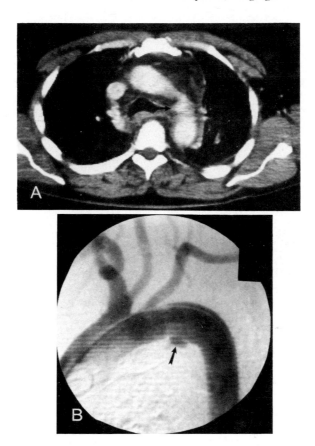

Figure 4.6.   Ruptured thoracic aorta (CT). **A,** axial CT scan with intravenous enhancement demonstrates a focal bulge *(arrow)* projecting medially from the aortic arch. Mediastinal fat is streaked with fluid density suggesting hemorrhage. **B,** corresponding digital subtraction arteriogram confirms an aortic pseudoaneurysm arising from the inferior aspect of the aortic arch *(arrow).* (From Mirvis SE, Kostrubiak I, Whitley NO, Goldstein LD, Rodriguez A. Role of CT in excluding major arterial injury after blunt thoracic trauma. AJR 1987;149:601–605).

faster than conventional methods, required less iodinated contrast, could be performed with smaller caliber catheters, and could be used to rapidly assess other vascular territories such as the neck or upper arms without requiring catheter exchange. My colleagues and I currently perform IADSA using a high-resolution (1024 × 1024) matrix and 9-inch image intensifier. The aorta is studied in two projections after injection of 36 ml of 60% contrast in 2 sec through a no.4 French high-flow pigtail catheter. For large patients, additional images at the level of the diaphragm may be required to include this region of the aorta. The high-contrast volumes and flow rates required for conventional aortography rarely cause acute rupture of a traumatic aortic pseudoaneurysm (27). In my experience, intravenous DSA lacks sufficient resolution in many cases to adequately exclude subtle vascular injuries and requires greater intravenous contrast loads than IADSA.

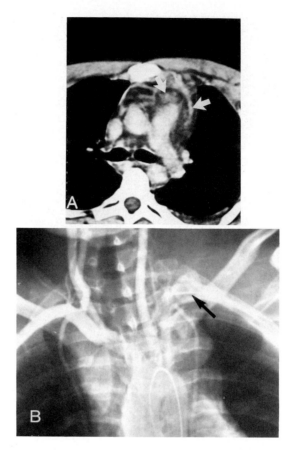

Figure 4.7. Mediastinal hemorrhage (CT). **A,** axial CT image at the level of the aortic root obtained after blunt chest trauma. Blood outlines parietal pleura and infiltrates mediastinal fat *(arrows).* **B,** arteriogram reveals avulsion of the left subclavian artery with extravasation of contrast into soft tissues *(arrow).* (From Mirvis SE, Kostrubiak I, Whitley NO, Goldstein LD, Rodriguez A. Role of CT in excluding major arterial injury after blunt thoracic trauma. AJR 1987;149:601–605).

MAGNETIC RESONANCE IMAGING

MRI provides detailed anatomic images of the body through any anatomic plane desired. MRI has far greater contrast resolution, but less spatial resolution, than CT scanning. MRI in clinical use images hydrogen protons within the body. Image intensity in each small tissue volume is determined by the number of hydrogen atoms present (predominantly in the form of fat and water), the restoration of alignment of proton spins with an external magnetic field after a radiofrequency perturbation (determined by relaxation time constants T1 and T2), and relative motion of protons through the imaged tissue volume. Since proton spins in flowing blood that were excited or flipped by radiofrequency exit the imaged volume prior to relaxation, their signal is not registered in the imaged volume, resulting in a characteristic flow void. This property permits MRI to directly visualize blood vessels carrying rapidly flowing blood without intravenous contrast agents. To date, MRI has been employed to demonstrate congenital anomalies of the aorta as well as chronic pseudoaneurysm resulting from aortic rupture. MRI can

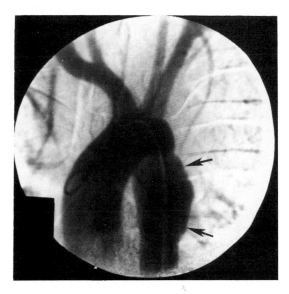

Figure 4.8.   Aortic pseudoaneurysm (DSA). Pseudoaneurysm of descending aorta after blunt decelerating chest trauma *(arrows)*. In my experience, DSA has proven to be a highly reliable way to document great vessel injury and is faster and safer than conventional serial film arteriography. (From Mirvis SE. Traumatic disruption of the thoracic aorta: imaging diagnosis. Trauma Q 1988;4:49–60.)

also be employed to assess the aorta following surgical repair of thoracic aortic ruptures.

Currently, MRI is limited in application to the acutely injured patient because of difficulties with hemodynamic monitoring and support in the magnetic field around the MRI device. Further developments in MRI-compatible physiologic support and monitoring devices and increasing availability of fast-imaging techniques and motion suppression techniques will undoubtedly permit direct MRI imaging of the great vessels in appropriately selected patients (28).

Pneumomediastinum
RADIOGRAPHIC APPEARANCE

Pneumomediastinum, a common sequela of blunt and penetrating thoracic injury, is recognized radiographically by demonstration of the parietal pleura. Normally, the pleura forms a border with the air-filled lung, but the introduction of air into the mediastinum leads to air density on either side of the parietal pleura, thus creating a line of soft-tissue density dividing the air-filled lung laterally and the air-filled mediastinum medially. The parietal pleural line is best appreciated along the superior left mediastinum and is often visualized paralleling the left cardiac border and fading below the midleft hemidiaphragm (Fig. 4.9). The parietal pleural to the right of the superior mediastinum can be visualized but is less consistently seen. It is important to observe that the parietal pleural line created by pneumomediastinum does not continue around the heart, as would be seen with pneumopericardium (see below). The presence of air density in the mediastinum leads to other important radiologic signs. The descending aorta is sharply outlined by air and can usually be followed into the upper abdomen

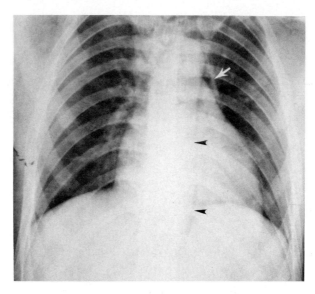

Figure 4.9. Pneumomediastinum (radiography). An AP chest radiograph demonstrates the parietal pleural line adjacent to the left superior mediastinal *(arrow)*. Note the sharp demarcation of the descending aorta due to adjacent mediastinal air *(arrowheads)*.

because of the adjacent air density (Fig 4.9). The space separating the aortic arch from the main pulmonary artery segment, the aorticopulmonary window, is sharply defined due to the contrast created by the adjacent air density (Fig. 4.9). Air in the inferior mediastinum will outline the base of the heart and the underlying diaphragm, producing an appearance of a "continuous diaphragm" across the thorax (Fig. 4.10). The presence of pneumomediastinum can best be appreciated on the lateral chest radiograph as retrosternal lucency and as streaks of air density in the middle mediastinum paralleling the trachea and esophagus (Fig. 4.11).

Air within the mediastinum can, on occasion, track into the retroperitoneum (Fig. 4.12) through transdiaphragmatic fascial communication or rupture into the intraperitoneal compartment, raising the specter of a primary pneumoperitoneum. In most cases in my experience, pneumomediastinum presents simultaneously with cervical soft-tissue emphysema.

CT APPEARANCE

Computed tomography is exquisitely sensitive to the detection of small quantities of air in the mediastinum due to its extended contrast range. Pneumomediastinum appears as lucency in the retrosternal area, with intervening streaks of mediastinal fat, and around the aorta and esophagus in the middle mediastinum. The laterally displaced parietal pleural is frequently visualized on the left side (Fig. 4.13).

ETIOLOGY
Macklin Effect/Barotrauma

In my experience, the most common etiology of pneumomediastinum seen in the acute setting is the Macklin effect in which air escapes from ruptured alveoli following blunt

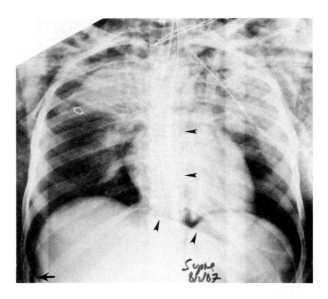

Figure 4.10. Pneumomediastinum (radiography). An AP chest radiograph after severe blunt chest trauma reveals marked bilateral subcutaneous emphysema, right upper lobe atelectasis *(open arrow),* left upper lobe contusion, and pneumomediastinum as indicated by the sharp outline of the descending aorta and the "continuous diaphragm sign" *(arrowheads).* Bilateral pneumothoraces are present with a deep sulcus sign on the right *(arrow).* The patient had a ruptured upper thoracic trachea and tracheoesophageal fistula at surgery.

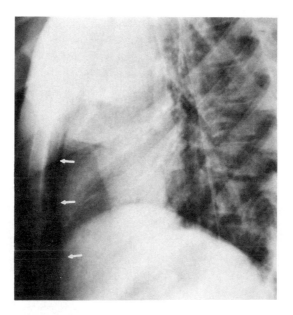

Figure 4.11. Pneumomediastinum (radiography). Radiolucency in retrosternal space represents anterior mediastinal air *(arrows).*

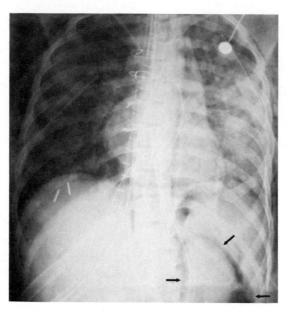

Figure 4.12. Retroperitoneal dissection of pneumomediastinum (radiography). AP chest radiograph reveals air surrounding the left kidney *(arrows)* that is believed to represent dissection of air from the mediastinum in a patient on long-term positive pressure ventilatory support. A primary gas-forming retroperitoneal process or colonic source of gas cannot be excluded as etiologic.

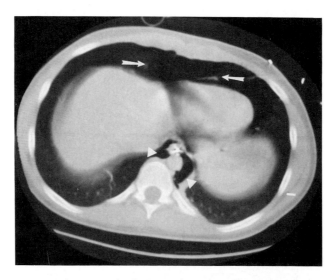

Figure 4.13. Pneumomediastinum (CT). An axial CT scan at the level of the diaphragm reveals anterior mediastinal air in the retrosternal space *(white arrows)* and air surrounding the descending aorta and esophagus *(white arrowheads)*. CT density windows were optimized to search for gas density.

thoracic trauma and dissects along the pulmonary interstitium into the hilum and mediastinum. Pneumomediastinum can result from, or be exacerbated by, positive pressure ventilatory support, especially in the presence of emphysema and pulmonary blebs. Several other etiologies, however, must be considered, including tracheobronchial rupture, esophageal rupture, or (less commonly) ascent from a retroperitoneal air leak (perforated colon, duodenum) or descent from the cervical region as after tracheostomy. Certainly, air can be introduced into the mediastinum from outside the body following penetrating injury by a knife or bullet, but perforation of the air-containing mediastinal structures should always be considered (see below).

Tracheobronchial Rupture

Tracheobronchial rupture (TBR) is an uncommon injury following blunt trauma; it occurs in about 1.5% of patients with major blunt thoracic trauma and is frequently initially masked by other injuries. Several theories have been suggested to explain the biomechanics of this injury: (*a*) sudden AP compression of the thorax with lateral displacement of the lungs and mainstem bronchi laterally exceeding the elasticity of the mainstem bronchi, (*b*) compression of the air-containing tracheobronchial tree against the closed glottis producing increased intraluminal pressure, (*c*) shearing forces of deceleration between the pendulous lung and fixed trachea, and (*d*) hyperextension of the cervical spine placing traction on the trachea and fixing its position more firmly (29, 30). About 80% of TBRs occur within 2.5 cm of the carina (30), with a slight predominance of right mainstem injury (29).

Radiologic signs of TBR include pneumomediastinum (61%), which is often severe, persistent, and progressive with widespread dissection of air into the neck and subcutaneous tissues; unilateral or bilateral pneumothorax (70%), typically unrelieved by thorascostomy tube evacuation; and interstitial gas in the lung paralleling the mainstem bronchi. Atelectasis may develop acutely or in delayed fashion in the lung distal to the interrupted bronchus due to partial or complete obstruction on the bronchus and is likely to persist (29, 30). In about 10% of patients with TBR, no radiologic signs are evident acutely that may indicate either partial or complete transection with an intact peritracheal or peribronchial adventia maintaining continuity of the airway (30–33). Such patients may present with delayed, persistent atelectasis following occlusion of the airway by fibrosis. If transection of the bronchus is complete, then the lung may collapse away from the mediastinum and settle into the posterior thorax or inferior thorax, depending on patient position—the so-called "fallen" lung sign (Fig. 4.14). The disrupted end of the bronchus may be sharp (Fig. 4.15) or tapering ("bayonet" sign) and can be visualized radiologically or, more frequently, by tomography. Fractures of the first through third ribs accompany TBR in 90% of patients (30, 31). TBR is diagnostically confirmed best by bronchoscopy but can often be demonstrated by bronchography or chest tomography. Early diagnosis of TBR improves the opportunity for successful primary surgical reanastomosis and offers the best chance for a successful long-term outcome (30).

Esophageal Disruption

Isolated esophageal rupture from blunt trauma is very rare (30, 34). Trauma, both blunt and penetrating, accounted for 10% of esophageal perforations occurring in 127 patients over a 47-year period reviewed by Bladergroen et al. (35). In most cases, esophageal rupture is accompanied by other significant intrathoracic injuries (34). A

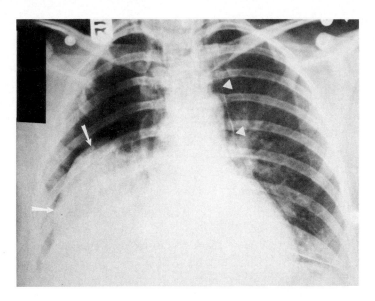

Figure 4.14. "Fallen lung sign" (radiography). An AP radiograph after blunt thoracic injury reveals a collapsed lung in the lower half of the right hemithorax and surrounding pneumothorax *(white arrows)*. Note the parietal pleural line on the left indicating pneumomediastinum *(white arrowheads)*.

variety of mechanisms account for acute esophageal injury following blunt thoracic trauma, including crushing between the spine and trachea, tearing due to extension, particularly at the level of the diaphragmatic hiatus, and direct penetration by cervical spine fracture fragments (Fig. 4.16). Radiologic signs include persistent pneumomediastinum and cervical emphysema (60%) (34), left pleural effusion, and abnormal mediastinal contour due to leakage of fluid or mediastinum hemorrhage. Develop-

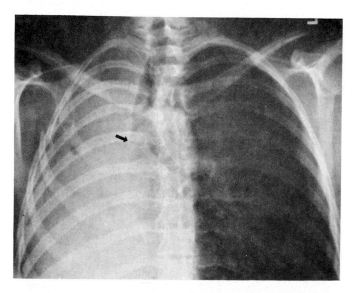

Figure 4.15. Bronchial "cut-off" sign (radiography). An AP radiograph after blunt trauma to the right hemithorax reveals opacification of the hemithorax. Note the abrupt cutoff of the right mainstem bronchus *(arrow)* indicating transection of the bronchus.

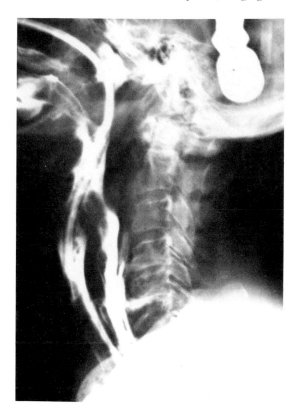

Figure 4.16. Ruptured cervical esophagus secondary to cervical spine fracture (contrast esophagogram). A barium esophagogram performed via a nasogastric tube in the hypopharynx obtained in a patient with hyperextension fracture-dislocation of C5/C6 reveals extravasation of contrast material from the esophagus into precervical soft tissue and ruptured disk space between C5 and C6. (From Reddin A, Mirvis SE, Diaconis JN. Rupture of the cervical esophagus and trachea associated with cervical spine fracture. J Trauma 1987;27:564–566.)

ment of esophageal rupture could be delayed by the presence of delayed breakdown of an ischemic segment of the esophagus or periesophageal hematoma (30). Iatrogenic causes, including nasogastric tube placement, esophageal intubation, and manipulation of esophagoscopy tubes, should also be considered as etiologic agents (30).

Once suspected, esophageal rupture can be confirmed radiologically. Contrast esophagoscopy, initially performed with water-soluble contrast media and then, if negative, with barium sulfate (Fig. 4.17), is about 90% sensitive in establishing the diagnosis (35), with greater diagnostic accuracy reported in the thoracic than in the cervical esophagus (34). Esophagoscopy has similar diagnostic sensitivity. Both studies together probably offer better diagnostic accuracy than either alone. CT scanning may demonstrate small air bubbles adjacent to the esophagus, indicating perforation with far greater sensitivity than plain radiographs.

Trauma to the Lung
PULMONARY CONTUSION

Pulmonary contusion, the most common primary lung injury secondary to nonpenetrating trauma, occurs in 30–70% of blunt chest trauma victims (36). The injury is

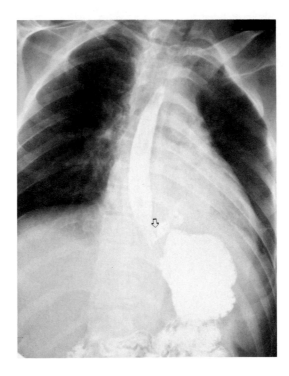

Figure 4.17.   Ruptured thoracoabdominal esophagus (contrast esophagogram). A barium swallow performed after a difficult endoscopy reveals contrast extravasation at the junction of the stomach and the distal esophagus *(arrow)* that led to left empyema of the thorax.

produced by direct transmission of energy through the chest wall to the underlying lung (30). Lung contusion is usually present on the initial admission chest radiograph, but its appearance may be delayed up to 6 hr (31). The lesion appears as a fluffy, air-space occupying process, which is typically nonsegmental, "geographic," and frequently peripheral in its distribution (Figs. 4.18 and 4.19). Contusions tend to occur adjacent to solid structures such as the ribs, sternum, and vertebral bodies. Contusion patterns often reflect the site and area of blunt impact upon the thoracic cage. The lesions may be unilateral or bilateral, focal, multifocal, or diffuse. The opacified lung results from hemorrhage and edema in the alveoli secondary to disruption of small blood vessels and damage to the alveolar-capillary membrane with increased fluid leakage into the alveolar space (29, 36). Air bronchograms may be seen within lung contusions but, in my experience, are frequently not present due to filling of the adjacent bronchi with blood or secretions. Although adjacent rib fractures may accompany lung contusion, they are not present in most cases (32).

Radiographic clearing of contusions is usually detected within 48–72 hr but may not appear for 5–7 days with more extensive injuries. Complete resolution usually requires 10–14 days (31). Failure of the density of the contusion to resolve during this time suggests either the wrong initial diagnosis or superimposition of another pathologic process such as pneumonia, aspiration, atelectasis, or adult respiratory distress syndrome (ARDS). The impaired ability of contused lung to clear secretions, regional diminished lung compliance, and the presence of intraalveolar blood and edema fluid

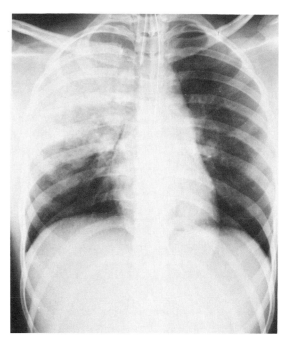

Figure 4.18. Pulmonary contusion (radiography). An admission anteroposterior chest radiograph demonstrates confluent, nonsegmental alveolar consolidation involving right mid and upper lung zones consistent with contusion.

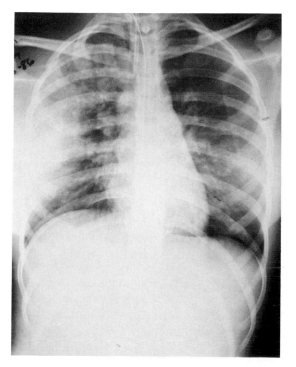

Figure 4.19. Pulmonary contusion (radiography). An admission anteroposterior chest radiograph reveals peripheral, nonsegmental alveolar, homogeneous consolidation typical of pulmonary contusion. No overlying rib fracture was present.

provide a nidus for the development of infection and sepsis (29). Although local, discrete contusions do not appear to have a significant impact on morbidity and mortality, diffuse pulmonary contusions often lead to severe ARDS, possibly due to extensive damage to alveolar-capillary membranes (36).

LACERATIONS, PNEUMATOCELES, AND HEMATOMAS

Pulmonary lacerations have been considered unusual sequelae of blunt chest trauma, but recent studies have suggested that they are in fact quite common, although frequently overlooked (37). A variety of mechanisms have been proposed to explain the production of pulmonary laceration. A concussion wave from blunt trauma may produce a shearing injury due to differential inertia between different lung segments, sudden closure of the glottis or compression of a bronchus may produce high intraluminal pressures that rupture distal alveoli, rib fractures can penetrate directly into the lung, posterior paraspinal segments of the lung can be compressed by the lower ribs and impact into adjacent vertebral bodies, and pleural adhesions may avulse peripheral portions of the lung (31, 37). Pulmonary lacerations generally occur in patients under 30 yr of age, when the elasticity of the ribs and lung is optimal (31).

Pulmonary lacerations may communicate with the visceral pleura, leading to pneumothorax. When intraparenchymal in location, lacerations of the lung are often masked by surrounding contusion and may not become radiographically visible until the contusion begins to resolve (31). Lacerations of the lung, although initially linear in configuration, tend to assume an ovoid or elliptical shape due to the elastic recoil of the lung. Pathologically, lacerations are lined by a pseudomembrane composed of alveolar remnants and may be single or multilocular, generally varying from 2 to 14 cm in diameter.

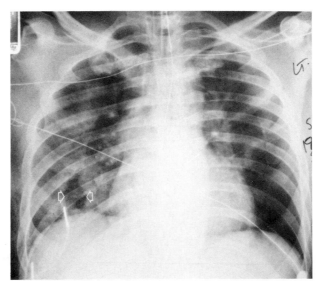

Figure 4.20.   Pulmonary laceration (radiography). An AP chest radiograph reveals ovoid radiolucency *(arrows)* at the right lung base. The surrounding area of pulmonary contusion is resolving.

Radiographically, lacerations appear as ovoid radiolucencies (cysts) surrounded by a thin 2- to 3-mm density representing the pseudomembrane. When hemorrhage occurs into the cavity, an air-fluid level may appear. When a clot forms, a thin crescent of air may persist over the clot, producing a so-called air-meniscus sign (Figs 4.20–4.23). The laceration may completely fill with clotted blood (a pulmonary hematoma) and present as a uniform mass on chest radiograph. Lung lacerations usually resolve over 3–5 weeks but may persist for months as a slowly shrinking "coin lesion" on the chest radiograph. It is important to note such a development prior to discharge to prevent misidentification of the resolving contusion as a potential malignancy. Lung lacerations may persist for months in the presence of continued pulmonary pathology such as ARDS and positive pressure ventilation (Fig. 4.21).

Although generally benign processes, pulmonary lacerations can, on occasion, produce complications. A laceration may communicate with an adjacent bronchus and

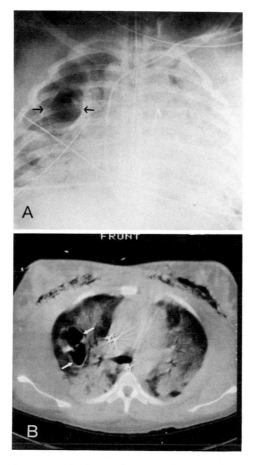

Figure 4.21. Pulmonary laceration (radiography and CT). **A,** AP chest radiograph in a patient with severe ARDS reveals a cystic lung laceration in the right upper lobe with a pseudomembrane border *(arrows).* **B,** corresponding CT scan again demonstrates bilateral changes of ARDS with diffuse air bronchograms. A biloculated traumatic lung cyst with a pseudomembrane is clearly defined on the right *(arrows).*

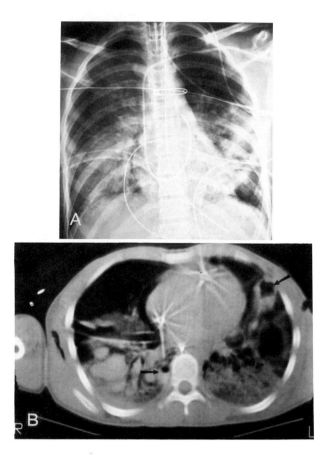

Figure 4.22. Pulmonary lacerations with hematoma (radiography and CT). **A,** AP chest radiograph reveals nonspecific multifocal patchy areas of consolidation in both lower lobes in a patient with gross hemoptysis. **B,** corresponding CT scan in the same patient reveals multiple areas of lung hematoma with some cavitating lesions *(arrows).* The thoracostomy tube is in a minor fissure. (From Mirvis SE, Tobin KD, Kostrubiak I, Belzberg H. Thoracic CT in detecting occult disease in critically ill patients. AJR 1987;148:685–689).

the visceral pleural, producing a bronchopleural fistula and a persistent air leak (see below). My colleagues and I have rarely noted the development of infection within a pulmonary laceration leading to abscess formation (Fig. 4.23). Large lung lacerations can expand under positive airway pressure and produce compression of adjacent normal lung by their mass effect. Traumatic lung lacerations can be diagnostically confused with congenital lung cysts or pulmonary sequestrations, lung abscesses, postpneumonia pneumatocele, and cavitations secondary to fungus or tuberculous infection.

PARENCHYMAL LUNG INJURY: COMPUTED TOMOGRAPHY

Recent studies have suggested that CT offers a greater sensitivity in identifying parenchymal lung injuries and extent of disease than does radiography (37–39). Wagner

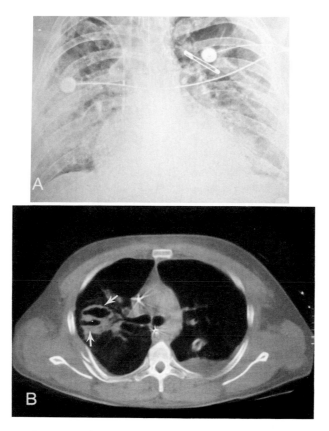

Figure 4.23.   Infected traumatic lung cyst (radiography and CT). **A,** AP chest radiograph reveals a patchy area of increased density in the right mid-lung zone in a febrile patient. **B,** corresponding CT the same day reveals a biloculated lung cyst with fluid level in the mid right lung *(arrows)*. Purulent drainage was aspirated from this region at bronchoscopy. (From Mirvis SE, Tobin KD, Kostrubiak I, Belzberg H. Thoracic CT in detecting occult disease in critically ill patients. AJR 1987;148:685–689).

et al. (37) have demonstrated that CT can detect pulmonary lacerations with far greater accuracy than radiography. In their series of 85 consecutive chest trauma victims, CT detected 99 lung lacerations compared to 5 detected by radiography. They suggest, based on these observations, that lung lacerations are so frequently present in nonpenetrating chest trauma that they probably constitute the major underlying lesion accompanying lung contusion, rather than the more commonly held view that contusions represent only lung "bruises" and are only manifestations of interstitial injury and disruption of the alveolar-capillary membrane.

In my experience, CT has been very valuable in the detection of lung lacerations and hematomas not visible on concurrent chest radiographs (Figs. 4.22–4.23); it generally depicts a greater extent of lung pathology than is suggested radiographically in most cases of parenchymal injury. On occasion, CT findings have been crucial in explaining the clinical presentation and in directing appropriate therapy.

Assessment of the Pleural Space
SIMPLE AND COMPLICATED PNEUMOTHORAX
Radiography

Pneumothorax represents a common and potentially life-threatening complication of penetrating or blunt chest trauma, respiratory support, particularly with positive pressure ventilation, and insertion of tracheostomy tubes and central venous lines from either a subclavian or jugular approach. Even a small pneumothorax may result in significant respiratory or cardiovascular compromise if unrecognized before mechanical assisted ventilation or general anesthesia (40). Delayed diagnosis or misdiagnosis may lead to a potentially fatal hypoxemia or tension pneumothorax. In a study by Tocino et al. (41) of 112 pneumothoraces in 88 critically ill patients, 30% of the pneumothoraces were not initially detected by the clinician or radiologist and half of these progressed to tension pneumothorax. Recognition of pneumothorax, which often requires an active "search" of the chest radiograph, may be underdiagnosed due to overexposure of the chest radiograph. A "bright light" is essential when evaluating chest radiographs for signs of pneumothorax.

In the erect or semierect patient, air in the pleural space collects over the apical and lateral portion of the hemithorax (41). The visceral pleura is visualized as a sharp white line beyond which no lung markings are detected (Fig. 4.24). An expiratory chest radiograph, if obtainable, accentuates the contrast between the lung and adjacent pleural air, increasing the detectability of the pneumothorax. Skin folds, tubes, and various monitoring lines outside the patient can, on occasion, be confused with a

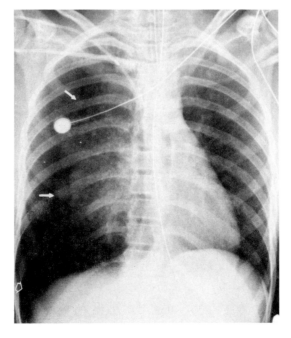

Figure 4.24.   Tension pneumothorax (radiography). An AP chest radiograph demonstrates collapse of the right lung. Note the visceral pleural edge *(arrows)* and displacement of the mediastinum to the left due to the tension component. Also note the depression of the right hemidiaphragm and deep costophrenic sulcus *(open arrow)*.

pneumothorax. Skin folds tend to be less sharply defined than the visceral pleura since air is seen only on one side of the line (42) and lung markings can be seen to project beyond the edge of a skin fold. If findings are uncertain, then a repeat chest radiograph should be obtained with the patient in a different position, such as the lateral decubitus with the side of the suspected pneumothorax elevated. All lines and tubes should be positioned away from the chest wall if possible.

Recognition of pneumothorax is markedly different in the supine patient. In this position, air in the pleural space collects at the highest portion of the thorax, which is the anterior costophrenic sulcus that runs laterally from the seventh costal cartilage in an oblique and inferior direction to the midaxillary line of the eleventh rib. Air in this location will produce hyperlucency of the upper abdominal quadrants and lower thorax. Air will outline the inferior margin of the anterior costophrenic sulcus, creating a "double diaphragm" contour (Figs. 4.25, 4.26) (43, 44). The diaphragm may also be depressed inferiorly. The lateral costophrenic sulcus will also contain air, producing a deep costophrenic sulcus appearance (Fig. 4.27) (45). Pleural air in the supine patient tends to lie in a subpulmonic location and may outline the visceral pleura of the lung base. Finally, pleural air in the supine patient surrounds the cardiac apex and may produce sharply defined pericardial fat tags and a distinct cardiac apex (43).

Pneumothorax can also present in unusual locations, such as the major or minor fissures (41, 46) and behind the inferior pulmonary ligament (41, 47). Adhesions of the visceral and parietal pleural surfaces can restrict the migration of pleural air and lead to loculation of air collections within the pleural space. Lobar collapse or consolidation may also alter the usual appearance of a pneumothorax. The diseased lobe exhibits a

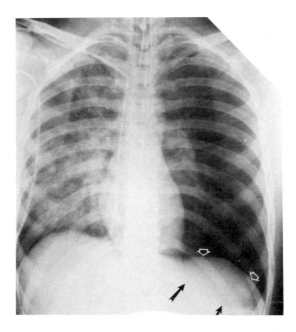

Figure 4.25.   Pneumothorax in supine patient with "double diaphragm" sign (radiography). A supine AP chest radiograph reveals increased lucency over the left hemithorax, a slight shift of the mediastinum to the right, and double diaphragm contours consisting of dome *(open arrows)* and anterior aspects *(black arrows)* of the left hemidiaphragm.

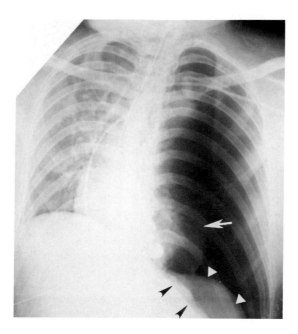

Figure 4.26. Tension penumothorax (radiography). A supine AP chest radiograph demonstrates a marked shift of the mediastinum to the right, hyperlucency of the left hemithorax, collapse of the left lung *(arrow),* and a double diaphragm contour *(arrowheads).*

greater retractile tendency and pleural air is more likely to collect around the collapsed lobe. Thus, even in an upright patient with lower lobe disease, the pneumothorax often collects in a subpulmonic location, potentially making chest tube evacuation difficult (42).

Tension pneumothorax (Figs. 4.24, 4.25) will produce flattening or inversion of the hemidiaphragm, contralateral shifting of the mediastinal structures, flattening of the ipsilateral cardiomediastinal contour, and spreading of the ipsilateral ribs. The ipsilateral lung may exhibit considerable collapse and may not be visible at all. The presence of a chest tube does not exclude the possibility of a tension pneumothorax since the tube may be improperly positioned in the pleural space or the pleural space may be loculated by adhesions, preventing relief of the pneumothorax (42).

Pneumothorax can be confused with subpleural air cysts accompanying emphysema, subcutaneous emphysema, traumatic lung cysts in a subpleural location, and pneumoperitoneum. Generally, movement of air to the uppermost portion of the thorax with a change in patient position will support the diagnosis of pneumothorax.

Computed Tomography

Although CT scanning is not recommended as a routine screening procedure for the detection of pneumothorax, this technique is exquisitely sensitive to small amounts of air in the pleural space. Wall et al. (40) reported that, of 35 patients with pneumothorax detected on abdominal CT after blunt trauma, 10 were recognized only by CT scan. Others have reported similar experiences in the detection of unsuspected pneumothorax by CT scanning (38, 39). Tocino et al. (41) has recommended using limited thoracic CT in all major trauma patients requiring emergency surgery or mechanical

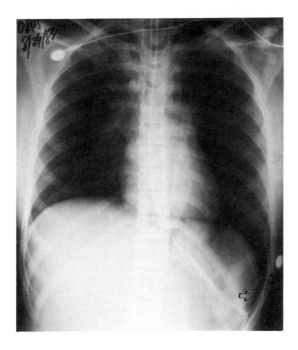

Figure 4.27. Deep sulcus sign of pneumothorax in supine patient (radiography). A supine AP chest radiograph reveals increased radiolucency in the left lower hemithorax and deep left costophrenic sulcus produced by a pneumothorax *(arrows)*.

ventilation to screen for occult pneumothorax. Tocino et al. (48) have detected unsuspected pneumothoraces utilizing a limited screening thoracic CT following cranial CT scanning. My colleagues and I routinely perform abdominal CT scanning beginning at the lung bases and photograph the lung bases at windows (level, -500 to -600 Hounsfield units; width, 100 Hounsfield units) designed to enhance detection of small pneumothoraces. At the Shock Trauma Center, unsuspected pneumothoraces are detected in about 5% of patients referred for abdominal CT scanning (Fig. 4.28).

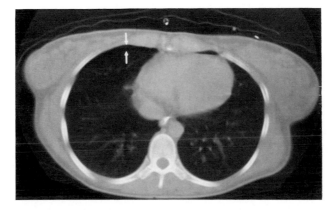

Figure 4.28. Pneumothorax (CT). An axial CT image at the lung bases performed as part of an abdominal CT scan demonstrates a small anterior pneumothorax on the right *(arrows)*. The photographic windows and level were optimized for detection of air density.

PLEURAL EFFUSION/HEMOTHORAX

Pleural effusions developing in the acute setting usually represent hemothorax. A small amount of hemorrhage often accompanies traumatic pneumothorax and will appear as an air-fluid level on an erect chest radiograph. Isolated hemothorax may be the result of injury to the visceral pleura or laceration or contusion of the lung. Bleeding of pulmonary venous origin is of low pressure and is likely to be self-limited. A rapidly expanding pleural effusion in the setting of acute thoracic injury is more likely to arise from higher pressure arterial sources, such as the intercostal, internal mamillary, or great vessels in the mediastinum.

A simple pleural fluid collection in an erect patient is typically manifested radiographically as a fluid meniscus crossing the lower thorax with widening of the lateral pleural stripe and blunting of the lateral costophrenic sulcus. Accumulation of

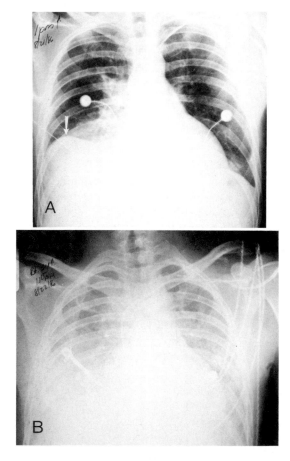

Figure 4.29.   Subpulmonic pleural effusion (radiography). **A,** erect AP chest radiograph demonstrates apparent elevation and lateral peaking of the right hemidiaphragm, suggesting pleural effusion under the right lung *(arrow)*. **B,** repeat radiograph on the same day in the supine position indicates the presence of large bilateral effusions layering posteriorly. Note that the vascular shadows of the lung are preserved since the fluid is pleural-based and not parenchymal in location.

fluid in the medial pleural space may appear as a triangular paraspinal mass. Fluid may also be visualized extending into the major and minor fissures. In the supine patient, a unilateral pleural fluid collection may produce only a uniform increase in density across the entire hemithorax as fluid layers in the posterior pleural space. Since pleural effusions are outside the lung, the normal bronchovascular markings are preserved despite increased density over the hemithorax (Fig. 4.29). Although very large effusions may be expected to produce a contralateral shift of the mediastinum by mass effect, this is partially offset by concurrent compressive atelectasis in the ipsilateral lung.

In the erect or semierect patient, fluid collections can become trapped under the lung base as subpulmonic collections. Theoretically, lower lobe atelectasis acts as a suction to draw and entrap fluid between the lung and hemidiaphragm. Radiographically, the subpulmonic fluid collection produces a pseudodiaphragm contour that mimics an elevated hemidiaphragm. The pseudodiaphragm has a flat surface contour adjacent to the heart but then inclines gradually upward laterally, producing a peak lateral to the usual high point of the hemidiaphragm (Fig. 4.29). Expiration tends to accentuate this appearance (49). In addition, since the lung in the posterior costophrenic sulcus is elevated upward by the subpulmonic fluid, the vascular shadows in the lower lobe will appear to end abruptly at the effusion-lung interface instead of projecting below the hemidiaphragm (49) on the frontal view as is normally seen. A decubitus view of the thorax will help quantitate pleural effusion and expose the underlying lung and hemidiaphragm.

Air and fluid collections in the pleural space may result from hydro-, hemo-, or pyopneumothorax. Such collections are made apparent as a result of air-fluid levels. Collections of air and fluid may be loculated in the pleural space by adhesions, making drainage difficult. The use of decubitus views is helpful in confirming whether fluid in the pleural space is free flowing or loculated. Persistent air collections in the pleural space that defy evacuation by chest tube may represent bronchopleural fistulas. Such an abnormal communication between the pleural space and airway can result from necrotizing pneumonias, pulmonary infarction, granulomatous and fungal infections such as aspergillosis, breakdown of bronchial surgical closure, thoracostomy tube insertion, lung biopsies, and deep, peripheral lung lacerations (29). Bronchography or instillation of methylene blue dye in the suspected bronchus can confirm a bronchopleural communication.

COMPUTED TOMOGRAPHY AND SONOGRAPHY OF PLEURAL FLUID COLLECTIONS

CT and sonography are more sensitive than radiographs to the presence of pleural fluid collections. In patients with fluid collections loculated at the bases or in patients with noncompliant lungs (such as develop with ARDS or chronic infection), large effusions, particularly if symmetric and bilateral, may not be apparent by chest radiographs obtained in the supine patient (Fig. 4.30). The fluid tends to be trapped behind and beneath the stiff lung. Both CT and sonography can identify these collections as well as guide aspiration and/or drainage of loculated pleural collections by catheter or thoracostomy tube. Sonography has the convenience of bedside evaluation of the pleural space and "real-time" monitoring of interventional procedures. CT can better evaluate the underlying lung parenchyma and cardiac and mediastinal structures while imaging the pleural space (Fig. 4.31).

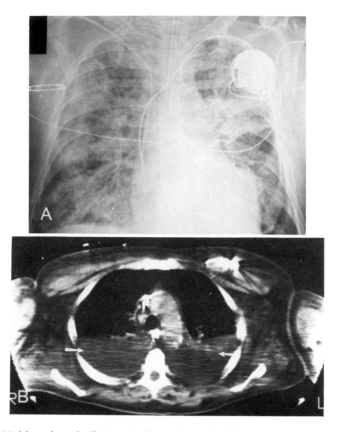

Figure 4.30.   Hidden pleural effusion (radiography and CT). **A,** supine AP chest radiograph in a patient with long-standing ARDS reveals chronic parenchymal sequelae of ARDS bilaterally, but no indication of pleural effusion. **B,** axial CT scan at the level of the aortic arch on the same patient on the same day reveals large symmetric pleural effusions trapped behind stiff, noncompliant lungs *(arrows)*. (From Mirvis SE, Tobin KD, Kostrubiak I, Belzberg H. Thoracic CT in detecting occult disease in critically ill patients. AJR 1987;148:685–689.)

Diaphragm Injury
DIAPHRAGM RUPTURE FROM BLUNT TRAUMA

Rupture of the hemidiaphragm is present in about 3–5% of patients undergoing celiotomy after blunt abdominal trauma (50, 51) and occurs in 0.008–3% of patients with major blunt thoracic injury (52). Left hemidiaphragm rupture predominates in blunt injury, representing 75% of 44 diaphragm injuries diagnosed at thoracotomy by Morgan et al. (50). Herniation of abdominal viscera into the thorax occurs through the left hemidiaphragm in 95% of cases (32). Presumably, increased intraabdominal pressure occurring at the time of blunt injury is transmitted through the abdominal viscera to the abdominal wall. The left hemidiaphragm is relatively unprotected by abdominal viscera, such as the liver, on the right side and represents an area of relative weakness among the structures containing the abdominal viscera. Most tears in the hemidiaphragm are radially oriented and occur in the area of the central tendon or at the musculotendinous junction. Avulsion of the diaphragm can occur at the insertion of the muscular

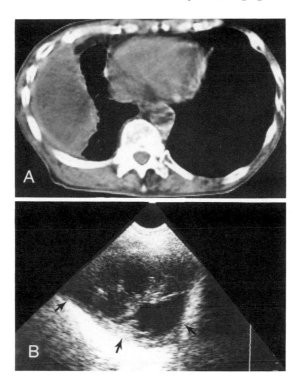

Figure 4.31.   Loculated pleural fluid (CT and sonography). **A,** axial CT scan demonstrates a large loculated right pleural fluid collection compatible with empyema. **B,** sonography of same area reveals a complex fluid with multiple loculations *(arrows)* within a collection not indicated by the CT scan. Both procedures can be used to guide drainage of the collection percutaneously.

attachments to the ribs, or rib fragments can directly lacerate the adjacent muscular portion of the hemidiaphragm. Cardiac subluxation through a simultaneous tear in the diaphragm and pericardium has been described (51).

Unfortunately, the clinical diagnosis of rupture of the diaphragm is difficult. Morgan et al. (50) established the diagnosis preoperatively in only 43% of 44 patients with this injury. Physical findings are nonspecific, consisting primarily of chest and abdominal wall contusions seen only in 16% of patients (50). The force required to produce tearing of the hemidiaphragm often produces significant associated injuries. In the series of Morgan et al. (50), 59% of patients had major intraabdominal visceral injury and 45.5% had major intrathoracic injury. These injuries may draw attention away from and delay recognition of diaphragm rupture.

IMAGING DIAGNOSIS OF DIAPHRAGM RUPTURE
Chest Radiography
Practically all radiologic modalities have been advocated for the diagnosis of traumatic diaphragmatic rupture, but the chest radiograph serves as the initial and most helpful imaging tool in evaluating the integrity of the hemidiaphragm after trauma (52). Unfortunately, previous studies have reported that 20–50% of patients with diaphragm laceration will have normal chest radiographs. This is particularly likely when there is

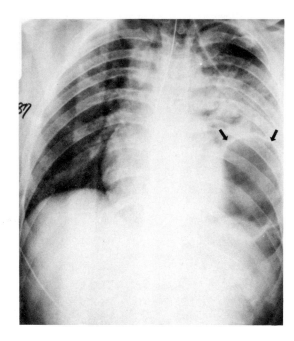

Figure 4.32.   Ruptured left hemidiaphragm with gastric herniation (radiography). An AP chest radiograph demonstrating the elevation of gastric fundus into the left hemithorax *(arrows)*, left perihilar lung contusion, and rightward mediastinal shift.

no herniation of abdominal contents through the tear in the hemidiaphragm (53). Wienecek et al. (53) have reported that a preoperative diagnosis based on plain radiographs alone could be made in only 24 (15%) of 165 patients with this injury. Beal and McKennan (54) reported preoperative radiologic diagnosis of diaphragmatic rupture in only 12 (32%) of 32 patients.

Apparent elevation of the hemidiaphragm, obliteration or distortion of its contour, and displacement of the mediastinum to the contralateral side are suggestive, but nonspecific, radiologic findings (Figs. 4.32, 4.33). Superimposed pathology at the lung base, including atelectasis, pleural effusions, pulmonary contusion, aspiration pneumonia, total or segmental eventration of the hemidiaphragm, posttraumatic phrenic nerve palsy, subphrenic fluid collections, and acute gastric distention, can mask or mimic findings of diaphragm rupture with herniation of abdominal contents. The demonstration of multiple air-fluid levels in the lower thorax is a more suggestive finding of herniation of air-containing viscera but can be mimicked by multiple traumatic lung cysts, loculated hemopneumothorax, and chronic esophageal and paraesophageal nontraumatic hernias. The demonstration of a focal constriction or waist-like band across the air-containing bowel should be considered pathognomonic of diaphragm rupture with partial constriction of herniated bowel by the torn edges of the diaphragm (Fig. 4.34).

In my experience, serial chest radiography is often very helpful in establishing the diagnosis of diaphragm rupture. Negative intrathoracic pressure will pull abdominal contents through the torn segment and reveal a more suggestive radiologic appearance. In addition, use of decubitus chest radiographs may help clarify radiologic findings in

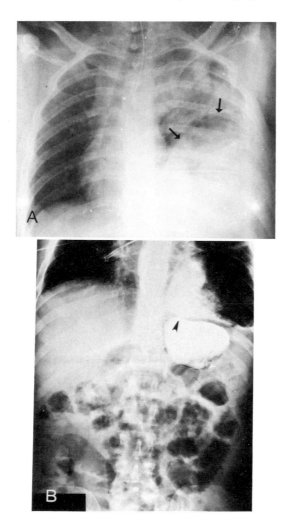

Figure 4.33. Transdiaphragmatic gastric herniation (contrast upper gastrointestinal study). **A,** AP chest radiograph reveals an apparent elevation of the left hemidiaphragm *(arrows)*, a left upper lung contusion, and a rightward mediastinal shift. **B,** instillation of contrast into the stomach via a nasogastric tube in a different patient confirms herniation of gastric fundus through the torn diaphragm. Note the constriction of the stomach at the point of herniation *(arrowhead)*.

the lower thorax by displacing pleural effusions, allowing better demonstration of the hemidiaphragm and helping to distinguish the nature of lower lung opacities. On occasion, my colleagues and I have found fluoroscopy valuable by demonstrating the position and function of the hemidiaphragms and the relationship of air-fluid levels to the diaphragm (Table 4.4).

Gastrointestinal Contrast Studies

The introduction of an esophagogastric tube may be very helpful in diagnosing intrathoracic gastric herniation; the tube serves to outline the location of the gastric fundus in relation to the hemidiaphragm. The addition of barium contrast by hand

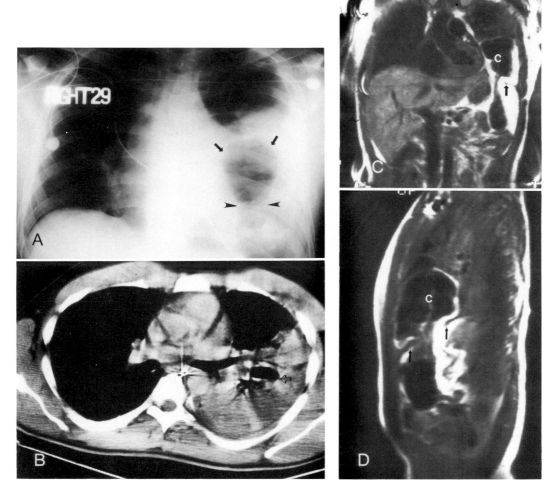

Figure 4.34. Transdiaphragmatic colonic herniation (radiography, CT, MRI). **A,** AP chest radiograph in a patient involved in a motor vehicle accident with left-sided impact reveals a gas pattern with haustral markings in the lower chest *(arrows)*. Note the constriction of the colon by edges of the hemidiaphragm proving herniation *(arrowheads)*. **B,** axial CT image obtained earlier in the same patient at the level of the left mainstem bronchus reveals lung consolidation and air-fluid level *(arrow)*. Differential diagnosis included herniated bowel or traumatic lung cyst. **C** and **D,** coronal and sagittal MRI scans in the same patient clearly demonstrate herniation of the colon into the left hemithorax through a diaphragm tear. Note the edges of the torn hemidiaphragms *(arrows)*. C = colon. (From Mirvis SE, Keramati B, Buckman R, Rodriguez A. MR imaging of traumatic diaphragmatic rupture. J Comput Assist Tomogr 1988;12:147–149.)

injection into the stomach through the esophagogastric tube will outline the stomach in relation to the lower thorax and can occasionally reveal constriction of the stomach at the level of the torn hemidiaphragm (Fig. 4.33B). Of course, barium should be suctioned from the stomach after the diagnostic study to prevent aspiration. If air-fluid levels are detected in the lower thorax by radiography and are not attributed to the stomach or proximal small bowel after upper gastrointestinal contrast study, a barium enema should follow to exclude herniation of the colon.

Table 4.4.
Imaging Algorithm for Suspected Diaphragmatic Rupture[a]

Anteroposterior Chest Radiography			
Normal	Positive	Positive (pathognomonic)	Suggestive
Does not exclude injury[a]	Air-fluid levels in lower thorax	Localized constriction of herniated bowel at the site of diaphragm rupture	Poorly defined diaphragm contour
Suggests no herniation	Clearly elevated hemidiaphragm		Mediastinal shift
↓	↓		
Follow-up chest radiograph	Confirm with nasogastric tube/ contrast studies		? air-fluid levels in lower thorax

✓

Serial radiography/decubitus chest
 radiographs
Place nasogastric tube and instill barium
Consider barium enema if upper
 gastrointestinal series is negative[b]
(if nondiagnostic)

↓

Fluoroscopy
Localize diaphragm
(if nondiagnostic)

↓

Computed tomography/sonography/nuclear
 scintigraphy[c]
(if nondiagnostic and patient stable
 hemodynamically)

↓   (or)

Magnetic resonance imaging with cardiac
 and respiratory gating

[a]Diagnostic imaging will generally not detect rupture without herniation.
[b]Use of barium contrast will preclude computed tomography until barium is removed.
[c]Depends on experience and expertise in institution.

Cross-sectional Imaging

The literature reports use of other imaging modalities, including sonography and CT, to diagnose traumatic diaphragmatic rupture (55–58). Sonography may be limited by the presence of gas in the splenic flexure and stomach, creating an acoustic barrier to the more frequently injured left hemidiaphragm. In several instances in my own experience, subcutaneous emphysema accompanying chest trauma has limited the use of sonography in imaging either hemidiaphragm. Ideally, if the hemidiaphragm contour can be imaged sonographically, then a defect and/or herniation can be detected. Of course this method is highly dependent on the skill and expertise of the examiner. Computed tomographic studies of the hemidiaphragm are limited to axially oriented images. Although reformation of images in the coronal and sagittal plane is possible, they typically lack the resolution of the axial images. Diagnosis of herniated abdominal

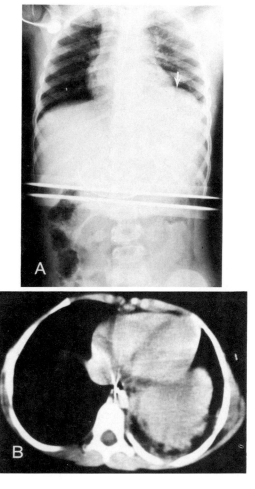

Figure 4.35.   Suspected ruptured left hemidiaphragm (radiography and CT). **A,** initial AP chest radiograph in an 8-year-old child admitted after being struck by a motor vehicle. The left hemidiaphragm is slightly elevated *(arrow)*. **B,** CT scan in the same patient at the midcardiac level reveals only elevation of the left hemidiaphragm.

contents depends on the demonstration of abdominal fat (omentum) or air-containing hollow viscera external (lateral or posterior) to the hemidiaphragm and, thus, within the thoracic cavity. My colleagues and I have observed that superimposed atelectasis, effusions, and pneumothorax produce difficulties in reliably identifying the margins of the hemidiaphragm after thoracic trauma. CT of two patients with left hemidiaphragm rupture revealed only elevation of the left-side abdominal viscera compared to the right side without detection of transdiaphragm herniation (Fig. 4.35).

MRI permits direct acquisition of coronal and sagittal images, which are ideal for displaying the relationship of the abdominal viscera to the essentially axially oriented hemidiaphragms. However, MRI is compromised by respiratory and cardiac motion near the diaphragm and is restricted by the severely traumatized patient's need for sophisticated physiologic monitors and life support apparatus, which is incompatible with the surrounding magnetic field. Recently, MRI proved diagnostic in demonstrating a left diaphragmatic rupture with herniation of colon into the chest (59) (Fig. 4.34, **C** and **D**) and in excluding diaphragm rupture in two other patients. The development of

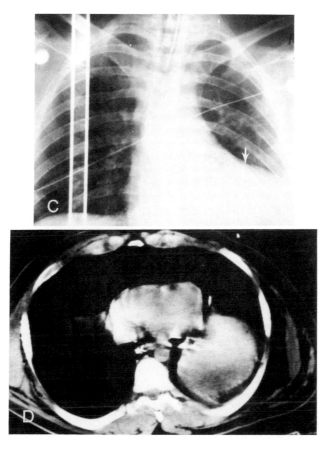

Figure 4.35 (Continued). **C,** admission chest radiograph in an adult male performed after blunt thoracic trauma reveals a slight elevation of the left hemidiaphragm *(arrow).* **D,** axial CT image at the cardiac base reveals an elevation of the hemidiaphragm without evidence of herniation of the abdominal viscera. Both patients had left diaphragmatic ruptures at celiotomy.

MRI-compatible monitors and support devices, shorter imaging times, and motion suppression techniques should permit a more thorough evaluation of MRI as diagnostic for diaphragm injuries in the near future.

Nuclear Scintigraphy

Isotopic techniques are available for imaging the lung, liver, and spleen in detecting transdiaphragm herniation. Injection of ^{99m}Tc-sulfur colloid will demonstrate the location of the liver and spleen and may detect either constriction of the parenchyma at the site of herniation or displacement of either organ into the thorax. Injection of ^{99m}Tc-macroaggregated albumin will permit simultaneous localization of the lung bases, liver, and spleen (liver-spleen-lung scan). Currently at the Shock Trauma Center, nuclear scintigraphy is seldom used for diagnosing diaphragm rupture.

Chest Wall Injury

Isolated fractures of the ribs, clavicle, or scapula alone seldom represent significant injuries, but they do reflect the magnitude of injury, particularly in older patients with noncompliant chest walls. Fractures of the first three ribs in particular indicate significant energy transfer. Fractures involving the thoracic outlet are significant in that they may be accompanied by brachial plexus or vascular injury in 3–15% of patients (37, 60). Although subclavian vascular injury should be suspected with fractures of the first three ribs, clavicle, and scapula, such injuries are usually accompanied by significant fracture displacement, extrapleural hematoma, brachial plexus neuropathy, or radiologic evidence of mediastinal hemorrhage (see above). Angiography in the absence of these signs produces a low yield of significant vascular injuries and is probably not warranted on an emergency basis (37, 61). Fractures of the lower ribs should increase suspicion of splenic, hepatic, or renal injury, confirmation of which should then be sought by appropriate diagnostic investigations.

Double fractures in three or more adjacent ribs or adjacent combined rib and sternal or costochondral fractures can produce a focal area of chest wall instability (Fig. 4.36). Paradoxical motion of a "flail" segment during the respiratory cycle can impair respiratory mechanics and promote atelectasis and impair pulmonary drainage. Although usually recognized by physical inspection, a flail segment involving the upper ribs may be hidden by the chest wall musculature (29). Rib fractures are often accompanied by extrapleural hematomas that present as focal lobulated areas of increased density on the chest radiograph. Due to their extrapleural nature, such hematomas indent the parietal pleura focally and maintain a convex margin toward the lung. Development of extrapleural hematomas over the apices may accompany fractures of the upper ribs or hemorrhage from the subclavian vessels from blunt trauma or iatrogenic causes (Fig. 4.37). Extrapleural hematomas will not change their configuration with changes in patient position as will free pleural space fluid collections. Bleeding from intercostal arteries after chest wall trauma can lead to exsanguinating hemorrhage. Both diagnosis and therapeutic embolization can be performed using angiographic techniques (Fig. 4.38).

Rarely, a segment of lung may herniate through a defect in the chest wall created by the flail segment. Transthoracic lung herniation increases in likelihood with positive pressure ventilatory support and with rupture of the internal thoracic fascia, parietal pleura, and pectoral and intercostal musculature. The diagnosis may be made by plain radiographs, but the defect is easier to detect by CT (Fig. 4.39). Although the herniated

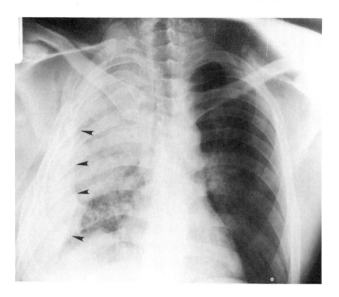

Figure 4.36. Flail chest/extrapleural hematoma (radiography). An AP chest radiograph demonstrates multiple, comminuted, displaced right rib fractures. A large fluid density extrapleural hematoma surrounds the right lateral hemithorax *(arrowheads)*. A right upper lung contusion is also noted.

portion of lung can be entrapped and strangulated, in my experience no significant sequelae generally occur with expectant management.

Fractures of the sternum are infrequent, occurring in 8% of major thoracic trauma admissions at one institution (62). Diagnosis requires both lateral and oblique views of the thorax. Concurrent injury to the great vessels can occur in association with sternal fracture (62) and should be sought in the presence of radiographic evidence of abnormal mediastinal contour. Laceration of the innominate artery secondary to a displaced fracture of the sternum has been reported but appears to be quite rare (63). Demonstration of a sternal fracture should always increase suspicion of myocardial contusion, which should be sought by appropriate diagnostic studies. Most sternoclavicular dislocations are anterior and of no major clinical significance. However, posterior dislocations of the clavicle relative to the manubrium can damage the great vessels, superior mediastinal nerves, trachea, and esophagus. Although sternoclavicular dislocations are demonstrable using angled chest radiographs (tube angled 35° cranially), they are most easily diagnosed using axial CT (Fig. 4.40).

Scapulothoracic dissociation is a rare injury characterized by a lateral displacement of the entire forequarter with intact overlying skin, complete acromioclavicular separation, and, usually, multiple fractures of the ipsilateral upper extremity (64). Avulsion injuries to the brachial plexus and subclavian nerves always accompany the injury.

Trauma to the Heart/Pericardium
PNEUMOPERICARDIUM

Pneumopericardium is a well-recognized clinical and radiologic entity. Causes include transsternal surgery, penetrating and (rarely) blunt thoracic trauma, infectious

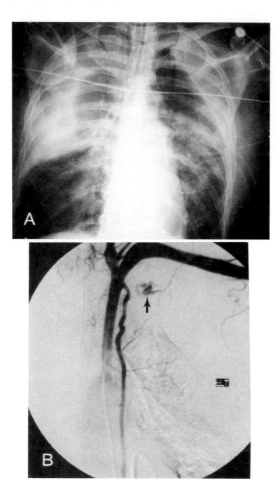

Figure 4.37. Bilateral iatrogenic extrapleural hematomas (radiography and DSA). **A,** erect AP chest radiograph obtained after multiple attempts to place a subclavian central line reveals large bi-apical fluid density masses. The failure to layer in a dependent position suggests loculation in the pleural space or an extrapleural location. **B,** selective left subclavian arteriogram reveals active bleeding from a small branch of the left subclavian artery *(arrow)*. A similar bleeding vessel was noted on the right side, explaining the source of extrapleural density.

pericarditis with gas-forming organisms, and fistula formation between the pericardium and adjacent air-containing structures such as the esophagus or stomach (65). Other etiologies include severe asthma, difficult labor, obstructive laryngitis, and therapeutic or diagnostic interventions such as sternal bone marrow biopsy and tracheostomy. Pneumopericardium may develop as a consequence of prolonged positive airway pressure, in which case air under pressure probably enters the pericardium around the pulmonary perivascular connective tissue. Direct communication from a ruptured trachea with the adjacent pericardium may result from blunt or penetrating trauma (65).

The identification of pneumopericardium by chest radiography was described by Wenckebach in 1910 and elaborated upon by Cimmino (66) more recently. Chest

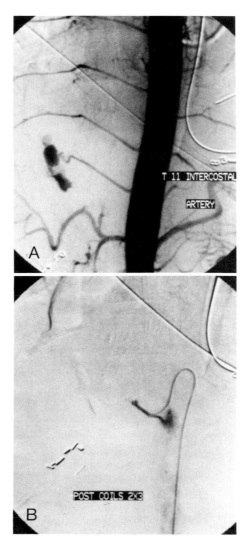

Figure 4.38.   Intercostal artery bleeding (angiographic embolization). **A,** thoracic angiogram performed to evaluate the aorta demonstrates extravasation of blood (contrast) from the ruptured right eleventh intercostal artery. **B,** selective intercostal arteriogram, obtained following placement of three Gianturco coils into the proximal artery, demonstrates complete occlusion of the bleeding vessel.

radiographs obtained in either posteroanterior or lateral projections show the heart partially or completely surrounded by air with the pericardium sharply outlined by air density on either side (Figs. 4.41, 4.42). Pneumopericardium can usually be distinguished from pneumomediastinum, since air in the pericardial sac should not rise above the anatomic limits of the pericardial reflection on the proximal great vessels. On radiographs obtained with the patient in the decubitus position, air in the pericardial sac will shift in location immediately, whereas air confined to the mediastinum will not

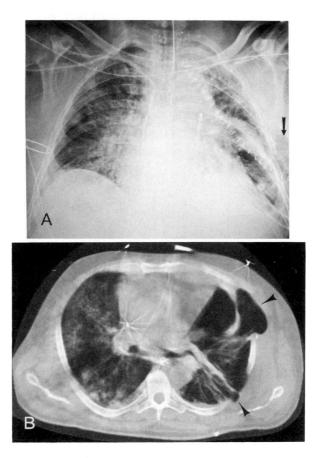

Figure 4.39. Transthoracic lung herniation (CT and radiography). **A,** AP chest radiograph in an elderly man with a left flail chest. Note the recent repair of a thoracic aortic rupture and air density adjacent to the left lateral chest wall *(arrow)* representing a herniated lung. **B,** axial CT through the midcardiac level confirms herniation of the lung through the chest wall. Note the smaller posterior herniation of the lung *(arrowheads)*. Residual infiltrates can be seen in the right lung. (From Mirvis SE, Tobin KD, Kostrubiak I, Belzberg H. Thoracic CT in detecting occult disease in critically ill patients. AJR 1987;148:685–689.)

move during a short interval. On occasion, it may not be possible to distinguish between pneumopericardium and pneumomediastinum with certainty.

Pneumopericardium, although generally innocuous, can lead to sufficient intrapericardial pressure to produce cardiac tamponade, so-called tension pneumopericardium (65). Presumably, under conditions of elevated airway pressure, air can be forced into the pericardium through connective tissue around the pulmonary veins, but it may not egress, as in a one-way valve mechanism. Mirvis et al. (65) have described five patients who developed tension pneumopericardium following closed-chest trauma. Each patient exhibited a global decrease in the area of the cardiac silhouette on chest radiography and at least a 2.0-cm decrease in the transverse cardiac diameter from base-line measurement at the time of physiologic cardiac tamponade after correction for target-film distance (Figs. 4.41, 4.42). Higgins et al. (67) have shown that symptoms

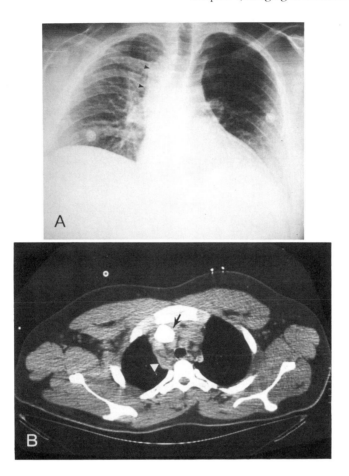

Figure 4.40. Posterior sternoclavicular dislocation (radiography and CT). **A,** AP chest radiograph on admission reveals increased soft-tissue density to the right of the trachea suggestive of mediastinal hematoma *(arrowheads)*. **B,** axial CT at the level of the sternoclavicular joint reveals posterior dislocation of the right clavicular head into the anterosuperior mediastinum *(arrow)*. Increased density to the right of the trachea probably represents hemorrhage *(arrowhead)*.

of severe hemodynamic compromise from tension pneumopericardium are accompanied by a perceptible decrease in the size of the cardiac silhouette in neonates with respiratory distress syndrome receiving positive pressure ventilatory support.

Clinical signs of cardiac tamponade, such as pulsus paradoxus, tachycardia, low-voltage electrocardiogram, increasing central venous pressure with decreasing cardiac output, muffled heart sounds, and worsening pulmonary function, may indicate developing cardiac tamponade. However, concurrent conditions, such as cardiac contusion, shock lung, intravascular volume depletion, tension pneumothorax, and sepsis may confuse the clinical picture. Furthermore, measures to maintain the blood pressure (e.g., vasopressors and volume support) can potentially mask early hemodynamic indicators of cardiac tamponade. In the presence of pneumopericardium, the development of a "small heart" sign should raise the specter of cardiac tamponade.

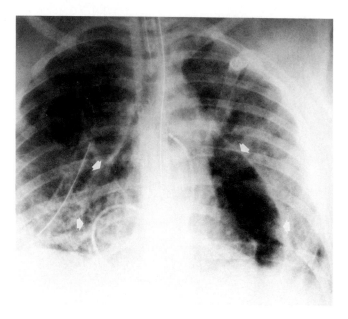

Figure 4.41. Tension pneumopericardium (radiography). An AP chest radiograph obtained on a patient on long-term positive pressure ventilatory support for ARDS. The pericardium *(arrows)* is markedly distended and the heart appears uniformly small. Impaired cardiac output necessitated pericardiotomy resulting in clinical improvement. (From Mirvis SE, Indeck M, Shorr RM, Diaconis JN. Posttraumatic tension pneumopericardium: the "small heart" sign. Radiology 1986;158:663–669.)

HEMOPERICARDIUM AND TAMPONADE

Hemopericardium may develop acutely as a direct consequence of blunt trauma to the anterior chest and severe crush injuries, but it more typically follows penetrating injury to the heart. A rapid accumulation of blood in the pericardial space often causes cardiac tamponade and severe hemodynamic compromise without altering the radiologic appearance of the cardiac silhouette, but it may be manifest as a nonspecific enlargement of the cardiopericardial contour (68). When time permits, a bedside sonographic evaluation of the heart rapidly and noninvasively permits detection of even small quantities of pericardial fluid and is the study of choice (68). Simultaneously, cardiac function, chamber size, and valvular integrity can be assessed. CT is also very sensitive for diagnosing fluid accumulation in the pericardial space. Pericardial hemorrhage (as indicated by high CT density) may be detected incidentally during CT evaluation of the thorax. Cardiac tamponade is reflected on CT by distension of the inferior vena cava and the hepatic and renal veins and by development of periportal vein edema within the liver (Fig. 4.43). CT and sonography are also more sensitive than radiography in the detection of chronically developing pericardial effusions, as may occur with postpericardiotomy syndrome or pericardial empyema (see below).

PERICARDIAL RUPTURE

Pericardial rupture represents a rare consequence of serious thoracic trauma (69). Rupture may involve the diaphragmatic pericardium and/or the pleuropericardium.

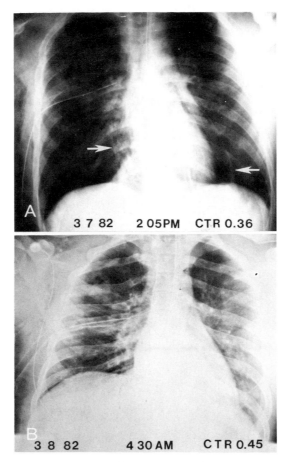

Figure 4.42. Tension pneumopericardium (radiography). **A,** AP chest radiograph on admission reveals a distended pericardium *(arrows)* with a uniformly small cardiac contour. Pathophysiology of cardiac tamponade is present. **B,** cardiac contour restored to normal with evacuation of the pneumopericardium by pericardiotomy (tube not visible) resulting in improved hemodynamics. (From Mirvis SE, Indeck M, Shorr RM, Diaconis JN. Posttraumatic tension pneumopericardium: the "small heart" sign. Radiology 1986;158:663–669).

Typically, the diagnosis is established surgically or at autopsy, but pericardial rupture can be indicated by chest radiograph with herniation of air-containing abdominal viscera into the pericardium accompanying diaphragmatic rupture. Pneumopericardium may appear in the presence of pneumothorax as air enters through the pericardial disruption. Finally, cardiac luxation into the pleural cavity (predominantly left) may occur after large pericardial tears and present as gross cardiac displacement (Fig. 4.44). Combined pericardial and diaphragmatic tears can lead to cardiac subluxation into the pleural cavity (51).

CARDIAC CONTUSION/DYSFUNCTION

Myocardial injury presents radiographically as a spectrum of findings related to the injury of the heart and chest. The cardiac findings may be similar to those occurring

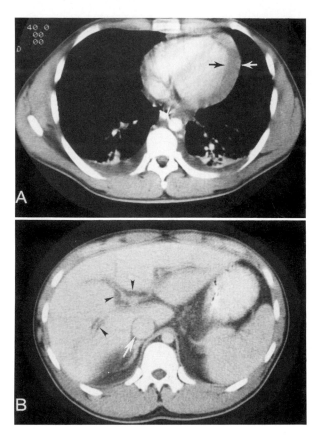

Figure 4.43. Acute pericardiac tamponade secondary to hemopericardium after blunt chest trauma (CT). **A,** axial CT with intravenous enhancement at the midcardiac level reveals fluid in the pericardial space *(arrows)*. The CT density measurement is compatible with blood. Pleural effusions and hemomediastinum are present. **B,** axial CT through liver reveals distension of the inferior vena cava *(arrow)* and lymphedema around portal venous tracts *(arrowheads)*. The findings are suggestive of tamponade and were confirmed at surgery, revealing a ruptured right atrial appendage. (From Goldstein L, Mirvis SE, Kostrubiak I. CT diagnosis of acute pericardial tamponade after blunt chest trauma. AJR 1989;152:739–741).

from acute myocardial infarction, such as congestive heart failure, ventricular aneurysm, or massive cardiac enlargement. The presence of anterior rib fractures and sternal fractures should raise suspicion of myocardial injury, although there is no clear relationship between the extent of chest wall injury and the degree of underlying cardiac damage. Myocardial injury can range from mild cardiac contusion to severe transmural contusion. Pathologically, blunt myocardial trauma produces a wide spectrum of injury, ranging from small, subepicardial, or subendocardial petechiae or ecchymoses to full-thickness contusion (70). The right ventricle is most frequently injured since it has almost 3 times more exposed anterior surface than does the left ventricle.

Clinically, mild myocardial dysfunction can produce low cardiac output and acute cardiac arrhythmias, whereas more severe injury can lead to congestive failure or cardiac rupture. Cardiac dysfunction after blunt chest trauma is one of the most

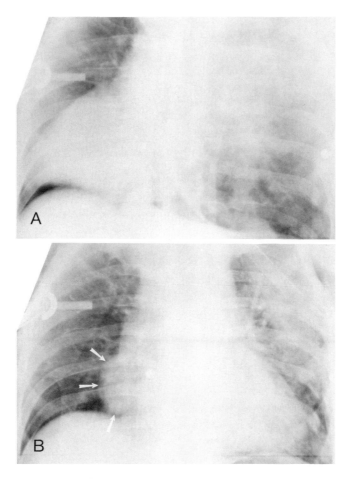

Figure 4.44.   Right pericardial rupture with cardiac subluxation (radiography). **A,** admission AP chest radiograph demonstrates gross displacement of cardiac silhouette into the right hemithorax. Numerous left lateral rib fractures occurred after a 30-foot fall onto the left side. **B,** follow-up chest radiograph obtained 15 min later reveals spontaneous return of the heart into the pericardial sac, with improvement in cardiac output. Note the rounded right cardiac contour *(arrows),* suggesting persistent herniation of the right atrium through the pericardial defect. At surgery a 6-cm right pericardial tear was repaired.

frequently missed or delayed diagnoses after severe injury and is frequently masked by more obvious injury (70).

At the Shock Trauma Center, cardiac contusion is diagnosed by radionuclide scintigraphy using first-pass radionuclide ventriculography followed by gated equilibrium imaging for assessment of ventricular wall motion. My colleagues and I consider this method the simplest and most accurate study to assess right ventricular ejection fraction. In a recent 8-month study at the Shock Trauma Center, 26 (48%) of 54 patients with multisystem injury and blunt chest trauma had abnormalities of ventricular wall motion. Abnormalities were confined to the right ventricle in 92% of cases and included right ventricular dilatation, localized wall motion abnormalities, and diffuse hypokinesia. Patients with wall motion abnormalities exhibited significantly lower right ventricular ejection fractions than those without. Follow-up nuclear scintigraphy was valuable in demonstrating significant improvement in cardiac function by 3 weeks after injury (70). Radionuclide ventriculography allows identification of trauma victims who warrant the most intensive monitoring for arrhythmias, guidance of fluid balance, and respiratory therapy for hypoxemia. Results of radionuclide ventriculography may influence the timing of surgery and the type of intraoperative monitoring and anesthesia used.

Although nuclear isotopic imaging with ^{99m}Tc pyrophosphate (infarct avid agent) may detect severe myocardial injury, it may not detect smaller areas of damage.

Two-dimensional echocardiography is useful for evaluating cardiac valve function, cardiac wall function, cardiac chamber size, papillary muscle function, and the anatomy of the aortic valve and root. Cardiac sonography may be particularly useful in settings in which the cardiac silhouette remains unchanged radiographically but clinical signs of severe hemodynamic embarrassment are present (34).

IATROGENIC COMPLICATIONS IN THE THORAX

Management of critically ill patients typically requires placement of both diagnostic and therapeutic devices into the thorax. Chest complications arising from such interventions are frequently sought and are first recognized radiographically.

Endotracheal/Transtracheal Intubation

Maintenance of adequate ventilatory support frequently requires placement of endotracheal or transtracheal tubes. It is estimated that complications resulting from these procedures carry a 0–8% mortality (71). The termination of the endotracheal tube should lie between 5 and 7 cm above the carina on the AP supine chest radiograph to allow maximal tube excursion in flexion and extension. The location of the carina, if not visible on an underexposed radiograph, lies between T5 and T7 in 90% of patients (72). Malpositioning of the endotracheal tube occurs in about 10% of all intubations (72) and typically involves right mainstem bronchial intubation (Figs. 4.45, 4.46). If unrecognized, such placement can lead to atelectasis or overinflation of the left lung, occlusion and atelectasis of the right upper lobe, and pneumothorax on the right. Esophageal intubation is usually recognized clinically and may be difficult to recognize on the AP supine radiograph. Radiographic signs include termination of the endotracheal tube below the level of the carina and gastric distension with air.

Uncommon complications of endotracheal intubation include (*a*) overdistention of the balloon cuff (Fig. 4.47), recognized by distension of the airway by the balloon, (*b*) hypopharyngeal or tracheal rupture, recognized by development of subcutaneous emphysema, pneumomediastinum, or pneumothorax and by distal migration of the cuff balloon to the endotracheal tube tip or ectopic position of the tip to the right of the tracheal lumen, and (*c*) aspiration, estimated to occur in 8% of intubations and recognized by development of alveolar infiltrates predominantly in the lower lung fields. Esophagography is recommended to evaluate for possible hypopharyngeal perforation. Tracheitis and ischemic necrosis of the tracheal cartilages can result from prolonged intubation or persistent elevated cuff pressures. Resulting inflammatory granuloma, tracheomalacia, or tracheal stenosis can be recognized bronchoscopically or by using radiographic tomography or bronchography (Fig. 4.48).

Tracheostomy can produce hemorrhage, which may present as mediastinal

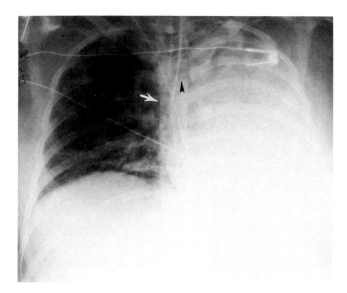

Figure 4.45.   Intubation of right mainstem bronchus (radiography). An AP chest radiograph reveals termination of the endotracheal tube in the right mainstem bronchus *(arrow)*. Complete atelectasis has developed in the obstructed left lung. *Arrowhead* indicates carina.

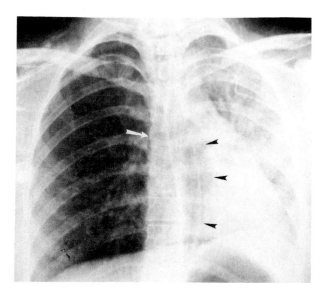

Figure 4.46.   Intubation of right mainstem bronchus (radiography). An AP chest radiograph demonstrates the endotracheal tube in the right mainstem bronchus *(arrow)* with a resulting overexpansion of the right lung and herniation across the mediastinum *(arrowheads)*.

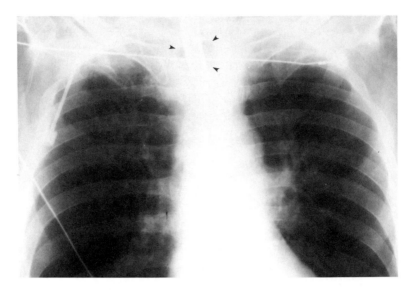

Figure 4.47. Overinflated endotracheal cuff (radiography). An AP chest radiograph reveals an overexpanded cuff on the endotracheal tube *(arrows)*. The balloon should not distend the trachea. Note the malpositioned central venous line on the right.

widening radiographically. Following tracheostomy, subcutaneous emphysema and pneumomediastinum are recognized radiographically in 5 and 2% of cases, respectively. Persistence of these findings or increasing gas dissection should prompt inspection of the tracheostomy site to detect the site of air leak.

Esophagogastric Tubes

Esophagogastric tubes, placed for aspiration of gastric contents or for feeding purposes, can generally be clinically confirmed to be intragastric. Unfortunately, malpositioning can occur, particularly in obtunded individuals (Fig. 4.49). Generally, malpositioned esophagogastric tubes are coiled in the esophagus or positioned in the tracheobronchial tree. Enteric feeding tubes are generally identified by a radiodense tip, and positioning in the duodenum or proximal small bowel is easily confirmed with an abdominal radiograph centered at the diaphragm to include both the distal esophagus and proximal small bowel. Perforation of the esophagus by esophagogastric tubes is most rare, but has been reported in up to 5% of patients in whom Sengstaken-Blakemore tubes are placed for management of esophagogastric hemorrhage (72). Perforation may present radiographically as loss of normal mediastinal contours, pneumomediastinum, and hydropneumothorax. Confirmation by esophagography with water-soluble agents is recommended.

Thoracostomy Tubes

Thoracostomy tubes are required for relief of pneumothorax and for drainage and monitoring of pleural fluid collections. Although a single AP radiograph is usually obtained to confirm chest tube position, this single view is quite inadequate for this purpose (38, 73, 74). At least two projections, preferably including a lateral thoracic

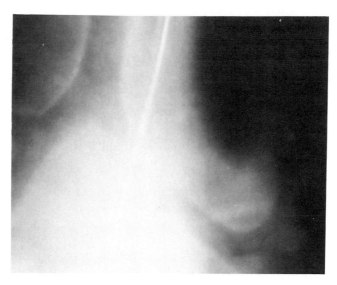

Figure 4.48. Bronchial stenosis complicating prolonged independent lung ventilation (tomography). A linear tomogram demonstrates near occlusion of the left mainstem bronchus following prolonged independent lung intubation for severe ARDS.

view, are needed to accurately define chest tube position radiographically. Frontal radiographs alone identified only 1 of 21 malpositioned tubes in a series of patients described by Stark et al. (74). Ideally, thoracostomy tubes should be placed into the anterior-apical region to drain pleural air and the posterior-inferior location to drain pleural fluid collections. Reported sites of chest tube malposition include the extrapleural soft tissues, pleural fissures, intraparenchymal, and transdiaphragmatic

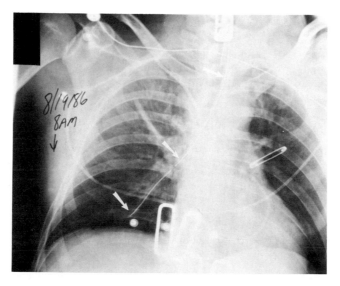

Figure 4.49. Malpositioned nasogastric tube (radiography). An AP chest radiograph obtained after the placement of a nasogastric tube reveals placement into the periphery of the descending right lower lobe bronchus *(arrows)*.

(75). CT has been shown to be highly accurate in demonstrating improperly positioned or occluded chest tubes (38, 74) (Fig. 4.50). CT is also very helpful in guiding chest tube positioning for loculated pleural fluid collections.

After chest tube removal, a residual site of pleural reaction may persist radiographically, appearing as two parallel radiodense lines along the site of chest tube insertion. Alternatively, a single small curvilinear residual density may appear, representing a loculated pleural-based fluid collection that has accumulated in the chest tube tract. These appearances should not be confused with a residual or recurrent pneumothorax.

Central Venous/Pulmonary Artery Catheters

Intensive care management requires placement of central venous and pulmonary arterial lines to provide physiologic monitoring and venous access for infusions. A wide variety of complications can result from initial attempts at placement and improper positioning of these lines.

Pneumothorax occurs in 1–12% of central venous line placements, depending largely on the skill and experience of the physician (73). Follow-up radiography is best obtained with the patient in the erect position in deep expiration. Unfortunately, only supine radiographs are obtainable in critically ill patients. Subtle pneumothorax will present as radiolucency in the costophrenic angles or subpulmonic location (see above).

Hemothorax or hemomediastinum can result from arterial or venous laceration at the time of catheter insertion and is frequently unrecognized. Radiographically, this complication may present as pleural effusion or extrapleural soft-tissue density (see

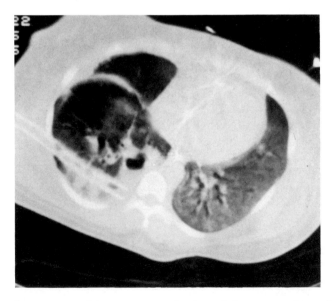

Figure 4.50.   Malpositioning of thoracostomy tube through lung parenchyma (CT). An axial CT image through the lower lungs reveals a diffuse parenchymal pattern consistent with ARDS. Note the thoracostomy tube traversing lung parenchyma. Noncompliant lungs, as may occur with ARDS, may predispose to such occurrences.

extrapleural hematoma above) such as an apical pleural cap (Figs. 4.4, 4.37). Loss of normal contours of the mediastinal silhouette will suggest mediastinal hemorrhage (Figs. 4.3–4.5, 4.40**A**).

Malpositioning of central venous lines occurs in 23–38% of insertions (72, 76). Termination of the catheter tip outside the thorax, as in the contralateral internal jugular vein, will result in inaccurate central venous pressure readings. Termination in a small caliber branch vein can lead to thrombus formation around the catheter tip and thrombophlebitis from instillation of hyperosmolar or toxic substances without dilution by high-volume blood flow (Fig. 4.47). Ideally, the central venous line tip should lie in the superior vena cava (SVC), parallel to the cava and above the level of the azygos vein. Termination in the right atrium can produce arrhythmias and is not recommended. Tocino and Watanabe (76) have described perforation of the SVC by catheters placed into the left subclavian and left innominate vein. Pressure by the catheter against the right lateral wall of the SVC is produced by the relative sharp right angle turn between the left innominate vein and the SVC. A slight bending at the terminal portion of the catheter is suggested by Tocino and Watanabe (76) as a sign of subintimal dissection of the catheter and impending perforation. Perforation may present radiographically as hydrothorax or distortion and widening of the mediastinal contour, particularly in the right paratracheal region.

Central venous catheters can terminate in a wide variety of suboptimal locations within the thorax, including the internal mamillary veins, cardiophrenic veins, azygos arch, and superior intercostal veins. They can also terminate in a variety of congenital anomalous venous channels, such as a persistent left SVC (persistent left cardinal vein) (Fig. 4.51). An abnormal catheter course on the frontal chest radiograph will usually suggest an aberrant placement but will often require a lateral view for confirmation.

Excessive advancement of central venous or pulmonary catheters without fluoroscopic guidance can lead to looping in the heart and subsequent knotting (Fig. 4.52). Should this complication be suggested by postplacement radiographs, removal should be attempted only with fluoroscopic control. If an intracardial knot forms, it can often be removed via percutaneous interventional catheterization techniques. Catheters may be sheared when withdrawn through a sharply beveled needle. Catheter fragments can embolize to the pulmonary artery and can lead to pulmonary infarction, sepsis, arrhythmias, and vascular perforation (72). Failure to remove these fragments has been reported to produce serious or fatal complications in 71% of cases (72). Prompt removal of catheter fragments is imperative.

Thrombosis around central venous catheters is detectable in 7–28% of patients, increasing to 71% after 7 days, and is more likely to develop with polyvinylchloride catheters than with silicone catheters such as the Hickman-Broviak catheter (72). Symptomatic occlusions in the SVC may be recognized clinically. Radiographically, SVC occlusion will produce an enlarged SVC shadow if proximal in location, dilatation of collateral venous channels (such as the azygos system and superior intercostal veins), and pleural effusions.

Swan-Ganz pulmonary artery catheters are usually placed without incident. For pulmonary arterial wedge pressure to reflect the left atrial pressure and left ventricular end diastolic pressure, there must be a continuous column of blood between the catheter tip and the left atrium. This circumstance occurs only in zone 3 (of West), where both the pulmonic artery and venous pressure exceed the pulmonary alveolar pressure. In the supine patient, zone 3 is in the lower lobe. A catheter placed in zone 1

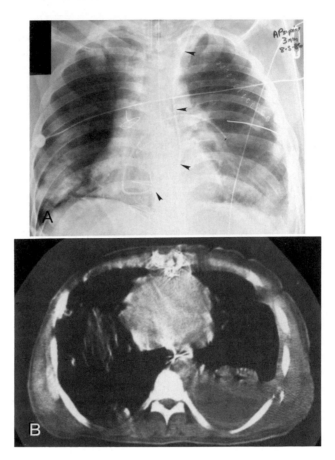

Figure 4.51. "Occult" empyema in recovery phase of trauma (CT). **A,** AP chest radiograph reveals a patchy infiltrate at the right lung base. Note the pulmonary artery catheter entering the heart via the persistent left superior vena cava and coronary sinus *(arrows)*. There is no indication of empyema or abscess. **B,** axial CT through the lung bases demonstrates well-encapsulated left posterior pleural fluid collection, which represented empyema on aspiration.

or 2 will record alveolar pressure, not left atrial pressure (72). A Swan-Ganz catheter placed in the upper or middle lobe must be repositioned for an accurate reading. The tip should always be distal to the pulmonic valve. Too peripheral placement or failure to deflate the balloon may lead to segmental arterial occlusion and pulmonary infarction. As a rule of thumb, positioning by chest radiography with the tip of the catheter within the middle third of the thorax will be satisfactory. Perforation of the pulmonary artery from the Swan-Ganz catheter is rare but results in a 53% mortality rate. Perforation can result in pulmonary hemorrhage, pericardial hemorrhage, or mediastinal hemorrhage. Perforation can be confirmed by contrast injection through the distal Swan-Ganz port.

DELAYED COMPLICATIONS OF TRAUMA MANIFEST IN THE THORAX
Adult Respiratory Distress Syndrome
Adult respiratory distress syndrome (ARDS) is a common pathologic consequence of a number of conditions that occur in victims of major trauma. ARDS may develop as a

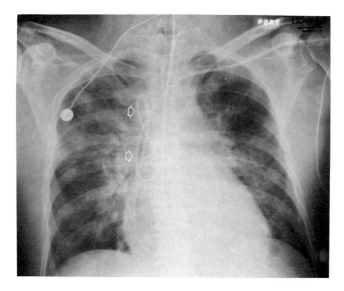

Figure 4.52. Excessive advancement of pulmonary artery catheter with looping in the superior vena cava (radiography). Note the figure-eight loop *(arrows)* of the left subclavian catheter in the superior vena cava. Although the tip is in the pulmonary artery, such looping could lead to intravascular knotting on removal.

result of systemic shock, sepsis, severe pulmonary contusion, massive aspiration, multiple blood transfusions, fat embolism, oxygen toxicity, burns, or coagulation abnormalities, among other etiologies. Although the precise pathophysiology of ARDS is beyond the scope of this discussion, toxic metabolites released in the pulmonary capillary bed injure the alveolar capillary membrane, leading to interstitial and alveolar edema and hemorrhage, microvascular thrombosis and pulmonary infarction, hyaline membrane formation, and proliferation of type II pneumocytes, that in turn lead to impairment of gas exchange and interstitial fibrosis (36).

Typically, ARDS does not manifest radiographically until 24–48 hr after trauma, but radiologic alterations may lag behind the clinical development of hypoxia and tachypnea. Initially, high-quality radiographs will reveal a diffuse interstitial pattern. Over the next 12–24 hr, a diffuse alveolar pattern appears with development of air bronchograms. Superimposed areas of parenchymal consolidation in a patchy distribution are frequently evident (Figs. 4.21, 4.30, 4.50, 4.53). My colleagues and I have frequently noted instances in which the distribution of lung opacities in ARDS is multifocal rather than diffuse, appearing to spare large areas of both lungs or an entire lung. The diminished compliance of the lung resulting from pathogenic changes of ARDS can produce a radiographic appearance of diminished lung volumes with elevation of the hemidiaphragms. The pulmonary parenchymal changes of ARDS are established rapidly, usually by 48 hr after onset, and remain very static for days to weeks afterwards. As ARDS changes resolve, the alveolar predominant pattern of lung opacity is replaced by a coarse interstitial pattern that slowly resolves over weeks to months.

The development of superimposed processes, such as pneumonia, aspiration, abscess or emphyema, and partial lobar atelectasis, may be difficult to detect radiographically on a background of diffuse lung opacity from ARDS. Frequent comparison with both recent and more remote past chest radiographs is necessary to

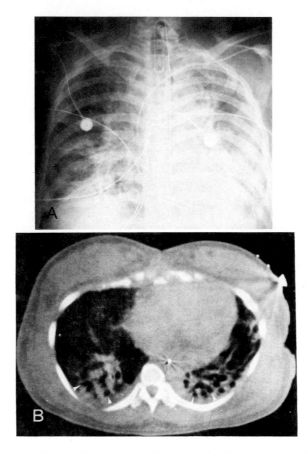

Figure 4.53. ARDS with complicating bronchiectasis (radiography and CT). **A,** AP chest radiograph reveals diffuse, patchy, persistent interstitial and alveolar density compatible with ARDS requiring long-standing ventilatory support. **B,** corresponding CT through the lung bases reveals dilated distal lower lobe bronchi *(arrows)* suggestive of bronchiectasis resulting from recurrent infection and high airway pressures.

detect new pulmonary opacities. Since ventilatory support for patients with ARDS frequently requires high airway pressures, frequent radiographic surveillance is necessary to detect development of pneumothorax, pneumatocyst formation, and interstitial emphysema as well as to ensure proper positioning of endotracheal and tracheostomy tubes. At the onset of positive pressure ventilatory support, the resulting increase in lung volumes may initially falsely suggest early resolution of lung opacities.

Lung abnormalities due to ARDS may be mimicked by several other pathologic processes, including diffuse aspiration, bacterial or viral pneumonia, and pulmonary edema from cardiac and noncardiogenic causes. ARDS is typically not accompanied by pleural effusions or cardiomegaly. The time course of rapid onset and slow resolution of pulmonary changes of ARDS should help distinguish it from other etiologies of diffuse pulmonary parenchymal density. Measurement of central venous pressure and wedge pressure can help distinguish ARDS from cardiogenic etiologies of pulmonary edema. The diffuse nature of ARDS and its tendency to produce small-vessel thrombosis makes demonstration of pulmonary emboli by nuclear scintigraphy (ventilation/ perfusion scan) difficult. If pulmonary embolism is suspected clinically in patients with ARDS, my colleagues and ı usually proceed directly to pulmonary arteriography to establish the diagnosis.

Thoracic CT is usually not necessary to diagnose ARDS radiologically, but it can be helpful in demonstrating the true extent of pulmonary parenchymal involvement, which typically exceeds that suggested by chest radiograph. CT demonstrates a diffuse or multifocal ground-glass-appearing lung consolidation with well-formed air bronchograms (Figs. 4.21, 4.50, 4.53). Patchy areas of dense lung consolidation are revealed. My colleagues and I have noted a tendency for greater involvement of the lower (dependent) lung zones and sparing of the lung periphery in ARDS as depicted by CT. In addition, underlying abnormalities complicating ARDS and its treatment, such as pneumatoceles, pneumothorax, lung cavitation, pleural effusions, tension pneumopericardium, and bronchiectasis (Figs. 4.21, 4.30, 4.41, 4.48, 4.50, 4.53), are often revealed by CT alone (38).

Fat Embolism Syndrome

Fat embolism syndrome is an uncommon complication of lower extremity long-bone and pelvic fractures, occurring in 3% or less of major trauma victims. Clinically, the syndrome presents 24–48 hr after trauma with rapid onset of neurologic dysfunction, fever, petechiae, and respiratory insufficiency (30, 31, 34). The clinical syndrome often precedes radiologic manifestations in the thorax. The chest radiograph can remain normal or can initially reveal an interstitial and patchy alveolar infiltrate that tends to localize around the hila. The pattern progresses rapidly over 24–48 hr to a more diffuse and peripheral alveolar pattern. Typically, cardiomegaly and pleural effusions are not present. The breakdown products of fatty acids embolized to the pulmonary capillary bed incite an ARDS pattern of lung injury indistinguishable from other etiologies of ARDS. The association of long-bone lower extremity fractures, the clinical symptoms described above, and an ARDS pattern on chest radiography strongly suggest the diagnosis.

Pulmonary Infection (Abscess and Empyema)

Infection complicating massive trauma is second only to central nervous system injury as the leading cause of death in this population (77). Thoracic sources of infection may complicate both primary thoracic and primary extrathoracic trauma. Parenchymal lung injury, impaired pulmonary ventilatory mechanics, thoracic surgical interventions, prolonged intubation, prolonged bed rest, and indwelling catheters all contribute to pulmonary and thoracic sources of infection. The development of fever and leukocytosis is frequent in multitrauma victims and the thorax is often a suspected site of infection. Usually, chest radiography demonstrating a localized infiltrate combined with sputum analysis is sufficient to diagnose parenchymal pneumonia. Unfortunately, lung abscesses or infected parenchymal lung hematomas, empyema, and pericardial empyema may escape easy detection by conventional radiography, particularly when only supine portable chest radiographs are obtainable or when diffuse parenchymal abnormalities (such as lung contusion or ARDS) are present.

In a recent study of 37 septic trauma patients (78), my colleagues and I found CT to be very useful in detecting occult pulmonary infections with a 95% accuracy rate for detection of lung abscess and 72% accuracy rate for detection of empyema. CT findings

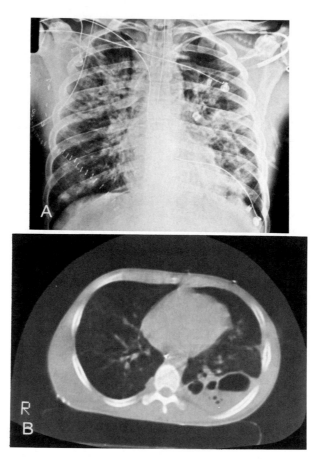

Figure 4.54. "Occult" empyema in recovery phase of trauma (CT). **A,** AP chest radiograph demonstrates patchy diffuse interstitial density compatible with resolving ARDS. No abscess or pleural fluid is suggested. **B,** corresponding axial CT scan at the midcardiac level reveals loculated pleural fluid of the left posteriorly with air-fluid levels. Purulent fluid was aspirated and drained using CT guidance. (From Mirvis SE, Tobin KD, Kostrubiak I, Belzberg H. Thoracic CT in detecting occult disease in critically ill patients. AJR 1987;148:685–689.)

of loculation, air bubbles in the pleural fluid, and enhancement and thickening of the adjacent pleura (split pleura sign) helped distinguish infected from noninfected pleura fluid collections (Figs. 4.51, 4.54). CT has also proven valuable in distinguishing peripheral lung abscess from empyema (79). Stark et al. (79) detected 100% of 70 inflammatory lesions in the thorax in 63 patients and obtained diagnostic information not available from chest radiography in 43% of the patients; CT defined the extent of the disease more accurately in an additional 34% of the patients. In a similar study of 56 critically ill patients at the Shock Trauma Center, CT frequently detected evidence of pericardial or pleural empyema not suggested or confirmable by conventional radiography (Figs. 4.43, 4.51, 4.54) (38).

Delayed Presentation of Aortic Pseudoaneurysm

About 2–5% of patients with traumatic aortic rupture without recognition and treatment will survive to develop a chronic pseudoaneurysm (80). Many such patients may remain

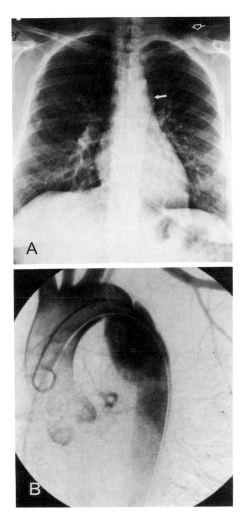

Figure 4.55. Chronic pseudoaneurysm following missed aortic rupture (radiography and DSA). **A,** posteroanterior chest radiograph obtained for screening reveals an abnormal bulge in the aortic arch contour with a rim of calcification *(arrow)*. A remote healed left clavicle fracture *(open arrow)* was sustained 10 years earlier in a motor car accident. **B,** aortic pseudoaneurysm verified by digital subtraction angiography. The patient underwent successful elective repair of the aorta.

symptom-free for months to years, but about 50–65% eventually develop symptoms related to an enlarging chest mass such as chest pain, dysphagia, or hoarseness due to recurrent laryngeal nerve involvement, cough, or dyspnea (30, 80). Chest radiographs play an essential role in detection of chronic pseudoaneurysms. Typically, an unusual bulging contour of the aorta is noted at or below the arch. Sometimes a discrete rim of calcification is noted surrounding the contour abnormality by radiography or, more precisely, by CT scanning (Fig. 4.55). Serial radiography will detect progressive enlargement of the pseudoaneurysm in about 20% of patients (30). Often, indications of past thoracic trauma, such as rib fractures, are evident on the chest radiograph. The diagnosis of aortic pseudoaneurysm can be confirmed by angiography or MRI (81). Since long-term follow-up of untreated chronic aortic pseudoaneurysms demonstrates frequent ruptures as long as 27 yr after injury, elective operative management is usually selected once the diagnosis is established (80).

CONCLUSIONS

Recent years have seen a proliferation of new imaging modalities that can be used to establish or confirm clinical diagnoses. CT, DSA, sonography, and MRI can all provide valuable information in selected clinical circumstances. The clinician and imaging specialist treating the acute trauma victim with major thoracic injury face a significant challenge to smoothly and efficiently integrate resuscitation, rapid and accurate diagnosis, and management to maximally benefit the patient. Although thoracic injury is the focus of this chapter, such injuries often occur in association with injuries to other body systems that may require diagnostic imaging priority. The increasing complexity, variety, and cost of available imaging modalities, as well as the myriad of diagnostic pathways that can be pursued in a given patient, make close cooperation and consultation between the clinical trauma physician and the diagnostic imaging specialist imperative.

REFERENCES

1. Ovenfors C, Hedgcock MW. Intensive care unit radiology: problems of interpretation. Radiol Clin North Am 1978;16:407–439.
2. Mirvis SE, Fritz SL, Siegel JH, Ramzy A. Radiographic unit for use in emergency and intensive care units. AJR 1988;150:691–692.
3. Stark P. Traumatic rupture of the aorta: a review. CRC Crit Rev Diagn Imaging 1984;21:229–255.
4. Parmley LF, Mattingly TW, Marion WC, Jahnke EJ. Non-penetrating traumatic injury of the aorta. Circulation 1958;17:1086–1101.
5. Symbas PN, Tyras DH, Ware RE, Diorio DA. Traumatic rupture of the aorta. Ann Surg 1972;178:6–12.
6. Kirsh MM, Behrendt DM, Orringer MB, et al. The treatment of acute traumatic rupture of the aorta: a 10-year experience. Ann Surg 1976;184:308–316.
7. Barcia TC, Livoni JP. Indications for angiography in blunt thoracic trauma. Radiology 1983;147:15–19.
8. Ayella RJ, Hankins JR, Turney SZ, Cowley RA. Ruptures of the thoracic aorta due to blunt trauma. J Trauma 1977;17:199–205.
9. Schwab CW, Lawson RB, Lind JF, Garland LW. Comparison of supine and upright portable chest films to evaluate the widened mediastinum. Ann Emerg Med 1984;13:896–899.
10. Mirvis SE, Bidwell JK, Buddemeyer EU, Diaconis JN, Pais SO, Whitley JE, et al. Value of chest radiography in excluding traumatic aortic rupture. Radiology 1987;163:487–493.
11. Marsh DG, Sturm JT. Traumatic aortic rupture: roentgenographic indications for angiography. Ann Thorac Surg 1976;21:337–340.
12. Sturm JT, Marsh DG, Bodily KC. Ruptured thoracic aorta: evolving radiologic concepts. Surgery 1979;85:363–367.
13. Seltzer SE, D'Orsi C, Kirshner R, DeWeese JA. Traumatic aortic rupture: plain radiographic findings. AJR 1981;137:1101–1014.
14. Marnocha KE, Maglinte DDT, Woods J, Goodman M, Peterson P. Mediastinal-width/chest-width ratio in blunt chest trauma: a reappraisal. AJR 1984;142:275–277.
15. Applebaum A, Karp RB, Kirklin JW. Surgical treatment of closed thoracic aortic injuries. J Cardiovasc Surg (Torino) 1976;71:458–460.
16. Gerlock AJ, Muhletalen CA, Coulan CM, Hayes PT. Traumatic aortic aneurysm-validity of esophageal tube displacement sign. AJR 1980;135:713–718.
17. Wales LR, Morishima MS, Reay D, Johansen K. Nasogastric tube displacement in acute rupture of the thoracic aorta: a post-mortem study. AJR 1982;138:821–823.
18. Dart CH, Braitman HE. Traumatic rupture of the thoracic aorta: diagnosis and management. Arch Surg 1976;111:697–702.
19. Simeone JF, Minagi H, Putman CE. Traumatic disruption of the thoracic aorta: significance of the left apical extra-pleural cap. Radiology 1975;117:265–268.

20. Simeone JF, Deren MM, Cagle F. The value of the left apical cap in the diagnosis of aortic rupture. Radiology 1981;139:37–39.
21. Peters DR, Gamsu G. Displacement of the right paraspinous interface: a radiologic sign of acute traumatic rupture of the thoracic aorta. Radiology 1980;134:599–603.
22. Heiberg E, Wolverson MK, Sundaran M, Shields LB. CT in aortic trauma. AJR 1983;140:1119–1124.
23. Goodman PC. CT of chest trauma. In: Federle MP, Brant-Zawadski M, eds. Computed tomography in the evaluation of trauma. 2nd ed. Baltimore: Williams & Wilkins, 1986:168–190.
24. Charkravarty M. Utilization of aortography in trauma. Radiol Clin North Am 1986;24:383–396.
25. Mirvis SE, Kostrubiak I, Whitley NO, Goldstein LD, Rodriguez A. Role of CT in excluding major arterial injury after blunt thoracic trauma. AJR 1987;149:601–605.
26. Mirvis SE, Pais SO, Gens DR. Intra-arterial digital subtraction angiography (IADSA) in the diagnosis of aortic rupture. AJR 1986;146:987–991.
27. Jeffrey RB. Aortic lacerations: fatal complications of thoracic aortography. Radiology 1987;165:367–369.
28. Mirvis SE, Borg U, Belzberg H. MR imaging of ventilator-dependent patients: preliminary experience. AJR 1987;149:845–846.
29. Henry DA. Thoracic trauma: radiologic triage of the chest radiograph. Proceedings of the American Roentgen Ray Society, April 1987;13–22.
30. Maltby JD. The post-trauma chest film. CRC Crit Rev Diagn Imaging 1980;14:1–36.
31. Goodman LR, Putman CE. The SICU chest radiograph after massive blunt trauma. Radiol Clin North Am 1981;19:111–123.
32. Putman CE, Goodman LR. Thoracic trauma. In: Teplick JG, Haskin ME, eds. Surgical radiology. Philadelphia: Saunders, 1981:1105–1132.
33. Pratt LW, Guitee LA, Smith RJ, Tryzelaar JF. Blunt chest trauma with tracheobronchial rupture. Ann Otol Rhinol Laryngol 1984;93:357–363.
34. Van Moore A, Ravin CE, Putman CE. Radiologic evaluation of acute chest trauma. CRC Crit Rev Diagn Imaging 1983;19:89–110.
35. Bladergroen MR, Lowe JE, Postlethwait RW. Diagnosis and recommended management of esophageal perforation and rupture. Ann Thorac Surg 1986;42:235–239.
36. Greene R. Lung alterations in thoracic trauma. J Thorac Imaging 1987;2:1–11.
37. Wagner RB, Crawford WO, Schimpf PP. Classification of parenchymal injuries of the lung. Radiology 1988;167:77–82.
38. Mirvis SE, Tobin KD, Kostrubiak I, Belzberg H. Thoracic CT in detecting occult disease in critically ill patients. AJR 1987;148:685–689.
39. Roddy LH, Unger KM, Miller WC. Thoracic computed tomography in the critically ill patient. Crit Care Med 1981;9:515–518.
40. Wall SD, Ferderle MP, Jeffrey RB, Brett CM. CT diagnosis of unsuspected pneumothorax after blunt abdominal trauma. AJR 1983;141:919–921.
41. Tocino IM, Miller MH, Fairfax WR. Distribution of pneumothorax in the supine and semirecumbent critically ill patient. AJR 1985;144:901–905.
42. Chiles C, Ravin CE. Radiographic recognition of pneumothorax in the intensive care unit. Crit Care Med 1986;14:677–680.
43. Ziter FMH, Westcott JL. Supine subpulmonary pneumothorax. AJR 1981;137:699–701.
44. Rhea JT, vanSonnenberg E, McCloud TC. Basilar pneumothorax in the supine adult. Radiology 1979;133:593–595.
45. Gordon R. The deep sulcus sign. Radiology 1980;136:25–27.
46. Spizarny DL, Goodman LR. Air in the minor fissure: a sign of right-sided pneumothorax. Radiology 1986;160:329–331.
47. Friedman PJ. Adult pulmonary ligament pneumatocele: a loculated pneumothorax. Radiology 1985;155:575–576.
48. Tocino IM, Miller MH, Frederick PR, Bahr AL, Thomas F. CT detection of occult pneumothorax in head trauma. AJR 1984;143:987–990.
49. Bryk D. Infrapulmonary effusion: effect of expiration on the pseudodiaphragmatic contour. Radiology 1976;120:33–36.
50. Morgan AS, Flancbaum L, Esposito T, Cox EF. Blunt injury to the diaphragm: an analysis of 44 patients. J Trauma 1986;26:565–568.
51. Bogers AJJC, Zweers DJ, Vroom EM, Huysmans HA. Cardiac subluxation in traumatic rupture of diaphragm and pericardium. Thorac Cardiovasc Surg 1986;34:132–134.

52. Toombs BD, Sandler CM, Lester RG. Computed tomography of chest trauma. Radiology 1981;140:733–738.
53. Wienecek RG, Wilson RF, Steiger Z. Acute injuries of the diaphragms: an analysis of 165 cases. J Thorac Cardiovasc Surg 1986;92:989–993.
54. Beal SL, McKennan M. Blunt diaphragm rupture: a morbid injury. Arch Surg 1988;123:828–832.
55. Heiberg E, Wolverson MK, Hurd RN, Jagannaadharao B, Sundarum M. CT recognition of traumatic rupture of the diaphragm. AJR 1980;134:369–372.
56. Ammann AM, Brewer WH, Maull KI, Walsh JW. Traumatic rupture of the diaphragm: real-time sonographic diagnosis. AJR 1983;140:915–916.
57. Rao KG, Woodlief RM. Grey scale ultrasonic demonstration of ruptured right hemidiaphragm. Br J Radiol 1980;53:812–814.
58. Gurney J, Harrison WL, Anderson JC. Omental fat simulating pleural fluid in traumatic diaphragmatic hernia: CT characteristics. J Comput Assist Tomogr 1985;9:1112–1114.
59. Mirvis SE, Keramati B, Buckman R, Rodriguez A. MR imaging of traumatic diaphragmatic rupture. J Comput Assist Tomgr 1988;12:147–149.
60. Bowers VD, Watkins GM. Blunt trauma to the thoracic outlet and angiography. Am Surg 1983;49:655–659.
61. Fermanis GG, Deane SA, Fitzgerald PM. The significance of first and second rib fractures. Aust NZ J Surg 1985;55:383–386.
62. Harley DP, Mena I. Cardiac and vascular sequelae of sternal fractures. J Trauma 1986;26:553–555.
63. Ben-Menachem Y. Avulsion of the innominate artery associated with fracture of the sternum. AJR 1988;150:621–622.
64. Oreck SL, Burgess A, Levine A. Traumatic lateral displacement of the scapula: a radiologic sign of neurovascular disruption. J Bone Joint Surg 1984;66:758–763.
65. Mirvis SE, Indeck M, Shorr RM, Diaconis JN. Post-traumatic tension penumopericardium: the "small heart" sign. Radiology 1986;158:663–669.
66. Cimmino CV. Some radio-diagnostic notes on pneumomediastinum, pneumothorax, and pneumopericardium. Va Med 196/;94:205–213.
67. Higgins CB, Broderick TW, Edwards DK, Schumaker A. The hemodynamic significance of massive pneumopericardium in preterm infants with respiratory distress syndrome. Radiology 1979;133:363–368.
68. Grumback K, Mechlin MB, Mintz M. Computed tomography and ultrasound of the traumatized and acutely ill patient. Emerg Med Clin North Am 1985;3:607–624.
69. Aho AJ, Vantinnen EA, Nelimarka OI. Rupture of the pericardium with luxation of the heart after blunt trauma. J Trauma 1987;27:560–563.
70. Rosenbaum RC, Johnston GS. Posttraumatic cardiac dysfunction: assessment with radionuclide ventriculography. Radiology 1986;160:91–94.
71. Tuddenham WJ. Iatrogenic lesions of the lungs. In: Teplick JG and Haskin ME, eds. Surgical radiology. Philadelphia: Saunders, 1981;1332–1356.
72. Wechsler RJ, Steiner RM, Kinori I, Monitoring the monitors: the radiology of thoracic catheters, wires, and tubes. Semin Roentgenol 1988;23:61–84.
73. Maurer JR, Friedman PJ, Wing VW. Thoracostomy tube in an interlobar fissure: radiologic recognition of a potential problem. AJR 1982;139:1155–1161.
74. Stark DD, Federle MP, Goodman PC. CT and radiologic assessment of tube thoracostomy. AJR 1983;141:253–258.
75. Fraser RS. Lung perforation complicating tube thoracostomy: pathologic description of three cases. Hum Pathol 1988;19:518–523.
76. Tocino IM, Watanabe A. Impending catheter perforation of the superior vena cava: radiographic recognition. AJR 1986;146:487–490.
77. Caplan ES, Hoyt NJ. Infection surveillance and control in the severely traumatized patient. Am J Med 1981;70:638–640.
78. Mirvis SE, Rodriguez A, Whitley NO, Tarr RJ. CT evaluation of thoracic infections after major trauma. AJR 1985;144:1183–1187.
79. Stark DD, Federle MP, Goodman PC, Podrasky AE, Webb WR. Differentiating lung abscess and empyema: radiography and computed tomography. AJR 1983;141:163–167.
80. Heystraten FM, Rosenbusch G, Kingma LM, Lacquet LK. Chronic posttraumatic aneurysm of the thoracic aorta: surgically correctable occult threat. AJR 1986;146:303–308.
81. Glazer HS, Gutierrez FR, Levitt RG, Lee JKT, Murphy WA. The thoracic aorta studied by MR imaging. Radiology 1985;157:149–155.
82. Sturm JT, Olsen FR, Cicero SJ. Chest roentgenographic findings in 26 patients with traumatic rupture of the thoracic aorta. Ann Emerg Med 1983;12:598–600.

83. Sefzcek DM, Sefzcek RJ, Deeb ZL. Radiologic sign of acute traumatic rupture of the thoracic aorta. AJR 1983;141:1259–1262.

84. Gundry SR, William S, Burney RE, MacKenzie JR, Cho KJ. Indication for aortography: radiology after blunt chest trauma: a reassessment of radiologic findings associated with traumatic rupture of the aorta. Invest Radiol 1983;18:230–237.

85. Woodring JH, Loh FK, Kryscio RJ. Mediastinal hemorrhage: an evaluation of radiologic manifestations. Radiology 1984;151:15–21.

86. Akins CW, Buckley MJ, Daggett W, McIldruff JB, Austen WG. Acute traumatic disruption of the thoracic aorta: ten-year experience. Ann Thorac Surg 1981:31:305–309.

5 Anesthesia in Thoracic Trauma

John K. Stene, MD, PhD

Thoracic injuries profoundly affect the physiologic response of the patient to injury and thus cause some of the most difficult clinical challenges for the trauma anesthesiologist. Not only are these patients affected by direct injury to the cardiopulmonary systems but they also manifest indirect effects that complicate anesthetic care, such as shock and, occasionally, cerebral air embolism.

Uses for anesthesia in the patient with thoracic trauma include anesthetic induction to establish a patent artificial airway, surgical anesthesia for a corrective operation, anesthesia to assist the surgeon in diagnostic tests, anesthesia for radiologic procedures, and, finally, postinjury and/or postoperative analgesia. Thoracic trauma commonly impairs the patient's gas exchange mechanisms. Many of these patients require artificial mechanical ventilation to maintain appropriate alveolar and arterial blood gas tensions. Endotracheal intubation to facilitate artificial ventilation is most easily achieved with intravenous hypnotics and muscle relaxants (1). Among the indications for intubation are the need to compensate for rib fractures, chest wall instability, and reduced respiratory muscle work during shock resuscitation (2) and the need to control ventilation during surgery.

Intubation of the patient with chest trauma, as for other patients suffering from serious injuries, can be accomplished by direct laryngoscopy and orotracheal intubation following an induction dose of an intravenous hypnotic and an intravenous muscle relaxant.

Many trauma patients require ventilation for several days both to stabilize the chest wall and to provide adequate gas exchange with severely injured lungs. Prolonged analgesia and sedation are required to help these patients tolerate the endotracheal intubation as well as to relieve the pain from their injuries. A combination of an opioid, a benzodiazepine, and a muscle relaxant is extremely useful for these patients.

Other modalities of analgesia are useful for controlling the pain of thoracic injury in a patient who does not require mechanical assistance to maintain gas exchange. Continuous epidural analgesia through a catheter placed in either the thoracic or lumbar epidural space has proved to be extremely effective for postthoracotomy as well as posttraumatic pain relief (3). Epidural opioids with or without very dilute local anesthetic solutions will allow high-level (to the cervical region) analgesia without major sympathetic nervous system blockade. Judiciously applied anesthesia care can markedly enhance the management of the patient suffering from thoracic trauma (Table 5.1).

Table 5.1.
Anesthesia for Thoracic Trauma

Anesthetic	Use
General anesthesia	Provides positive pressure ventilation to manage impaired gas exchange; allows operations with an open hemithorax
Regional anesthesia	Provides excellent long-term analgesia postoperatively either with or without mechanical ventilation

DIRECT EFFECTS OF CARDIOPULMONARY INJURIES ON ANESTHETIC MANAGEMENT
Lung Injuries

Lung injuries produced by chest trauma, such as pulmonary contusion, lung laceration, and/or barotrauma to the lung, affect the patient's pulmonary gas exchange and the uptake and distribution of inhalational anesthetics. Contusion of the lung disrupts the alveolar capillary membrane and causes interstitial and alveolar filling with blood. The contused area will alter the exchange of oxygen and carbon dioxide between the alveolus and the blood. If the contusion is small, these effects may have minimal impact on patient care. However, large contusions will lead to marked impairment of oxygenation as well as carbon dioxide elimination. At the extreme, massive bilateral pulmonary contusion may require treatment with an extracorporeal membrane oxygenator (4). Classically, the contusion takes several hours to evolve fully on chest x-ray. The most prominent effect of lung contusion is to produce regions of low pulmonary ventilation to perfusion ratios (V/Q), frequently producing the extremely low V/Q ratio of 0 or a right-to-left shunt (5). This right-to-left shunt will have marked effects on oxygenation as well as on the uptake of inhalational anesthetics. The poorly soluble anesthetic nitrous oxide will demonstrate an accelerated rise of its end tidal to inspired concentration ratio. This is because the pulmonary contusion also causes relative overventilation of other lung regions. However, the venous admixture effect of the contusion will retard the rate of rise of the arterial nitrous oxide concentration and slow the anesthetic induction. Isoflurane, being of intermediate solubility, will also have an enhanced rate of rise of end tidal to inspired concentration ratio but will have minimal retardation of the rise of arterial concentration secondary to venous admixture because each liter of mixed venous blood contains more isoflurane than N_2O. Thus, the induction of anesthesia with isoflurane will be only slightly delayed by pulmonary contusions (6).

As lung contusions resolve, they frequently cause bullae or cyst formation in the lung (7, 8). These pulmonary cysts will act as dead space if they are ventilated and will have no effect in gas exchange if they are not ventilated. However, the cysts may be particularly sensitive to rupture secondary to barotrauma; therefore, the anesthesiologist must be careful to control ventilatory pressures in patients with such bullae. Lung lacerations complicate anesthetic management because of continued hemorrhage that can lead to hemorrhagic shock if not controlled. A lacerated lung also usually has a continuous air leak from the tracheobronchial tree, which, if relatively large, will require increased inspired ventilation to compensate for loss of alveolar gas exchange. If the bronchopleural fistula robs the lung of a significant portion of each tidal volume, a double-lumen endotracheal tube will have to be placed to isolate the lungs from each other (Table 5.2). The lung without laceration can then be ventilated with tidal volumes and rates high enough to compensate for poor CO_2 removal from the lung with a large

Table 5.2.
Use of Endobronchial Tubes in Chest Trauma

Condition	Tube
Thoracic aortic aneurysm	Left endobronchial tube—collapse left lung to facilitate exposure
Traumatic rupture of bronchus	Use endobronchial tube in contralateral bronchus
Unilateral lung contusion	Left endobronchial tubes are easier to insert and can effectively allow independent lung ventilation
Unilateral ARDS	Usually use left endobronchial tube; but use right endobronchial if high airway pressures will be required in right lung
Large bronchopleural fistula with massive air leak	Use endobronchial lumen in lung to be ventilated to avoid high endobronchial cuff pressures to prevent air leak through bronchopleural fistula
Intrapulmonary hemorrhage	Use left endobronchial tube to isolate blood to lung that is bleeding; provides improved gas exchange in contralateral lung

air leak. Unfortunately, the lacerated lung with air leak will continue to cause an increased venous admixture despite independent lung ventilation. This situation can be surgically corrected temporarily by cross-clamping the pulmonary hilum to stop both air and blood flow to that lung. The same considerations for gas exchange and anesthetic uptake as discussed above will apply to this right-to-left shunt.

One of the worst complications of pulmonary laceration or pulmonary penetration from any cause is a bronchial-venous fistula involving the pulmonary vein, leading to continuous entry of air into the pulmonary venous drainage and thus systemic air emboli (9). Such a bronchial-venous fistula may occur following penetrating lung trauma from knives or bullets and may occasionally be seen with sudden decompression in divers when alveolar units rupture to form a continuous path of air entry into pulmonary venous drainage. Treatment requires the discontinuation of both ventilation and perfusion to the lacerated lung. Again, a surgical clamp across the lung hilum will achieve this effect temporarily until the lung can be repaired. A double-lumen endotracheal tube can facilitate treatment by allowing full ventilation to the other lung. Any neurologic damage from the arterial air embolism can be improved by decompressing the patient in a hyperbaric chamber, which will dissolve the air bubbles into the bloodstream.

Chest Wall Injury

Thoracic trauma frequently causes instability of the chest wall secondary to multiple rib fractures or open pneumothoraces (sucking chest wounds). Multiple rib fractures destabilize the chest wall so that it becomes difficult for the patient to generate significant negative pleural pressure for ventilation. If the rib fractures are unilateral, the ventilation will tend to shift to the lung in the intact chest wall. However, blood flow will not be diverted away from the lung in the unstable hemithorax; therefore, the patient will develop marked venous admixture or right-to-left pulmonary shunting. The energy transfer from the blunt trauma that fractured the ribs usually contuses the underlying lung. This contused lung will become stiffer and less compliant than normal lung and will further aggravate the hypoventilation of the injured hemithorax. The sharp ends of the fractured ribs frequently lacerate the underlying lung and may also penetrate the skin, leading to an open pneumothorax.

Penetrating injuries of the lung will lead to some degree of open pneumothorax. A large defect in the chest wall will suck air in during each inspiration and expel some of it during expiration. If the resistance of air flow through the open pneumothorax is less than the resistance of air flow through the trachea and bronchus to the hemithorax, the underlying lung will collapse rapidly as changes in interpleural pressure with ventilation tend to pull air in through the pneumothorax. These chest wall defects must be covered with air-tight dressings and a chest tube inserted to evacuate the pleural air.

The treatment of an unstable chest wall requires intubation or tracheostomy and mechanical ventilation to splint the ribs while they heal. This treatment, described by Avery in 1956 (10), revolutionized the management of patients with injury-induced chest-wall instability. Prior to this treatment technique, attempts to operatively fixate the rib fractures were successful in stabilizing the ribs but frequently increased the patient's morbidity; however, this latter treatment modality is regaining some favor (see Chapter 9). Some clinicians have recently recommended continuous regional anesthesia to provide pain relief for the injured chest wall while allowing the patient to breathe spontaneously with a natural airway. Their contention is that the pain of the rib fractures leads to the splinting and hypoventilation, causing gas exchange abnormalities with chest trauma (3). Patients with massive chest-wall injury and/or multiple injuries will probably still need to be maintained on mechanical ventilation for a period of time following their injury, but the use of continuous regional anesthesia via an epidural, intercostal, or interpleural approach appears to be promising in the management of chest wall injuries (11–13).

Cardiac and Great Vessel Injuries

Blunt trauma to the anterior chest wall can easily lead to a myocardial contusion (14, 15). The contused myocardium is characterized by disrupted capillaries and hematoma surrounding the cardiac myocytes (16). A large transmural contusion will frequently lead to cellular disruption and necrosis of the cardiac myocytes and thus behave acutely like a transmural myocardial infarction, with the release of intracellular enzymes into the bloodstream and regional cardiac wall motion abnormalities. However, the contused myocardium is not surrounded by a zone of relative ischemia, as is the ischemic myocardium. Furthermore, the contused area will heal with a well-perfused scar, whereas the ischemically injured myocardium will heal with an avascular scar.

A small epicardial contusion will frequently cause only transient arrhythmias by acting as an irritable focus (17). Large transmural contused areas lead to dyssynergia of the ventricular wall and can impair cardiac ejection and stroke volume. The worst complication from large myocardial contusion is contusion through papillary muscles with disruption of the mitral valve (16). The acute mitral regurgitation that follows contusion through the left ventricular papillary muscles frequently leads to a fatal outcome unless it is possible to replace the valve with an artificial valve.

The natural history of myocardial contusion and the best method of treatment are still controversial (18, 19). Because it is so difficult to diagnose small myocardial contusions, it has been very difficult to identify patients with myocardial contusion and follow them to ascertain the natural history of the contusion as well as the best forms of treatment. Some traumatologists feel that a patient with a myocardial contusion must be treated as if he/she had a myocardial infarction, i.e., with rest and oxygen for several days. However, a patient with a contused myocardium does not need pharmacologic manipulations to decrease the zone of relative ischemia around the infarction. In the operating room, myocardial contusions seem to affect the anesthesia only if they are large enough to cause regional wall-motion abnormalities of the left ventricle. A patient who has a large transmural contusion should be monitored intraoperatively with a pulmonary artery (Swan-Ganz) catheter and treated appropriately to continuously optimize his/her hemodynamic status.

More serious injuries to the myocardium are lacerations secondary to either penetrating trauma or chamber rupture from blunt trauma (14). Large lacerations frequently are rapidly fatal. However, some patients can survive ventricular laceration since muscle edges of the laceration reapproximate as interchamber and extrachamber interpericardial pressures equilibrate. These patients are salvageable with rapid intraoperative repair. Penetrating trauma that punctures the coronary artery will lead to ischemic injuries of the myocardium distal to the penetrant injury. If the patient has relatively good collateral flow into this area, the ischemic damage may be minimal. However, lacerated coronary arteries frequently bleed briskly into the pericardium, leading to a hemopericardium with cardiac tamponade. A massive interstitial pulmonary air leak that leads to pneumomediastinum may cause air to dissect into the pericardium, causing pneumopericardium and tamponade. Tamponade of the pericardium is diagnosed by marked pulsus paradoxus with respiration. Tachycardia is associated with a decrease in arterial pressure and an increase in venous pressure. If a pulmonary artery catheter has been inserted, both the central venous pressure and the pulmonary capillary wedge pressure will be elevated and numerically equal. The cardiac output will be diminished. Echocardiography will demonstrate an enlarged pericardial space and small ventricular volumes with tamponade. Tamponade must be relieved rapidly to allow the heart to function normally. Pericardiocentesis may be performed both diagnostically and therapeutically in patients with suspected hemopericardium or pneumopericardium. If there is any question about pericardial tamponade reaccumulating, the patient should receive a pericardial window to vent the pericardium. The anesthetic management of the patient with pericardial tamponade is aimed at maintaining a rapid heart rate to minimize the need for ventricular filling and the avoidance of drugs that depress the myocardium (20). Furthermore, intravenous fluids should be administered to increase cardiovascular preload to the maximum. Useful drugs in these patients include benzodiazepines, such as midazolam, to induce unconsciousness and amnesia. In the absence of a closed head injury, ketamine hydrochloride can be very useful in this situation as it tends to perpetuate a tachycardia and might accentuate sympathetic stimulation to the myocardium. Judiciously utilized opioids can maintain the patient's level of analgesia without depressing the myocardium or venous return.

Blunt chest trauma can lead to an acute traumatic thoracic aortic aneurysm. These aneurysms frequently rupture and cause the patient to exsanguinate. However, the hemorrhage may be controlled temporarily by hematoma formation that allows the patient time to receive definitive medical therapy. The hemorrhage associated with an aortic injury will cause the upper mediastinum to be widened on an upright chest x-ray. Definitive diagnosis requires arteriography. Because of the high potential for temporarily sealed aneurysms to completely rupture and lead to sudden death, these patients need to undergo immediate surgical repair of the aortic injury. Aneurysms distal to the left subclavian takeoff may be managed with short-term cross-clamping and resection with grafting. Likewise, ventricular shunting or partial bypass from the left ventricle to the distal aorta may be used to reduce the afterload stress on the left ventricle during the repair. More proximal aneurysms, including the ascending aorta and the aortic arch, will require cardiopulmonary bypass for complete repair. The anesthetic management of the patient who requires cardiopulmonary bypass is similar to that used for the patient requiring anesthesia for cardiac surgery. For the patient who has distal thoracic aortic aneurysms repaired with cross-clamping and grafting, the anesthetic management is designed to maintain cardiac preload and venous return during cross-clamping, with potent arterial vasodilators used to minimize the acute afterload effects on the left ventricle. Consideration must be given to the trade-offs of reducing afterload by systemic vasodilatation and associated loss of perfusion pressure and volume to the spinal cord. Close communication and cooperation between the surgeon and anesthesiologist are crucial to successful management of circulation requirements in these cases.

It is important to stimulate renal diuresis prior to aortic cross-clamping and to attempt to replace the patient's blood volume to the point that the vasodilated bed distal to the aortic cross-clamp can be perfused adequately when the cross-clamp is released. Some surgeons prefer to administer mannitol (12.5 g intravenously) just prior to cross-clamping and to repeat it 15 min after cross-clamping begins. Metabolic acidosis occurs as the ischemic vascular bed is reperfused. Prophylactic hyperventilation will help buffer the effect of the metabolic acidosis. In severe cases, intravenous buffers, such as bicarbonate or tromethamine, may be needed. These patients should be monitored with intraarterial catheters, preferably in the right radial artery, as cross-clamping will decrease pressure in the femoral and left radial arteries. A pulmonary artery catheter should be placed preoperatively, if the patient's condition is sufficiently stable, to monitor cardiac output and the effects of cross-clamping on the left ventricle. While still a controversial modality, a lumbar subarachnoid catheter (spinal) has been reported to be useful experimentally to help reduce ischemia of the spinal cord during aortic cross-clamping (21). Aortic cross-clamping will lead to increased pressure in the carotid arteries proximal to the cross-clamp. This increased carotid arterial pressure will be transmitted to the intracerebral cerebrospinal fluid (CSF), which is in continuity with the spinal cord CSF. When the pressure in the distal spinal cord CSF is raised, the arterial perfusion pressure to the spinal cord is reduced by the aortic cross-clamp. If the mean arterial pressure in the spinal cord is reduced too much while CSF pressure rises, the perfusion of the spinal cord will be impaired and infarction may occur. Draining CSF through a continuous spinal catheter will reduce the rise in CSF pressure and help maintain an adequate spinal cord perfusion pressure, which may prevent acute paraplegia secondary to spinal cord infarction. Local anesthetics and opioids may be administered through a spinal catheter just as they are through an epidural catheter. Furthermore, a subarachnoid (spinal) catheter may be used safely up to 48 hr postoperatively. The doses of drugs administered directly into the CSF are 10–20% of the doses used with an epidural catheter.

INDIRECT EFFECTS OF CHEST INJURY ON ANESTHESIA

Hemorrhagic shock following chest trauma will complicate anesthetic management. The anesthesiologist must be careful to use drugs to provide adequate hypnosis, amnesia, and analgesia while optimizing cardiovascular homeostasis (1). Many of the anesthetic drugs are myocardial depressants. These drugs must be either avoided or used in very small, judiciously selected doses during hemorrhagic shock. Drugs such as thiopental sodium, fentanyl citrate, or sufentanil are highly lipophilic and will rapidly cross the blood-brain barrier. If these drugs are injected intravenously into a patient with a reduced blood volume from hemorrhagic shock, the concentration achieved in the bloodstream will be much higher than in an euvolemic patient. Therefore, very small doses of these drugs can be used to achieve the desired hypnosis or analgesia and, if carefully monitored, to avoid cardiovascular depression. Nalbuphine, an opiate agonist/antagonist, has some properties similar to high-dose naloxone when given in large doses in that it will temporarily increase cardiac output and blood pressure. Thus, nalbuphine may be used in relatively large doses to provide analgesia. Nitrous oxide should be avoided as it tends to accumulate in closed air spaces such as pneumothoraces. Furthermore, nitrous oxide and opioid combinations tend to be very depressing to the cardiac output (22). Therefore, air should be used to reduce the F_{IO_2} below 1. Although isoflurane and halothane are myocardial depressants and vasodilators, in low concentration they will improve the hypnosis and analgesia with minimal cardiac depression. An advantage of an inhalationally delivered drug is that if the patient shows excessive cardiovascular depression from the anesthetic, the drug can be eliminated rapidly through the lungs. Although pulmonary contusion will slow the rise and fall of inhalational gas tensions in the lung as described above, the change is still more rapid than the change of intravenous drug concentration.

Shock must be treated by restoring the intravascular fluid volume. Shock treatment priorities are to (a) restore the circulating volume, (b) restore hemoglobin concentration to a level adequate for oxygen consumption, and (c) restore coagulation. Initially, asanguinous fluids are used to establish open intravenous lines and to rapidly restore circulating volume. Colloid resuscitation protocols are more effective in rapidly restoring circulating volume than crystalloid resuscitation protocols. However, all patients will need a fair volume of crystalloid infusion following trauma to replace water lost from the extravascular interstitial compartments. Water is lost both in hemorrhagic blood loss and in edema that occurs in the region of traumatized tissues. Experimental animal preparations and some human experiments have demonstrated the superior capability of colloid resuscitation to rapidly restore circulating volume as well as cardiac output and oxygen consumption (23, 24). Since hypoperfusion of vascular beds during shock states leads to total obstruction of capillaries and a no-reflow phenomenon, it may be advantageous to rapidly restore circulating volume to prevent capillary beds from being massively shut down. Hemoglobin concentration must be maintained at levels adequate to support oxygen delivery and needed oxygen consumption. Since increased velocity of microcirculatory blood flow compensates for the loss of hemoglobin, hemoglobin and hematocrit levels do not have to be restored to normal values. Although the optimum postresuscitation hemoglobin concentration is unknown, it is known that a mild degree of hemodilution can enhance microvascular perfusion.

Air embolism was discussed above as a result of penetrating injuries to the lung. Nitrous oxide should be avoided at all costs in patients in whom systemic embolism is suspected, since it will be concentrated in the air bubbles and cause them to grow to larger volume; 100% oxygen ventilation may help reduce the size of the air bubbles, as it will lead to an increased gradient for nitrogen and other insoluble gases to diffuse out of the air bubble into the dissolved blood phase. An unsuspected arterial air embolism from a penetrating lung injury can lead to intraoperative neurologic dysfunction and even to the failure of the patient to wake up at the end of the anesthetic.

Prolonged hypoperfusion associated with traumatic tissue injury can lead to the adult respiratory distress syndrome (ARDS). ARDS is characterized by excessive interstitial edema with normal intravascular pressures. Excessive edema is the result of large leaks in the capillary membranes, which allow fluid to escape into the pulmonary interstitium. Frequently, this interstitial edema provides a focus for collagen to be laid down, leading to fibrotic areas of the lung. As the lung develops interstitial fibrosis, alveoli are also disrupted with a loss of the alveolar epithelium. The alveolar epithelium is replaced by proliferation of the type II pneumocytes that are sparsely represented in the normal lung. These cells secrete surfactant into the normal alveolus and also appear to be the embryonic alveolar cells. If the patient survives the hypoxia of ARDS and the lung injury ceases, the lung will begin to heal, and the type II pneumocytes will differentiate into the normal alveolar epithelium.

Since ARDS is caused by neutrophils damaging the pulmonary endothelium (leading to leaky capillaries) and is aggravated by the generalized inflammatory state, it frequently heralds further inflammatory damage to other organs. In patients who had prolonged ischemia secondary to hemorrhagic shock, ARDS frequently is the herald of a progressive multisystem organ dysfunction. Lung failure is followed by renal failure, hepatic failure, bone marrow failure, failure of the epithelial barrier in the intestine, and ultimately patient death in the full multisystem organ failure syndrome (25). Prevention of ARDS and multisystem organ failure requires rapid restoration of both circulating volume and adequate oxygen delivery to meet cellular demands. Mechanical ventilation of the lungs with relatively large tidal volumes and positive end-expiratory pressure levels high enough to prevent large areas of alveolar collapse also seems to help prevent ARDS, probably because the lung maintained in the well-ventilated state with normal anatomic relationships of alveoli and capillaries will not develop intravascular areas of relative hypoxia to aggravate the inflammatory attack on the capillary endothelium. Once ARDS occurs, efforts must be made to prevent further damage to the lung. Avoiding marked hypervolemic states will help prevent excessive fluid from leaking through the injured pulmonary capillaries. High oxygen ventilation should be avoided as oxygen itself injures the lung as well as causing absorption atelectasis from poorly ventilated regions. If the patient can be supported until the capillary endothelium stops excessive fluid leaking, then supportive care (maintaining oxygenation and ventilation with a mechanical ventilator) will usually lead to survival. The lungs that have been insulted by ARDS take a long time to totally heal, although many of these patients will return to relatively normal pulmonary function.

ANALGESIA
Epidural

Patients with multiple rib fractures and injuries to the chest benefit greatly from continuous epidural analgesia (Table 5.3). Epidural catheters can be placed into the epidural space at the cervical, thoracic, or lumbar level of the cord. Cervical epidural catheters are difficult to insert and have a high potential for complications; therefore, they are of little use in managing the patient with chest trauma. Thoracic or lumbar level epidural catheters, however, are quite useful in managing such patients. The catheters are inserted through an appropriate needle, usually a Tuohy needle, that is advanced from the skin into the epidural space. The entrance of the needle into the epidural space is indicated by negative epidural space pressure pulling air or fluid through the needle (loss of resistance). The catheter is then threaded through the needle a few centimeters into the epidural space, the needle is removed, and the catheter is taped in place. Both local anesthetics and preservative-free opioids can be injected through the catheter to provide analgesia. Because the spread of analgesia tends to be equally cephalad and caudad from the level of the tip of the catheter, it is probably advantageous to use thoracic-level epidural catheters in patients with chest trauma. Thoracic catheters will

Table 5.3.
Continuous Regional Analgesia for Chest Trauma[a]

Lumbar subarachnoid catheter	Very small doses of opioids (i.e., 0.25 mg of morphine) provide prolonged analgesia
Lumbar epidural catheter	Simple to insert; chest wall analgesia can be achieved with higher volumes and doses of drugs; typical dose, 5–10 mg of morphine every 4–12 hr; fentanyl infusion, 70–100 μg/hr; 0.0625–0.125% bupivacaine may be added to opioid, 15–25 ml/injection for intermittent injection or 5–12 ml/hr for continuous infusion
Thoracic epidural catheter	Excellent chest wall analgesia with small amounts of drug use; typical dose, 2.5–5.0 mg of morphine every 4–12 hr; fentanyl infusion, 50–70 μg/hr; 0.0625–0.125% bupivacaine may be added, 5–10 ml/injection for intermittent injection or 4–8 ml/hr for continuous infusion
Intercostal catheter	Good unilateral analgesia; typical dose, 0.25–0.50% bupivacaine, 20–25 ml/injection; also consider 2% 2-chloroprocaine, 20–25 ml/hr for continuous infusion

[a]The typical doses given here are based on extensive experience with acutely injured trauma patients and are larger than doses required for elective surgical patients. All patients should be monitored closely for signs of toxicity or inadequate analgesia and drug doses should be adjusted appropriately.

provide a band of anesthesia throughout the thoracic dermatomes. Local anesthetic solutions can anesthetize motor, sensory, and autonomic neurons in the spinal cord, whereas epidurally administered opioids bind to enkephalinergic receptors in the dorsal columns of the spinal cord and thus provide only sensory analgesia. Opioids and the local anesthetics appear to work synergistically when injected together into the epidural space (12, 26). However, the anesthesiologist must be careful when injecting the local anesthetic solutions epidurally to avoid sympathetic nervous system paralysis with a high (above T4) block. Very dilute solutions of bupivacaine (0.0625–0.125%) have been used to provide synergistic analgesia with opioids and to avoid profound sympathetic nervous system paralysis. Opioids can be used to achieve high levels of epidural analgesia without sympathetic paralysis. However, one must be careful with opioids; if they are given in a volume that extends the blockade above the cervical cord into the brain stem, profound respiratory depression will result (27). Furthermore, the systemic vascular absorption of the opioids will lead to appreciable blood levels following epidural injection; therefore, one must be careful when giving intravenous opioids along with epidural opioids.

Subarachnoid (spinal) injected opioids also provide prolonged analgesia. In this case, very small amounts, i.e., ≤1 mg, of morphine sulfate injected into the lumbar CSF will provide analgesia up to cervical levels of the spinal cord with almost no systemic absorption. Although subarachnoid catheters are useful in draining off CSF to reduce the lumbar CSF pressure during thoracic aorta cross-clamping, this form of continuous analgesia is more limited than epidural analgesia following chest trauma. A percutaneous catheter into the lumbar subarachnoid space can be used for up to 48 hr with minimal risk of CSF infection. However, leaving the catheter in place longer than 48 hr places the patient at risk for meningitis. Epidural catheters dwell in a space relatively resistant to infection and may be left in place for prolonged periods with minimal risk of systemic or local infection.

Another continuous regional anesthetic technique useful for thoracic trauma is the use of a continuous intercostal catheter—an epidural catheter placed in the subcostal neurovascular space. These catheters are inserted just caudad to the edge of the rib approximately 7 cm lateral to the midline and passed centrally into the neurovascular groove on the caudad surface of the rib. Large doses of local anesthetics injected through these catheters will result in bilateral chest-wall analgesia. For a patient with one or two isolated rib fractures, such a catheter may be more useful than an epidural catheter. Other investigators report great success by passing the catheter through the pleural membrane so that it remains in the pleural space and then injecting large doses of local anesthetics that, again, spread across the pleura and can even provide bilateral chest wall analgesia (28, 29).

Patient-Controlled Analgesia

For the patient who is alert and has moderate to minimal pain following chest trauma, an intravenously administered patient-controlled analgesia device is ideal. This device allows the patient to control the rate at which intravenously administered opioids are received. To prevent inadvertent overdose, the physician sets the limit on the maximum rate of opioid injection that the patient can receive each hour. It has been demonstrated many times that patients use fewer milligrams of morphine with the patient-controlled analgesia pump than when the drug is given on demand by the nurses. Furthermore, patients with patient-controlled analgesia pumps receive a more constant level of analgesia than they do when they have to demand injections from the nurses every 3 or 4 hr (30).

CURRENT POSTOPERATIVE PAIN MANAGEMENT PRACTICES AT THE MIEMSS SHOCK TRAUMA CENTER

The Maryland Institute for Emergency Medical Services Systems (MIEMSS) Shock Trauma Center experience with posttraumatic pain management in patients with thoracic trauma has demonstrated that continuous epidural analgesia maintained by intermittent injections is the technique of choice. Many of the posttraumatic patients required doses of epidural opioids far in excess of typical postobstetrical or postelective surgical analgesic requirements. Patients with extensive soft-tissue injuries as well as multiple rib fractures may require reinjection of the epidural catheter every 4–6 hr. Many of these patients received up to 60 mg of morphine/day epidurally with no signs of excessive narcotization. Lumbar epidural catheters have been the preferred route at the Shock Trauma Center; therefore, the patients required 15–25 ml/injection, usually with 0.125% bupivacaine plus morphine, to receive reliable chest wall analgesia. Bupivacaine clinically appears to act synergistically with the opioids to provide more satisfactory analgesia than opioids or local anesthetics alone. Occasionally, a patient required a demonstration of surgical level anesthesia by using 1.5% lidocaine through the catheter as psychologic proof that the epidural catheter was working. We also found that 100 μg of fentanyl citrate or sufentanil provided excellent analgesia when mixed with an appropriate volume of dilute bupivacaine.

Continuous infusions of fentanyl citrate and bupivacaine were difficult to manage in the trauma patients due to the extreme variation in noxious stimuli associated with various nursing procedures. Therefore, we found that the constant reassessing of the patients' analgesic requirements with intermittent bolus injections to be a very useful component of the pain management service.

Intercostal catheters provide excellent pain relief from posttraumatic chest wall pain. However, these catheters have proven difficult to maintain in position in an actively moving patient. Therefore, the more secure epidural catheter has been utilized more frequently to control posttraumatic chest pain. Culturing approximately 40 catheters that were removed after 1–8 days in the lumbar epidural space revealed no time-dependent pattern of bacterial contamination. Although a few catheters were colonized with the patients' skin flora, none of the patients with positive catheter culture had a fever or was infected with the same organism at a different site.

SUMMARY

Carefully administered anesthetic care for the patient with serious chest trauma will improve his/her outcome. The anesthesiologist must ensure the patient has an adequate airway, receives adequate ventilation, and is capable of adequate gas exchange despite the traumatic alterations to pulmonary physiology. The anesthesiologist also must ensure that the patient can maintain adequate cardiac output to meet homeostatic needs despite direct injury to the myocardium or great vessels. Anesthetic drugs must be administered carefully to avoid excessive cardiovascular depression and to allow monitoring of potential neurologic damage from thoracic trauma. Finally, posttraumatic/postoperative pain relief can be maintained by continuous regional anesthesia techniques or continuous patient-controlled analgesia administration.

REFERENCES

1. Stene JK. Anesthesia for the critically ill trauma patient. In: Siegel JH, ed. Trauma: emergency surgery and critical care. New York: Churchill Livingstone, 1987:843–862.
2. Peters RM. Fluid resuscitation and oxygen exchange in hypovolemia. In: Siegel JH, ed. Trauma: emergency surgery and critical care. New York: Churchill Livingstone, 1987:157–179.
3. Ullman DA, Fortune JB, Greenhouse BB, Wimpy RE, Kennedy TM. The treatment of patients with multiple rib fractures using continuous thoracic epidural narcotic infusion. Reg Anaesth 1989;14:43–47.
4. Snider MT, Campbell DB, Kofke WA, High KM, Russell GB, Keamy MF, Williams DR. Venovenous perfusion of adults and children with severe acute respiratory distress syndrome. Trans Am Soc Artif Intern Organs 1988;34:1014–1020.
5. Craven KD, Oppenheimer L, Wood LDH. Effects of contusion and flail chest on pulmonary perfusion and oxygen exchange. J Appl Physiol 1979;47:729–737.
6. Eger EI II. Anesthetic uptake and action. Baltimore: Williams & Wilkins, 1974.
7. Grenning R, Kynette A, Hodes PJ. Unusual pulmonary changes secondary to chest trauma. AJR 1957;77:1059–1065.
8. Cochlin DL, Shaw MRP. Traumatic lung cysts following minor blunt chest trauma. Clin Radiol 1978;29:151–154.
9. Graham JM, Beall AC Jr, Mattox KL, Vaughan GD. Systemic air embolism following penetrating trauma to the lung. Chest 1977;72:449–454.
10. Avery EE, Morch ET, Benson DW. Critically crushed chests: a new method of treatment with continuous mechanical hyperventilation to produce alkalotic apnea and internal pneumatic stabilization. J Thorac Surg 1956;32:291–311.
11. Abouhatem R, Hendrickx P, Titeca M. Thoracic epidural analgesia in the treatment of rib fractures. Acta Anaesthesiol Belg 1984;35 (suppl):271–275.
12. Rankin APN, Comber REH. Management of fifty cases of chest injury with a regimen of epidural bupivacaine and morphine. Anaesth Intensive Care 1984;12:311–314.
13. Worthley LIG. Thoracic epidural in the management of chest trauma. Intensive Care Med 1985;11:312–315.
14. Getz BS, Davies E. Steinberg SM, Beaver BL, Koenig FA. Blunt cardiac trauma resulting in right atrial rupture. JAMA 1986;255:761–763.
15. Sutherland GR, Calvin JE, Driedger AA, Holliday RL, Sibbald WJ. Anatomic and cardiopulmonary responses to trauma with associated blunt chest injury. J Trauma 1981;21:1–12.
16. Saunders CR, Doty DB. Myocardial contusion. Surg Gynecol Obstet 1977;144:595–603.
17. Dolara A, Morando P, Pampaloni M. Electrocardiographic findings in 98 consecutive non-penetrating chest injuries. Dis Chest 1967;52:50–56.
18. Doty DB, Anderson AE, Rose EF, Go RT, Chiu CL, Ehrenhaft JL. Cardiac trauma: clinical and experimental correlations of myocardial contusion. Ann Surg 1974;180:452–460.

19. Brantigan CO, Burdick D, Hopeman AR, Eiseman B. Evaluation of technetium scanning for myocardial contusion. J Trauma 1978;18:460–463.
20. Lake CL. Anesthesia and pericardial disease. Anesth Analg 1983;62:431–443.
21. Hollier LH. Protecting the brain and spinal cord. J Vasc Surg 1987;5:524–528.
22. Eisele JH. Cardiovascular effects of nitrous oxide. In: Eger EI II, ed. Nitrous oxide/N_2O. New York: Elsevier, 1985:125–156.
23. Hankeln K, Radel C, Beez M, Przemislaw L, Bohmert F. Comparison of hydroxyethyl starch and lactated Ringer's solution on hemodynamics and oxygen transport of critically ill patients in prospective crossover studies. Crit Care Med 1989;17:133–135.
24. Schott U, Lindbom LO, Sjostrand U. Hemodynamic effects of colloid concentration in experimental hemorrhage: a comparison of Ringer's acetate 3% dextran-60, and 6% dextran-70. Crit Care Med 1988;16:346–352.
25. DeCamp MM, Demling RH. Posttraumatic multisystem organ failure. JAMA 1988;260:530–534.
26. Olsson GL, Leddo CC, Wild L. Nursing management of patients receiving epidural narcotics. Heart Lung 1989;18:130–137.
27. Etches RC, Sandler AN, Daley MD. Respiratory depression and spinal opioids. Can J Anaesth 1989;36:165–185.
28. Murphy DF. Intercostal nerve blockage for fractured ribs and postoperative analgesia. Reg Anaesth 1983;8:151–153.
29. Reiestad F, Stromskag KE, Holmqvist E. Intrapleural administration of bupivacaine in postoperative management of pain. Anesthesiology 1986;65:A204.
30. Harmer M, Rosen M, Vickers MD. Patient-controlled analgesia. Oxford: Blackwell Scientific Publications, 1985.

6 Critical Care of Chest Trauma

Charles E. Wiles III, MD

Mikulicz invented scientific critical care for chest surgery when, in 1903, he sent Ferdinand Sauerbruch to the laboratory to discover a way to safely enter the thoracic cavity (1). Since then, some of the greatest challenges to intensivists and anesthesiologists have been posed by the difficulties of surgery in a negative-pressure environment. Many of the solutions to these problems, such as positive-pressure ventilation (PPV), are practical measures that are the complete antithesis of normal physiology.

The art of critical care in chest surgery and chest trauma involves the balance between normal human physiology and the demands of injury and illness. All of the sophisticated paraphernalia of intensive care have their own problems and complications that must be minimized or controlled to effect a positive patient outcome. This chapter reviews the general principles of critical care as applied to chest trauma, addresses the special problems presented by specific chest injuries, and considers the complications of chest injury.

CRITICAL CARE GOALS

As a general rule, the sooner support systems can safely be removed from a patient with chest injury, the better that patient's prognosis. The intensivist's role is to determine when support systems are needed and when they can be safely removed. Successful critical care in this scenario encompasses four specific goals: optimal cardiac performance, optimal lung function, prevention/treatment of infection, and limitation of damage to other organ systems.

Optimize Cardiac Performance

Successful critical care is a balancing act in which effects, positive or negative, on one organ system must be evaluated in terms of the rest of the patient. Cardiac performance is a central concern because all organ systems require oxygen for normal aerobic function and oxygen delivery requires appropriate cardiac function (2). Furthermore, deficiencies in oxygen uptake from pulmonary failure or failure of oxygen extraction in advanced sepsis may, to a certain extent, be ameliorated by extraordinary cardiovascular output and oxygen-carrying capacity. Cardiac injury, on the other hand, may require special support, such as arrhythmia control or intraaortic counterpulsation, to achieve minimal satisfactory oxygen delivery.

The techniques of cardiac optimization are fairly straightforward (2, 3). Hemodynamically significant arrhythmias must be corrected with cardioversion or drugs as appropriate. Although major conduction disturbances may require a mechanical pacemaker, many simple arrhythmias may require only oxygen or electrolyte (K^+) correction to return the patient to normal sinus rhythm. Patients with ischemic myocardial injury may benefit from prophylactic lidocaine or other drugs. Trauma patients with cardiac disease prior to injury will generally require their usual cardiac medications.

The oxygen-carrying capacity of the blood must be evaluated:

$$CaO_2 = (Hb \times 1.39 \times SaO_2) + (0.0031 \times PaO_2)$$
$$C\bar{v}O_2 = (Hb \times 1.39 \times S\bar{v}O_2) + (0.0031 \times P\bar{v}O_2)$$

where CaO_2 = arterial oxygen content, Hb = hemoglobin, SaO_2 = arterial oxygen saturation, PaO_2 = arterial oxygen tension, $C\bar{v}O_2$ = mixed venous oxygen content, $S\bar{v}O_2$ = mixed venous oxygen saturation, and $P\bar{v}O_2$ = mixed venous oxygen tension.

Hemoglobin is the essential element. How much hemoglobin is desirable for ideal oxygen transport? How much "sludging" of capillary beds will excessive hemoconcentration produce? There are no definite answers. A hemoglobin of 11 to 12 g is felt by many to produce optimal oxygen-carrying capacity with acceptable rheologic effects. The need for hemoglobin must be weighed carefully against the risks of transfusion (acquired immune deficiency syndrome, hepatitis, cytomegalic inclusion virus, etc.) and against an individual patient's ability to compensate for suboptimal oxygen-carrying capacity (anemia). Older patients require more hemoglobin than younger ones as a general rule.

Factors that adversely affect oxyhemoglobin dissociation, such as alkalosis, must also be corrected, and competitive inhibitors of hemoglobin oxygenation, such as methemoglobin, must be eliminated.

The next step in cardiac performance optimization is volume loading. Adequate intravascular volume is particularly important for right ventricular performance. Some measure of cardiac filling is necessary to evaluate cardiac preload. The central venous pressure may be used as a rough approximation, but the pulmonary capillary occlusive or wedge pressure is thought to be a better indicator, especially for the left ventricle. Complicated patients with multiple system dysfunction may require more direct measurements of intravascular volume (4). A quick practical method of ensuring adequate preload is to administer a volume of crystalloid or colloid solution as a rapid challenge until a sustained rise in filling pressure(s) is produced. For example, 500 ml of colloid solution is administered rapidly. The fluid challenge is repeated 5 min later, unless a 5-torr rise in pulmonary capillary occlusion or wedge pressure has been noted.

The heart's efficiency in circulating blood also depends on the resistance against which it must pump; this relationship may be expressed as the systemic vascular resistance, the total peripheral resistance, or an index related to the patient's size (e.g., systemic vascular resistance index). Excessive vasoconstriction may produce some degree of myocardial compromise. Once adequate volume and oxygen-carrying capacity (Hb) have been determined, it is frequently desirable to reduce cardiac afterload to some optimal level (e.g., 1000 dyne sec cm^{-5}) to facilitate oxygen delivery. Short-acting drugs, such as nitroprusside or nitroglycerine delivered by continuous intravenous infusion at a rate titrated to produce the desired effect, are preferred (5).

Many patients will then need some additional inotropic support to ensure adequate oxygen delivery to the appropriate organs. As many as one-third of trauma patients will show some quantifiable depression in myocardial performance due to shock or cardiac injury despite the absence of previous cardiac disorders (6). The physiologic end-point for inotropic support is a plateau in the oxygen consumption ($\dot{V}O_2$) versus cardiac output curve (Fig. 6.1).

Of the inotropic agents available, a pure inotrope, such as dobutamine, is preferred over vasoconstrictor drugs such as dopamine (in high doses), epinephrine, or norepinephrine. Isoproterenol in very small doses (0.25–1.0 mg/min) may be added when vasodilation or bronchodilation is desired. Higher doses of isoproterenol may lead to tachyarrhythmias. Physiologically meaningful end-points for cardiac support, such as the plateau in the oxygen consumption curve illustrated in Fig. 6.1, are recommended as indices of successful cardiac resuscitation.

Optimize Lung Function

Gas exchange, i.e., oxygen uptake and carbon dioxide elimination, is the primary function of the lungs. These spongy, compliant honeycombs of alveoli are the interface between the atmosphere and the patient's bloodstream. They are delicate organs, and many of the routine procedures and practices of critical care medicine put them at risk. Chest trauma, such as lung laceration or pulmonary contusion, poses significant risks to the pulmonary system. The objective of critical care of the lungs is to ensure adequate gas exchange with minimal additional pulmonary damage.

Under ideal circumstances, patients with chest trauma require no special pulmonary support; this ideal, however, is often beyond reach. When pulmonary support is required, it should be limited to the minimal necessary support for the shortest possible time (7). Bed rest, oxygen, gas pressure, resuscitation fluid, and drugs are all potentially damaging to delicate pulmonary parenchyma. Mucus plugging the airways can lead to infection and barotrauma. The mediators of the inflammatory response may attack the lungs and produce the respiratory distress syndrome. Infection and superinfection are ever-present dangers.

Advanced pulmonary failure often requires a careful analysis of the specific pathophysiology of a particular patient's pulmonary insufficiency to devise a plan of support. Although negative-pressure ventilators based on the iron lung are still used, the

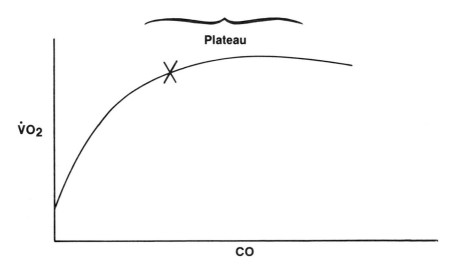

Figure 6.1.   The oxygen consumption ($\dot{V}O_2$) versus cardiac output (*CO*) curve.

current mainstay of pulmonary support is positive-pressure mechanical ventilation (PPMV).

Unless otherwise noted, mechanical ventilation is assumed to mean PPMV with some amount of positive end-expiratory pressure (PEEP).

The specific goals of mechanical ventilation are (*a*) $PaO_2 = 100$ torr, (*b*) $FIO_2 \leq 0.5$, (*c*) Qs/Qt $\leq 20\%$, and, (*d*) $PaCO_2 = 40$ torr. PEEP up to 10 cm of H_2O is usually well-tolerated and helps to reduce pulmonary shunt as well as improve oxygenation by maintaining the functional residual capacity. Higher levels of PEEP ("super PEEP") may be required to achieve minimal acceptable oxygenation and shunt, but high levels of PEEP have many cardiovascular side effects and may imperil other organs (8, 9). Inotropic and volume support of the cardiovascular system can compensate for some of the cardiovascular compromise caused by PEEP (4).

Ventilation is a function of the minute volume (tidal volume × respiratory rate). The $PaCO_2$ generally reflects the adequacy of the minute volume. Hypermetabolic patients sometimes require a large minute volume for CO_2 control. Head-injured patients may require hyperventilation ($PaCO_2$, 25–30 torr) to control cerebral edema. Controlled mechanical ventilation (CMV) usually provides a relatively high tidal volume (10–15 ml/kg) at a slow rate (10–12 breaths/min) to achieve a normal $PaCO_2$ of 40 torr. High airway pressure, reflecting increased lung stiffness, may be encountered in the adult respiratory distress syndrome, pulmonary fibrosis, and other conditions. High pressure is thought to be responsible for barotrauma to the lungs. Reducing tidal volumes and increasing respiratory rate can help to reduce airway pressures, as can altering the inspiratory/expiratory time. Changing the pattern of inflation from square wave to an up slope may also permit better ventilation at lower pressures (10). The use of high-frequency ventilation (HFV) alone or in combination with CMV may improve oxygenation, ventilation, or both in some cases of advanced pulmonary failure (see below under "Current Modalities").

Prevent/Treat Infection

Infection is an ever-present hazard and a major complication in chest trauma. Foreign bodies, such as endotracheal, tracheostomy, and thoracostomy tubes, may place the patient at risk to bacteria by bypassing the body's normal defenses. Mechanical ventilators can become contaminated and introduce bacteria into the airway line.

Damaged or dead tissue (pulmonary contusion) and undrained blood (hemothorax) provide ideal media for bacterial growth. Meticulous sterile technique and timely removal of support systems help minimize the risk of infection (11).

Limit Damage

One of the trade secrets in the critical care of patients with chest trauma is to limit damage to thoracic and extrathoracic organs caused by therapeutic devices and procedures. Patients with pulmonary resections or lacerations benefit from early weaning from PPV support so as to protect, as much as possible, resection stumps and damaged pulmonary parenchyma. Control of blood pressure is a major concern in patients with aortic anastomoses. High thoracic pressures from PEEP may be transmitted through the vena cava and impair perfusion of the liver, kidneys, and bowel, leading to impaired function of those organs (8, 9).

Other measures that contribute to limiting damage to chest trauma patients include the particular management of extrathoracic injuries. Orthopedic management is of particular importance. Early rigid stabilization of long-bone and pelvic fractures permits early mobilization and avoids the inevitable consequences of the enforced supine position such as atelectasis, pneumonia, venous thrombosis, and pulmonary embolism (12–14).

MAJOR INJURIES
Heart

Cardiac contusion is the primary blunt cardiac injury. Most myocardial contusions are benign. From a critical care perspective, arrhythmia monitoring and suppression (if needed) are the major concerns. A few patients with myocardial contusion develop hemodynamic instability requiring cardiac resuscitation as outlined above (15, 16).

Rupture of cardiac valves or papillary muscles must be considered when patients with blunt or penetrating chest trauma experience precipitous heart failure. Cardiac murmurs and typical pulmonary artery pressure tracings are clues to diagnosis. Emergency valve replacement may be lifesaving. These injuries are very rare (17). Echocardiography is the diagnostic method of choice, although cardiac catheterization may also be considered.

Patients with penetrating cardiac wounds are fairly common in urban trauma centers. Wounds inflicted by firearms tend to be rapidly fatal because the patient bleeds out rapidly, whereas those inflicted by sharp instruments often present with the signs of pericardial tamponade. Postoperative complications of penetrating cardiac wounds include arrhythmias, pericardial tamponade, and the postpericardiotomy syndrome, which may progress to restrictive pericarditis (18, 19).

The postpericardiotomy syndrome is characterized by fever, leukocytosis, and electroencephalographic evidence of pericardial inflammation. A pericardial rub can sometimes be heard. Young patients seem to be particularly at risk. Nonsteroidal antiinflammatory drugs are the treatment of choice.

Lungs

From a critical care viewpoint, pulmonary injuries can be characterized by the presence or absence of an air leak (see Chapters 9 and 10 for a comprehensive description of lung and tracheobronchial injuries). Mechanical ventilation may aggravate or perpetuate the air leak. High priority must therefore be given to reducing airway pressures and PEEP to allow closure of the airway injury.

Complex arrangements involving ventilation-triggered valves and chest tubes have been reported. I have had minimal success and some aggravation with those devices. HFV has been particularly successful in managing bronchopleural fistulas. Major leaks may require surgical repair, although a new technique using fibrin glue injected through an occluding catheter passed via a bronchoscope has been recently described (20).

Patients without leaking airways pose other problems. A pulmonary contusion, for example, is characterized by blood in the alveolar and interstitial spaces. Not only may gas exchange be compromised, but necrotic material and pooled blood provide an optimum culture medium for bacterial growth and infection (21).

Diaphragm

Rupture of the diaphragm may present late in a patient's course. PPV to the thorax may prevent abdominal viscera from passing into the chest despite the presence of a diaphragmatic injury. Normal negative-pressure breathing restored when the ventilator is terminated may provoke herniation of the abdominal contents, thereby producing respiratory decompensation. Chest roentgenograms are often useful under these circumstances. More subtle diaphragmatic injuries may be recognized using magnetic resonance imaging or ultrasonography (22–24).

Esophagus

Delayed recognition of an esophageal injury may have disastrous consequences. The patient will present with sepsis due to mediastinitis. Surgical drainage is required and primary repair of the contaminated esophageal field is unwise. The diagnosis of esophageal perforation can be made using contrast radiography or flexible fiberoptic esophagoscopy. A combination of flexible fiberoptic esophagoscopy with contrast esophagography may produce the most accurate evaluation of the injured esophagus. To avoid late sepsis, particular attention should be paid to a thorough early evaluation of patients at risk for esophageal injury (25, 26).

COMMON COMPLICATIONS
Atelectasis

Atelectasis is one of the most common complications after abdominal or chest surgery. Collapse of the lung may represent either a few alveoli (microatelectasis), a segment of the lung (segmental atelectasis, plate-like atelectasis), a major anatomic division of the lung, or an entire lobe. Occasionally, the entire lung itself may become atelectatic. The collapse of any airspace, whether it be a few alveoli or an entire lung, predisposes the patient to infection from retained secretion and bacterial colonization. Left uncorrected for a relatively short time, atelectasis can lead to permanent loss of gas-exchange surfaces in the atelectatic area.

Prevention is the best means of dealing with atelectasis; deep breathing and coughing will maintain patent airways. Once atelectasis has developed, coughing and deep breathing will in some cases reexpand the airway, but nasotracheal or endotracheal suctioning may be required. Use of an incentive spirometer may have some therapeutic or prophylactic effect as well. Chest physical therapy, including positioning, percussion, and vibration, is often useful in mobilizing secretions and maintaining or opening airways. Dramatic effects have been seen with chest physical therapy and atelectatic segments (27). Bronchoscopy using the fiberoptic flexible bronchoscope may be required to reexpand atelectatic segments of the lung.

Pneumonia

One of the most serious complications after chest trauma is the development of pneumonia. In the trauma patient, pneumonia tends to be bacterial in nature and involve relatively commonly encountered bacteria. Compromised patients and patients who have been hospitalized for a long period may develop pneumonia with exotic organisms such as resistant Gram-negative bacteria and viruses.

The diagnosis of pneumonia depends on the appearance of an infiltrate on chest x-ray, sputum containing white blood cells and organisms (in the case of a bacterial pneumonia), and signs of a systemic infection, such as fever and leukocytosis. This institution requires that, since atelectasis may often be confused with pneumonia on roentgenogram, the x-ray must show persistent infiltrate after vigorous chest physical therapy to be diagnostic for pneumonia.

The mainstays of treatment for bacterial pneumonia include chest physical therapy, dependent drainage of the infected lung segments, and the application of specific antibiotic therapy. In the absence of definitive culture results, empiric therapy may be instituted using a selection of broad-spectrum antibiotics based on analysis of the Gram's smear of the sputum.

Early appropriate termination of ventilator support may be useful in preventing the development of nosocomial pneumonias. Rigorous evaluation of antibiotics for any purpose in the trauma patient may limit the development of resistant pneumonias. Resistant Gram-negative organisms are associated with a very high mortality in patients who develop these resistant pneumonias (7, 11).

Pneumothorax

Whether associated with an iatrogenic complication or with injury, pneumothorax is a very frequently encountered complication in the trauma critical care unit. Careful attention to technical detail and positioning for the placement of subclavian and other central intravenous lines may prevent the development of some pnuemothoraces, but this complication is unavoidable in many patients due to distorted anatomy, venous thrombosis, hyperinflated lungs, and other unanticipated causes. The appearance of a pneumothorax, usually found on chest x-ray but occasionally discovered on physical examination with the absence of breath sounds and hyperresonance and tympanitic percussion on the affected hemithorax, requires careful evaluation for immediate therapy. A simple pneumothorax may not be immediately life-threatening but, in a patient on PPMV, it may progress over time into tension pneumothorax. A simple pneumothorax by itself may also predispose the patient to the development of empyema in the affected chest. Tension pneumothorax, in which the air pressure within the chest cavity that collapses the lung produces hemodynamic changes in the cardiovascular system, is an acute emergency. The immediate relief of a tension pneumothorax is mandatory. The diagnosis of a tension pneumothorax is often made by the absence of breath sounds on the affected side, by the presence of hyperresonance to percussion, and particularly with deviation of the trachea away from the affected side. A needle inserted into the tension pneumothorax and vented to the atmosphere will produce immediate relief. Definitive therapy for either a simple or tension pneumothorax is accomplished with a tube thoracostomy.

Hemothorax

Hemothorax is defined as the presence of blood in the chest cavity outside the lung. Posttraumatic hemothoraces may develop from blood lost from rib fractures, from pulmonary injury, from injury to the heart and great vessels, or from other sources of hemorrhage within the chest. Enormous hemothoraces may produce a tension effect either by themselves or in combination with a pneumothorax (hemopneumothorax).

The risks associated with hemothorax include the development of an infection in blood retained in the chest cavity and the development of pulmonary fibrosis associated with the long-term presence of blood within the pleural space. Of particular concern to the intensivist and surgeon taking care of a patient with a hemothorax is ongoing hemorrhage from the chest. Beginning with the removal of the initial hemothorax, the blood shed should be measured. A significant amount of shed blood (approximately 2000–2500 ml) may signal the need for a thoracotomy to control hemorrhage. Equally important is the rate of ongoing blood loss from the chest. Blood loss in excess of 200–300 ml/hr for several hours is also considered an indication for surgical exploration of the chest (see Chapter 2 for more details).

Empyema

Infected pleural fluid is not an uncommon complication of patients with multiple trauma (28), particularly if they have sustained chest trauma. Our own hypothesis regarding the pathogenesis is that bacterias from the oropharynx are blown distally through the contused and lacerated lungs and seed the pleural cavity. Recently, with changes in the types of ventilators and improvements in oropharyngeal care, we have markedly reduced the incidence of empyema in our institution. The treatment continues to be proper antibiotic therapy, lung reexpansion, and proper drainage (see Chapter 9 for more extensive details of management).

Pneumomediastinum

Pneumomediastinum is the presence of air in the mediastinum. This condition is usually noted on chest roentgenograms and is usually benign. Under very rare circumstances, the pneumomediastinum may progress to the point of interfering with cardiovascular stability. Under these circumstances, tube decompression of the pneumomediastinum may be indicated.

Pneumopericardium

Pneumopericardium is also a rarely encountered condition. Like pneumomediastinum, it is frequently associated with some degree of barotrauma (the Macklin effect) (29). Under rare circumstances, pneumopericardium may lead to the signs and symptoms of pericardiotamponade. Relief of the pneumopericardium via a needle pericardiocentesis or a pericardial window reverses the hemodynamic effects of the tamponade (30).

Arrhythmia

Arrhythmias are relatively infrequent occurrences in the trauma patient unless there is some underlying coronary disease. The most common arrhythmia seen is sinus tachycardia. This tachycardia may indicate that the patient is hypovolemic. The treatment for hypovolemia, particularly in the trauma patient, is volume resuscitation. Other arrhythmias may be related to electrolyte imbalances, hypokalemia being a commonly encountered deficiency. Correction of the serum potassium level will remove this particular arrhythmia. Other arrhythmias may be related to the presence of monitoring devices such as the pulmonary artery catheter. These arrhythmias are usually encountered while the catheter is being placed. They frequently indicate some irritation of the ventricle and are usually easily controlled if necessary by the use of lidocaine.

Patients with head injuries may demonstrate any sort of cardiac arrhythmia, which may be due to uncoordinated central regulation. In patients with head injuries and in other trauma patients with arrhythmic disturbances, advanced life support protocols are recommended for the control of those arrhythmias that are hemodynamically significant. Arrhythmias that do not produce any hemodynamic compromise may not require definitive treatment (2).

Heart Failure

Overt cardiac failure in a trauma patient without preexisting myocardial insufficiency is relatively uncommon. Even patients who receive vigorous fluid resuscitation seldom show the classic signs of congestive heart failure. When heart failure occurs, diuresis is often effective in reducing cardiac preload and permitting efficient cardiac activity.

Subtle myocardial compromise can be detected in approximately one-fourth of all trauma patients. At least one-third of trauma patients in the geriatric category will present with measurable myocardial decompensation (6). They may not show the classic signs and symptoms of congestive heart failure, but force-velocity curves of ventricular performance will indicate occasionally substantial reductions in cardiac performance. PPMV may compound suboptimal cardiovascular performance measured in these patients (9). It is the policy of this institution to aggressively monitor cardiovascular performance in such patients and to institute myocardial support with inotropic agents (as outlined above) in any patient in whom myocardial decompensation of a significant degree is detected despite the absence of the overt classic signs of congestive heart failure. One must bear in mind that the signs of heart failure commonly associated with cardiac disease in nontrauma patients may indicate extracardiac cardiovascular events in the trauma patient. Pericardial tamponade and tension pneumothorax are two primary examples. Other tension phenomena, including tension pneumopericardium, tension hemopneumothorax, and other forms of mediastinal tamponade, may also present as "heart failure." The therapy of these problems should be directed at the underlying cause and may often require prompt intervention.

Tracheoesophageal Fistula

Tracheoesophageal (TE) fistula is a rare but devastating complication encountered in the trauma unit. It is an acquired communication between the esophagus and the trachea and may be regarded as a pressure sore or decubitus ulcer of the esophagus that has eroded into the trachea. It is usually located between the posterior wall of the trachea and the anterior wall of the esophagus at the level of the tracheostomy or endotracheal tube balloon. Inflation of the endotracheal balloon, together with a relatively rigid esophageal appliance such as a hard plastic nasogastric or oral gastric tube, is thought to produce sufficient pressure on the walls of these two structures to compromise their perfusion and to lead to the erosion. The use of high-volume, compliant, soft balloon cuffs on the tracheal tubes, together with small-caliber soft (Sylastic) transesophageal tubes, may contribute to prevention of the development of TE fistulas. The use of enterotomy tubes as gastrostomies and jejunostomies may also be helpful in appropriate patients. A TE fistula may be suspected when tube feedings appear in the tracheal suction aspirate. The diagnosis can usually be established by endoscopy of the trachea and/or esophagus. Therapy is surgical repair.

Other acquired TE fistulas may be related to undiagnosed injuries of the trachea and esophagus. Careful attention to the diagnostic work-up of patients at risk of having these problems will lead to their early recognition and prompt repair in most cases.

Tracheoinnominate Fistula

Another rare but deadly complication encountered in the trauma critical care unit is tracheoinnominate (TI) fistula. These lesions represent another erosion of the trachea, this time of the anterior surface. It is thought to be related to the tip of a tracheostomy tube or to its cuff. Low tracheostomy has been identified as a major risk factor for this condition. The tracheal erosion then progresses into the adjacent innominate artery and can produce exsanguinating hemorrhage. Bleeding from a TI fistula classically is heralded by a sentinel bleed. Although bleeding from the tracheostomy, endotracheal tube, or tracheostomy site is commonly encountered in a critical care unit, any significant bleeding must be investigated thoroughly and vigorously. The diagnosis of TI fistula is established by tracheobronchoscopy. Removal of the tracheostomy tube to inspect the area obscured by this appliance is recommended. An oral or nasal endotracheal tube may need to be placed to permit the examination.

The treatment of TI fistula is surgery; once a TI fistula is diagnosed, prompt intervention in the operating room is essential. Exsanguinating hemorrhage prior to definitive surgical control may occur. First aid for bleeding from a TI fistula includes hyperinflation of the tracheostomy balloon for tamponade. Other measures that have been recommended include removal of the tracheostomy tube and replacement with an endotracheal tube as well as digital simultaneous compression through the tracheostomy site of the innominate artery against the clavicle. Prompt direct surgical control of the innominate trunk is essential (31, 32) (see Chapter 20).

Lung Cyst

Traumatic lung cyst is a common complication. The availability of computed tomography scanning has revealed many traumatic lung cysts that would otherwise have gone undetected. These lesions represent barotrauma to the alveoli in which several alveoli break down to form a large cystic cavity. They usually do not have clinical significance unless they become infected. An infected traumatic lung cyst presents as a cystic cavity with an air fluid level. Therapy consists of antibiotics and chest physical therapy if the cyst communicates with the major airways. An infected traumatic lung cyst that does not communicate with the major airways may require percutaneous or open surgical drainage. Pulmonary resection for traumatic lung cyst is rarely required (33).

Arterial Laceration

Discussion of injuries to the vessels of the thorax encountered with original trauma is beyond the scope of this chapter; however, the arteries of the chest remain at risk in the critical care unit. An iatrogenic puncture of a thoracic artery during placement of a support device is a relatively common occurrence. The return of bright red pulsatile blood under pressure establishes the diagnosis. Treatment for this problem is removal of the needle or catheter and, if possible, direct digital compression for an appropriate length of time. Intercostal arteries may be injured during the placement of a thoracostomy tube or during thoracentesis. Removal of the needle is often sufficient. Direct compression may be effective. In the case of an intercostal artery injured during the placement of a chest tube, replacement of that tube with a large Foley catheter may be useful. The balloon (preferably 30-ml volume) is then inflated within the chest and the catheter is retracted under light traction. This maneuver may produce tamponade of a damaged intercostal artery. Occasionally, direct surgical control is required. Major hemothorax or significant hemorrhage from a chest tube may be encountered from time to time in the critical care unit; it can represent a complication or delayed bleeding from the patient's original injuries after clot lysis and retraction. Immediate evaluation is required. If the bleeding is significant (approximately 2000–2500 ml immediately or more than 200–300 ml/hr for 2–3 hr), surgical intervention may be required. Chest hemorrhage under these circumstances may be life-threatening.

Wound Infection

Infection in contaminated wounds is a common concern. Thorough surgical preparation and careful wound care will limit the development of this complication. Trauma patients, however, will continue to develop wound infections. Daily inspection of all traumatic wounds, including the thoracotomy wounds if present, should be a routine part of the critical care evaluation. Any local signs or symptoms of wound infection (rubor, calor, dolor, tumor) in the presence of such systemic signs of infections, such as fever and leukocytosis, raise the consideration of a wound infection.

Wound infections are best treated with evacuation of the infected wound in local wound care. Deep wound infections involving cartilage bone may be particularly difficult to care for. Excision of cartilage or bone may be required.

CURRENT MODALITIES AVAILABLE AT THE MIEMSS SHOCK TRAUMA CENTER
High-frequency Ventilation

HFV was developed in an effort to reduce high airway pressure in patients on mechanical ventilators and to improve cardiovascular performance in patients who require mechanical ventilation. Other indications include bronchopleural fistula, endoscopy, and the intraoperative requirement for a quiet surgical field in certain procedures (34).

Three variations of HFV have evolved: high-frequency jet ventilation, high-frequency oscillation, and combined high-frequency ventilation (CHFV). High-frequency jet ventilation is the delivery of a high number of small-volume jets of gas into the airway. High-frequency oscillation involves vibrating a continuous stream of inspired gases. CHFV superimposes pulses of HFV (50 H) on a base rate of ventilation provided by CMV (Fig. 6.2).

Borg et al. (35, 36) conducted a prospective study of CHFV at the Shock Trauma Center of the Maryland Institute for Emergency Medical Services Systems (MIEMSS) between 1983 and 1987. In a study group of 35 patients, compared with a well-matched control group (approximately 88), CHFV permitted better cardiovascular performance, better oxygen utilization, reduced pulmonary artery pressures, and improved gas exchange. There was a 23% improvement in survival. Problems encountered included humidification of the huge volume of gas involved in HFV and the problem of "auto-PEEP" encountered with HFV in the expiratory phase (37). As with any new

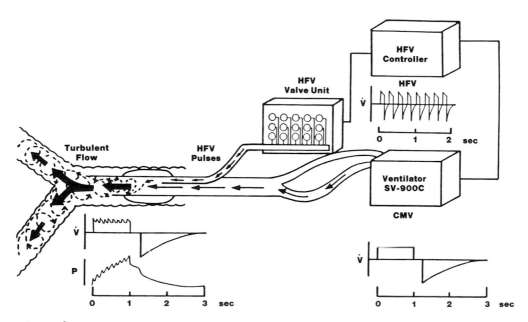

Figure 6.2.   Combined high-frequency ventilation. (From Borg UR, Stoklosa JC, Siegel JH, et al. Prospective evaluation of combined high frequency ventilation in posttrauma patients with ARDS refractory to optimized conventional ventilatory management. Crit Care Med 1989;17:1129–1142).

procedure, there is a "learning curve." Technical problems tend to decrease as personnel become familiar with new equipment.

Simultaneous Independent Lung Ventilation (SILV)

Trauma patients may have one damaged area in otherwise normal lungs. Pulmonary contusion and laceration are examples of such unilateral focal injuries. PPMV delivers the same pressures uniformly throughout both lungs. Since gases follow the path of least resistance, the higher pressures that may be required to ventilate damaged areas may put the normal pulmonary parenchyma at risk of barotrauma. Transbronchial aspiration of infected secretions from an area of lobar pneumonia may infect other areas of the lung as well.

These considerations led the MIEMSS group to pursue the concept of SILV. The original series of highly selected patients was reported by Siegel et al. (38) and Geisler et al. (39).

Alternatively, patients who might benefit from SILV may be selected on the basis of a localized unilateral process on chest roentgenogram. Once a double-lumen endotracheal tube is in place, compliance curves for each lung can be developed independently and, if a major difference is noted, SILV can be considered.

At MIEMSS, the equipment currently used includes the Bronchocath double-lumen double-cuff endotracheal tube (Fig. 6.3) and two Siemens 900C Servo mechanical ventilators. The Servo circuits permit one ventilator (master) to drive the other (slave) ventilator in a coordinated simultaneous pattern (Fig. 6.3).

The use of SILV permits the application of different tidal volumes to each lung. PEEP may be applied differently, thus minimizing its damage to the healthier lung and maximizing the benefit to the injured lung. Different patterns of ventilation such as different inspiratory/expiratory ratios can be applied to each lung. HFV can be applied selectively to one lung or the other. Problems encountered involve primarily the endotracheal tube. A double-lumen tube has two narrow channels that may hinder pulmonary toilet and bronchoscopy. Extra-long suction catheters are required. The distal (bronchial) cuff is a low-volume, low-compliance, high-pressure cuff that may damage the bronchus if left in situ for a prolonged time. The left-facing Bronchocath endotracheal tube is recommended for SILV since intubation of the right bronchus tends to obstruct the bronchus to the right upper lobe and to produce atelectasis.

The results with the initial series of patients demonstrated that, in some patients, gas exchange could be improved with SILV. Some patients who appeared to have unilateral disease on roentgenogram proved to have a bilateral process on critical evaluation. Some septic adult respiratory distress syndrome patients showed improvement in pulmonary function with SILV and positioning of the patient to optimize ventilation-perfusion relationships. Results were promising enough to lead to the initiation of a prospective randomized study of SILV applied within 24 hr of injury to patients with unilateral lung trauma. That study is currently underway.

Automated Respiratory Gas Monitoring

Multibed respiratory gas monitoring, developed over the past 19 yr, is available in four of the 12-bed intensive/critical care units in the R Adams Cowley Shock Trauma Center (40–42). Measurements made 24 hr/day are gas flow, volume, pressure, and composition (O_2, CO_2, N_2) in the airway common to inspiration and expiration (just to the patient side of the Y-piece). Breath-by-breath waveform analysis of these digitized signals

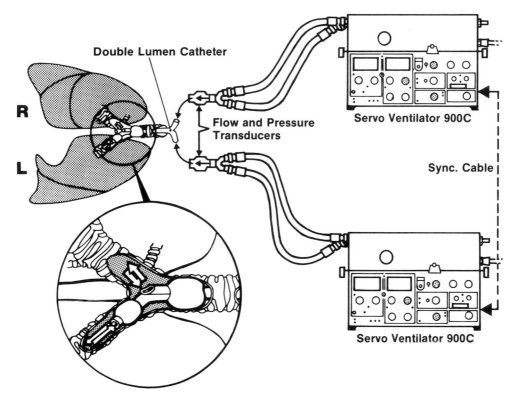

Figure 6.3. Computer-based analytic system for respiratory monitoring. (From Siegel JH, Stoklosa JC, Borg U, et al. Quantification of asymmetric lung pathophysiology as a guide to the use of simultaneous independent lung ventilation in posttraumatic and septic ARDS. Am Surg 1985;202:425–439).

permits real-time calculation of pulmonary mechanics (e.g., minute ventilation, inspired/expired volume and time ratios, pulmonary compliance, nonelastic airway resistance), alveolar gas composition (alveolar PO_2 and PCO_2), and metabolic gas exchange (oxygen consumption, carbon dioxide production, respiratory quotient, and caloric production ("indirect calorimetry")). Multibed respiratory gas monitoring data are sent directly to the MIEMSS clinical computer system for permanent storage and for immediate viewing at CRT terminals at each bedside. The data are averaged over 24 hr in the case of the metabolic parameters to give a true measure of metabolic rate for precise nutritional management decisions. For example, the 24-hr averaged caloric rate determines the total nonprotein calorie requirement, and respiratory quotient indicates the correct carbohydrate-to-fat ratio of the feeding. Pulmonary mechanics data are useful for diagnosis of pulmonary and airway problems and rapid assessment of the effects of management. Alveolar gas composition provides a measure of alveolar dead space to diagnose pulmonary emboli and to monitor alveolar PCO_2 during acute unstable periods, particularly in head-injured patients requiring precise control of CO_2 levels. Correlation of blood gas and airway gas measurements permits on-line automated calculation of cardiac output by the Fick principle, intrapulmonary shunt fraction, alveolar dead space, and oxygen delivery-to-consumption ratios.

CONCLUSIONS: OPTIMIZE AND MOBILIZE

Critical care support of patients with chest trauma is directed at supporting injured organ systems until spontaneous healing from injury or surgical repair can occur. In the process, further damage from life-support devices and procedures must be minimized by careful attention to detail. Optimization of cardiac performance can compensate for some degree of pulmonary insufficiency. Optimization of oxygenation may help an injured heart. Mobilization of secretions and blood from the tracheobronchial tube reduces the risk of secondary infection. Mobilization of the patient from the deadly enforced supine position reduces the risk of avoidable organ failures. The watch words of critical care in chest trauma patients are *optimize* and *mobilize*.

REFERENCES

1. Thorwald J. The triumph of surgery. Winston, Richard, Clara, trans. New York: Pantheon Books, 1960:365.
2. Siegel JH, Linberg SE, Wiles CE III. Hemodynamic evaluation and cardiovascular therapy of low flow shock state. In: Siegel JH, ed. Trauma: emergency surgery and critical care. New York: Churchill Livingstone, 1987:201–284.
3. McQuillen KA, Wiles CE III. Diagnosis and initial management of traumatic shock. In: Cardona VD, Hurn PD, Mason PJB, Scanlon AM, Veise-Berry SW, eds. Trauma nursing: from resuscitation through rehabilitation. Philadelphia: Saunders, 1988:106–183.
4. Siegel JH, Stoklosa JC, Borg U. Cardiorespiratory management of the adult respiratory distress syndrome. In: Siegel JH, ed. Trauma: emergency surgery and critical care. New York: Churchill Livingstone, 1987:581–613.
5. Cerra FB, Hassett J, Siegel JH. Vasodilator therapy in clinical sepsis with low output syndrome. Surg Res 1978;25:180.
6. Tacchino RM, Siegel JH, Emmanuele T, Wiles CE III, Cotter K. Incidence and therapy with myocardial depression in critically ill posttraumatic patients. Proceedings of the 43rd annual meeting of the Central Surgical Association, Chicago, 1986.
7. Seibel R, LaDuca J, Hassett J, et al. Blunt multiple trauma (ISS = 36) femur traction, and the pulmonary failure septic state. Ann Surg 1985;202:283–295.
8. Demling RH, Staub NC, Edmunds LH. Effect of end-expiratory airway pressure on accumulation of extravascular lung water. J Appl Physiol 1975;38:907–912.
9. Dorinsky PM, Whitcomb ME. The effect of PEEP on cardiac output. Chest 1983;84:210–216.
10. Tharratt RS, Allen RP, Albertson TE. Pressure controlled inverse ratio ventilation in severe adult respiratory failure. Chest 1988;94:755–762.
11. Hoyt NJ. Infection and infection control. In: Cardona VD, Hurn PD, Mason PJB, Scanlon AM, Veise-Berry SW, eds. Trauma nursing: from resuscitation through rehabilitation. Philadelphia: Saunders, 1988:224–262.
12. Bone LB, Johnson KD, Weigelt J, Scheinberg R. Early versus delayed stabilization of femoral fractures: a prospective randomized study. J Bone Joint Surg 1989;71:336–340.
13. Burgess AR, Brumback RJ. Early fracture stabilization. In: Cowley RA, Conn A, Dunham CM, eds. Trauma care: surgical management, vol I. Philadelphia: Lippincott, 1987:182–203.
14. Brumback RJ, Bosse MJ, Poka A, Burgess AR. Intramedullary stabilization of humeral shaft fractures in patients with multiple trauma. J Bone Joint Surg (Am) 1986;68:960–970.
15. Shorr RM, Crittenden M, Indeck M, Hartunian SL, Rodriguez A. Blunt thoracic trauma: analysis of 515 patients. Ann Surg 1989;206:200–205.
16. Soutter DI, Rodriguez A. Cardiac contusion: diagnosis and management. Trauma Q 1988;4:6–15.
17. Munim A, Chodoff P. Traumatic acute mutual regurgitation secondary to blunt chest trauma. Crit Care Med 1983;1:311.
18. Leonard DJ, Gens DR. Diagnosis of cardiac injury: pericardiocentesis versus diagnostic pericardial window. Trauma Q 1988;4:29–33.
19. Phillips T, Rodriguez A, Cowley RA. Right ventricular outflow obstruction secondary to right-sided tamponade following myocardial trauma. Ann Thorac Surg 1983;36:353–358.
20. Regel G, Sturm JA, Neumann C, Schueler S, Tscherne H. Occlusion of bronchopleural fistula after lung injury—a new treatment by bronchoscopy. J Trauma 1989;29:223–226.
21. Shin B. Lung contusion. In: Cowley RA, Conn A, Dunham CM, eds. Trauma care: medical management, vol II. Philadelphia: Lippincott, 1987:71–97.

22. Rodriguez-Morales G, Rodriguez A, Shatney CH. Acute rupture of the diaphragm in blunt trauma: analysis of 60 patients. J Trauma 1986;26:438–444.
23. Ammann AM, Brewer WH, Maull KI, et al. Traumatic rupture of the diaphragm: real time sonographic diagnosis. AJR 1983;140:915–916.
24. Mirvis SE, Keramati B, Buckman R, et al. MR imaging of traumatic diaphragmatic rupture. J Comput Assist Tomogr 1988;12:147–149.
25. Brotman S, Shatney CH, Cowley RA. False negative peritoneal lavage. Am Surg 1981;47:309–310.
26. Reddin A, Mirvis SE, Diaconis JN. Rupture of the cervical esophagus and trachea associated with cervical spine fracture. J Trauma 1987;27:564–566.
27. Imle PC, Mars MP, Eppinghaus CD, Anderson P, Ciesla ND. Effect of chest physiotherapy positioning on intracranial and cerebral perfusion pressure (Abstract). Crit Care Med 1988;16:382.
28. Caplan ES, Hoyt NJ, Rodriguez A, Cowley RA. Empyema occurring in the multiply traumatized patient. J Trauma 1984;24:785–789.
29. Macklin MT, Macklin CC. Malignant interstitial emphysema of the lungs and mediastinum as an important occult complication in many respiratory diseases and other conditions: an interpretation of the clinical literature in the light of laboratory equipment. Medicine 1944;23:281–358.
30. Shorr RM, Mirvis SE, Indeck MC. Tension pneumopericardium in blunt chest trauma. J Trauma 1987;27:1078–1082.
31. Boyd AD. Tracheostomy and cricothyroidotomy. In: Worth ME Jr, ed. Principles and practice of trauma care. Baltimore: Williams & Wilkins, 1982:32–39.
32. Courcy PA, Rodriguez A, Garrett HE. Operative technique for repair of tracheoinnominate artery fistula. J Vasc Surg 1985;2:332–334.
33. Dunne M, Rodriguez A, Brotman S. Traumatic lung cyst. Contemp Surg 1983;23:51.
34. Holzapfel L, Robert D, Perrin F, Gaussorgues P, Giudicelli DP. Comparison of high-frequency jet ventilation to conventional ventilation in adults with respiratory distress syndrome. Intensive Care Med 1987;13:100–105.
35. Borg UR, Stoklosa JC, Siegel JH, Wiles CE III, Belzberg H, Blevins S, Cotter K, Laghi F, Rivkind A. Prospective evaluation of combined high frequency ventilation in posttrauma patients with ARDS refractory to optimized conventional ventilatory management. Crit Care Med 1989;17:1129–1142.
36. Borg U, Belzberg H, Blevins S. Combined high frequency ventilation. Acta Anaesthesiol Scand 1989;33(suppl 90):155.
37. Benson MS, Pierson DJ. Auto-PEEP during mechanical ventilation of adults. Respir Care 1988;33:557–568.
38. Siegel JH, Stoklosa JC, Borg U, Wiles CE III, Sganga G, Geisler FH, Belzberg H, Wedel S, Goh K. Quantification of asymmetric lung pathophysiology as a guide to the use of simultaneous independent lung ventilation in posttraumatic and septic ARDS. Am Surg 1985;202:425–435.
39. Geisler FH, Siegel JH, Stoklosa JC, Borg U, Kung Y, Goh K, Wiles CE III, Belzberg H, Wedel S. Computer-based optimization of abnormal respiratory physiology in the critically ill trauma patient (Abstract). J Trauma 1984;24:659.
40. Turney SZ. Computerized multibed respiratory monitoring. In: Nair S, ed. Computers in critical care and pulmonary medicine, vol 3. New York: Plenum Publishing, 1983:9–25.
41. Fraser RB, Turney SZ. New method of respiratory gas analysis: light spectrometer. J Appl Physiol 1985;59:1001–1007.
42. Turney SZ. Respiratory monitoring. In: Applefeld JJ, Linberg SE, eds. Acute respiratory care. Boston: Blackwell Scientific Publications, 1988:107–134.

7 Infection in Thoracic Trauma

Steven Gitterman, MD, PhD
Ellis Caplan, MD

In trauma patients who survive the immediate postinjury phase, infectious complications are among the leading causes of death. Both lung and thoracic cage injury following thoracic trauma predispose the patient to pneumonia, the most common cause of infectious mortality in trauma patients. In this chapter, we emphasize the prevention and early recognition of infection as the primary means of reducing morbidity in the trauma patient. Although our initial focus is the care of the patient after thoracic trauma, the subsequent principles discussed represent our general approach to all critically injured patients.

OVERVIEW

The thoracic cavity can be conceptualized as a series of three anatomically separate spaces (pleural, parenchymal, and pericardial) with the esophagus traversing posteriorly. Microbiologic contamination and subsequent infection of these normally sterile areas can occur by four routes: (*a*) aspiration of material via direct continuity with the oropharynx (e.g., aspiration pneumonia or inhalation of organisms); (*b*) violation by direct injury, either by trauma itself or by iatrogenic manipulation such as chest tube insertion; (*c*) concomitant injury of a hollow viscus with contamination of the thoracic cavity by the endogenous gastrointestinal flora; and (*d*) hematogenous dissemination of bacteria from a nonthoracic source. Each of these potential mechanisms for bacterial invasion (which may exist simultaneously) requires a different approach to prophylaxis and therapy.

In contrast to abdominal trauma associated with intestinal spillage, contamination occurring in isolated penetrating thoracic injury usually involves inoculation of skin flora of low virulence; because of this, infection at the site of penetrating thoracic trauma is uncommon (1). It is the invasive aspects of modern critical care support that pose the greatest infectious risks after thoracic trauma. Our experience at the Shock Trauma Center of the Maryland Institute for Emergency Medical Services Systems (MIEMSS) has led us to the impression that infections following thoracic injury are similar to those that occur in most trauma patients. This does not ignore the importance of the nature of the injury in considering infectious sources but rather emphasizes that the most common sites of infection following trauma (respiratory tract, urinary tract, intravascular lines) are similar in all critically ill patients. We therefore apply the same principles to patients with thoracic trauma that we apply to all patients admitted to our center: identification of those at higher risk of infection, regular and continual laboratory surveillance of all patients, and careful assessment of patients' ongoing recovery.

Due to the unique mechanical and anatomic aspects of the thorax, infections after thoracic injury have been considered separately in several studies of trauma patients; similarly, the infectious risk for patients undergoing elective pulmonary surgery has also been the subject of separate investigations. Because we believe that the treatment of the major infectious complications of trauma is similar in all severely ill patients, we have deferred discussion of infections common after thoracic trauma to the section on general care of the patient. However, because of controversies regarding appropriate antibiotic prophylaxis (rather than treatment) in the setting of thoracic injury, we will discuss this area extensively under the heading "Infectious Issues Specific to Thoracic Trauma."

INFECTIOUS ISSUES SPECIFIC TO THORACIC TRAUMA

Antibiotic treatment for infections in the thorax has been less controversial than the use of antibiotics to prevent infection after thoracic injury. In the former, general principles of appropriate antimicrobial coverage with adequate surgical drainage and debridement apply. Although the need for open versus closed drainage is still evolving for certain specific entities (e.g., mediastinitis), therapeutic options exist for almost all specific pathogens that cause infection in the thorax. For empiric therapy, reasonable choices for broad-spectrum coverage can almost always be made.

The appropriate use of antibiotics for the prevention of infection in the thorax is less clear. Although a consensus strongly favoring prophylactic antibiotic use in surgery has arisen (3,4), these are primarily situations wherein the use of perioperative antibiotics has been shown to be effective in preventing postoperative wound infections (5). Prophylactic antibiotics have also been recommended for thoracic trauma, but in this setting they have been advocated as prophylaxis against pneumonia and empyema, as well as wound infections. Mechanical factors limiting thoracic expansion, the almost universal placement of thoracostomy tubes, and the frequent need for endotracheal intubation have all been cited as factors that place the patient with chest injury at particularly high risk of pulmonary infection and therefore justify liberal antibiotic prophylaxis. Unfortunately, only a small number of controlled studies have critically examined this issue, often with small sample sizes and different outcome criteria; not surprisingly, divergent conclusions about the need for prophylaxis have been reached. A summary of recent experimental trials examining this issue is presented in Table 7.1; each of these studies is discussed further under specific subsections below.

Wound Infection

In penetrating thoracic injury, the initial risk of wound infection in the absence of gross contamination is from direct inoculation of skin flora, primarily staphylococcal species (*S. aureus* and *S. epidermidis*). Infection at the primary site of injury is unusual with adequate debridement. The greater risk of "wound" infection after thoracic trauma is at the site of surgical intervention, either from operative intervention or from thoracostomy tube placement. Antibiotics administered after trauma or following emergency surgical intervention should be considered as treatment, rather than as prophylaxis, and should be continued for longer than a single dose. The decision to administer antibiotics after emergency intervention or after penetrating trauma should be considered on an individual basis but should rarely be necessary in the latter case.

In many trauma situations the opportunity to administer prophylactic antibiotics before surgery exists. The utility of prophylaxis to prevent wound infections in this setting (i.e., infections at the site of surgical incision) has been studied extensively in patients undergoing elective pulmonary surgery. Truesdale et al. (6) found no wound infections in 57 patients undergoing elective pulmonary surgery (28 receiving a first-generation cephalosporin and 29 randomized to placebo) and carefully documented a high incidence of adverse reactions to cephalosporin administration. Cameron et al. (7) found no efficacy for perioperative cephalothin in 171 patients randomized to antibiotic or placebo prior to elective pulmonary resection; however, the subsequent incidence of other infections with cephalothin-resistant Gram-negative bacilli was higher in the antibiotic-treated group.

Other investigators have obtained results favoring prophylactic antibiotic use before elective pulmonary surgery. Ilves et al. (8) described a statistically significant decrease in both "deep" and "superficial" wound infections with perioperative cepahlothin prophylaxis (7/118 treated patients versus 22/93 controls) in patients undergoing elective pulmonary procedures (although a high percentage of the complications were seen in surgical procedures with concomitant gastrointestinal tract involvement). Kvale et al. (9) noted two major wound abscesses in 34 placebo-treated patients versus none in 43 patients treated with a first-generation cephalosporin for 5 days. A prospective study by Frimodt-Moller et al. (10) also showed a decreased rate of wound infection with "prophylactic" antibiotic use (penicillin). In a noncontrolled, retrospective analysis, Bryant et al. (11) described a reduction in wound infection incidence from 18.4 to 4.8% after institution of a systemic prophylactic regimen with cephalothin. Each of these studies used prolonged administration of antibiotics; in contrast, Tarkka et al. (12) found no difference in the number of wound infections in patients undergoing elective pulmonary surgery when comparing doxycycline for 5 days with a single perioperative dose of cefuroxime. As an alternative strategy using "local" prophylaxis, Walker et al. (13) noted a reduction from a postoperative wound infection rate of 20% in elective pulmonary surgery to 2% following the instillation of cefuroxime at the thoracic incision site.

The results of the few studies of prophylactic antibiotic use in thoracic trauma are similarly contradictory. In a randomized study examining wound infection rates after chest tube placement for penetrating thoracic trauma, Mandal et al. (1) observed no wound infections in 80 patients randomized to either continuous doxycycline or a placebo control. In a trial comparing continuous cephapirin versus placebo, LeBlanc and Tucker (14) also concluded that antibiotics were not efficacious in the setting of penetrating trauma. LoCurto et al. (15) arrived at the opposite conclusion, finding significant benefit for prophylactic coverage for wound infections after tube thoracostomy for trauma.

Although not involving direct penetration of the thoracic cavity, a recent large multicenter study (15a) found a statistically significant decrease in the incidence of wound infections at the site of elective breast surgery with use of prophylactic cefonicid (a cephalosporin antibiotic with activity similar to that of cefazolin but with a longer half-life and slightly less antistaphylococcal activity). Twenty-six of 303 patients randomized to placebo had a definite or probable wound infection versus 17 of 303 randomized to cefonicid. In both groups, the incidence of readmission for wound complications (7 antibiotic and 11 placebo patients) and the incidence of incision and drainage of the wound (5 placebo and 7 antibiotic patients) was low.

The discrepancy of published results and the low incidence of wound infection make questionable any categorical statement of the utility of antibiotics in preventing

Table 7.1.
Antibiotic Therapy in Noncardiac Thoracic Surgery[a]

Reference	Surgery	Study Design	Antibiotic	Outcome	Conclusion
Truesdale et al. (6)	Lung carcinoma resection	Prospective, double-blind	First-generation cephalosporin × 48 hr versus placebo	5/29 infections in prophylaxis group versus 5/28 in placebo group. 8 infections were pneumonia (4 in each group). No benefit was seen for secondary parameters (e.g., length of stay).	"We conclude that a short course of cephalosporin prophylaxis is not more effective than placebo in preventing infections following noncardiac thoracic surgery."
Cameron et al. (7)	Elective pulmonary resection or surgery	Prospective, double-blind	First-generation cephalosporin beginning night before surgery and until 6 hr postop. Pleural space and wound were irrigated with antibiotic solution.	22 septic complications (16 patients) in 88 subjects receiving prophylaxis versus 26 (23 patients) in 83 placebo subjects. Gram-negative more common in prophylaxis, Gram-positive (*S. aureus*) in placebo.	"... it is our recommendation that patients undergoing pulmonary resection should not receive parenteral, prophylactic antibiotics."
Ilves et al. (8)	"Thoracotomy," primarily for lung cancer resection	Prospective, double-blind	First-generation antibiotic immediately pre-op and 4 hr after surgery	27 infections in 118 patients receiving antibiotic versus 42 in 83 patients receiving placebo. No increase in Gram-negative infections. Antibiotics reduced wound, pulmonary, and pleural infections.	"Our policy is to routinely employ prophylactic perioperative antibiotic coverage in clean contaminated major thoracic cases."

Study	Population	Design	Regimen	Results	Conclusion
Kvale et al.(9)	Elective thoracotomies with pulmonary resection	Prospective, double-blind	First-generation cephalosporin for 5 days	17 infections in 34 placebo patients versus 8 infections in 43 antibiotic-treated patients. 14 thoracic infections (pneumonia, bronchitis, empyema, wound abscess) in placebo versus 2 in prophylaxis group.	"We believe that the evidence gathered in this prospective controlled series gives strong support for the value of antibiotics in pulmonary resections."
Frimodt-Moller et al. (10)	Elective pulmonary resections	Prospective, double-blind	Penicillin G pre-op and for 1 day postoperatively	32 infections in 28/47 placebo patients versus 19 infections in 17/45 patients receiving antibiotics. Wound infection (9 in placebo, 2 in antibiotic group) accounted for differences.	"...our study demonstrated a significant effect of high-dose, short-term penicillin prophylaxis in pulmonary surgery...."
Bryant et al. (11)	Noncardiac thoracic surgery	Retrospective and prospective	First-generation cephalosporin for 5 days	14/76 patients with infection (6 empyema, 8 wound infections) in the year before prophylaxis; 4/84 patients (2 empyema, 2 wound infection) in the year after prophylaxis started.	Results "eliminated an intolerable rate of postoperative wound infections" but "we make no claim that this study documents a lower postoperative infection rate than might be achieved without antibiotics under other circumstances."

Table 7.1.
Antibiotic Therapy in Noncardiac Thoracic Surgery (Continued)[a]

Reference	Surgery	Study Design	Antibiotic	Outcome	Conclusion
Mandal et al. (1)	Chest tube insertion after penetrating chest trauma	Randomized, prospective study	Doxycycline at the time of surgery and continued until chest tube removal versus placebo	0/40 infections in the antibiotic group versus 1/40 (empyema) in control group	"Neither our retrospective study nor the present prospective study justifies the routine administration of antibiotic prophylaxis for knife or gunshot wounds of the chest in the patient population studied."
LeBlanc and Tucker (14)	Chest tube insertion (primarily after trauma)	Randomized, prospective study	First-generation cephalosporin until chest tube removal versus placebo	2/39 infections in patients receiving antibiotics, 10/46 in control group. 1 pneumonia in each group and 1 empyema in controls. Difference largely due to wound infections.	". . . our results failed to demonstrate the need for antibiotic prophylaxis. Technical problems have been identified as the cause of the largest number of infections."
Grover et al. (19)	Penetrating chest trauma	Randomized, double-blind	Clindamycin for duration of chest tube placement or 5 days (whichever was shorter) versus placebo	2/38 patients with infection (1 empyema) in antibiotic group versus 8/37 (6 empyema) in control. An additional 13 patients in the control group were described as having radiographic evidence of pneumonia versus 4 in the placebo group.	"Patients receiving clindamycin had statistically lower incidence of radiographic pneumonia, less fever, lower white blood cell counts; they acquired empyema less frequently. . . ."

Study	Setting	Study type	Intervention	Results	Conclusion
Stone et al. (20)	Chest tube insertion (38% after trauma)	Randomized, double-blind	Cefamandole for duration of chest tube placement versus placebo	1/60 "infections of the lung parenchyma or pleural space" in antibiotic group versus 9/60 in placebo	"... preventative treatment with cefamandole can be significantly effective in reducing the incidence of posttraumatic pulmonary and pleural sepsis in patients who have sustained penetrating thoracic trauma"
Lo Curto et al. (15)	Chest tube insertion after trauma	Randomized, prospective study	Cefoxitin for duration of chest tube placement	8/28 thoracic infections (empyema or pneumonia) in controls versus 1/30 in cefoxitin-treated group	"We conclude that antibiotic prophylaxis is a valuable adjunct in the setting of tube thoracostomy for thoracic injury and support its routine use."

Modified from Mandal AK, Montano J, Thadepalli H. Prophylactic and no antibiotic compared in penetrating chest trauma. J Trauma 1985;25:639–643.

wound infection after uncomplicated traumatic injury. As mentioned previously, the administration of antibiotic "prophylaxis" for penetrating wounds must occur after the acute injury, missing the ideal period for antibiotic activity; in studies with prolonged antibiotic use, "treatment," rather than prophylaxis, may be occurring. Even with the appropriate administration of antibiotics in studies of elective surgery, results are equivocal. Most studies showing benefit for antibiotic usage have started with initially high rates of wound infection, greater than would be expected for most thoracic surgeries when classified as "clean-contaminated" procedures and certainly higher than our experience at the MIEMSS Shock Trauma Center. As noted above, the majority of trials cited did not study what is currently believed to be the "ideal" characteristics for wound prophylaxis: high intraoperative levels and cessation postoperatively.

For prophylaxis prior to operative intervention other than chest tube placement, we agree with the approach advocated in *The Medical Letter* (18) and by other authorities (4), who recommend single-dose antibiotic administration before elective thoracic surgery and in the setting of surgical intervention after trauma. For newly hospitalized patients, a first-generation cephalosporin with good activity against *S. aureus* is preferred; in the patient hospitalized for longer than 3 to 4 days (and likely colonized with Gram-negative bacilli), a third-generation cephalosporin with antistaphylococcal activity (e.g., cefotaxime or ceftriaxone) may be superior. However, *S. aureus* strains that produce a beta-lactamase active against cefazolin have been associated with postoperative wound infections in patients who received prophylactic cefazolin (18a). If this report is confirmed and similar strains become more common, an antibiotic with activity against these strains (e.g., cefamandole) may be recommended in the future. We do not employ routine prophylaxis for uncomplicated thoracic trauma, an approach also advocated by Root et al. (16). In both our experience and the surgical literature, wound infection at the site of penetrating trauma is low and does not justify antibiotic use.

The treatment of an established wound infection in the thorax is similar to that of wound infections elsewhere and requires both appropriate antibiotic therapy and surgical debridement if necessary. *S. aureus* is the most common pathogen isolated from thoracic wound infections, but in all instances (especially in patients with prolonged hospitalization), an attempt should be made to obtain wound aspirates, drainage, or debrided material for Gram stain and culture. Uncommonly, costochondritis can complicate wound infection in the thorax and requires more prolonged therapy. Severe complications of wound infection (e.g., fasciitis) are also uncommon after isolated thoracic trauma but can occur with devastating consequences. These complications are discussed in greater detail in other texts (18b). Mediastinitis following cardiac surgery (or esophageal penetration) is discussed separately below.

Empyema

Empyema in the trauma patient is most commonly caused by organisms introduced at the time of chest tube insertion. Patients having thoracostomy tubes placed after injury are at greater risk of developing empyema than patients with tube insertion for spontaneous pneumothorax, due to a higher likelihood that undrained or loculated pleural collections could be seeded. Empyema occurring in the setting of a preexisting patent chest tube usually reflects an additional undrained collection. Less commonly, infection in the pleural space occurs by seeding from an adjacent pneumonia, and infection is established separately in the pleural space despite adequate drainage.

If empyema is suspected, material should be aspirated from the chest tube as proximal to the wound as possible and examined by Gram stain. Material should also be sent for culture. The presence of concomitant pneumonia should be assessed and sputum also examined by Gram stain and culture. We have found thoracic CT scan valuable for identifying undrained collections not apparent on x-ray and for discriminating intrapleural versus intraparenchymal disease. If polymicrobial infection is found or intestinal organisms are cultured soon after hospitalization, contamination from concomitant bowel and diaphragmatic injury should be suspected. Antibiotic therapy should be initiated based on Gram stain material, concomitant infection (e.g., pneumonia), and experience at individual intensive care units. If empiric coverage is necessary, the antibiotic chosen should always include activity against *S. aureus*. The site of chest tube insertion should always be examined if empyema is suspected, but this is an uncommon site of wound infection.

Although the prevention of empyema has been a major impetus for using prophylactic antibiotics in patients with thoracic trauma, few controlled studies have examined this issue. Studies in this setting have most often been designed to evaluate the utility of antibiotics in the prevention of empyema following closed-tube thoracostomy with or without trauma. Despite the lack of evidence supporting this practice, continuous antibiotic use for the duration of chest tube placement is routine in many institutions. In an early prospective trial of antibiotic use after simple penetrating thoracic trauma, Grover et al. (19) described a significant decrease in the incidence of empyema with the use of intravenous clindamycin, reporting a 2.6% (1/38) incidence of empyema in a group treated with 5 days of intravenous therapy versus 16.2% (6/37) in a double-blind placebo control. Stone et al. (20) found three empyemas in controls (and an overall incidence of pulmonary infection of 13.3%) versus none in patients receiving continuous cefamandole after chest tube placement for thoracic trauma. LoCurto et al. (15) noted similar findings after chest tube placement following thoracic injury: four empyemas occurred in 28 placebo-treated controls (14%); none occurred in an experimental group receiving continuous cefoxitin. These latter investigators also described significantly shorter periods of both hospitalization and pleural intubation in the group receiving cefoxitin. However, similar to the situation for wound infections, conflicting results have appeared. In the previously cited trial by Mandal et al. (1) of doxycycline versus placebo for the duration of chest tube placement, only one patient (randomized to placebo) of 80 developed empyema. LeBlanc and Tucker (14) also observed only one case of empyema in 85 patients, 39 of whom were treated with empiric cepharin (a first-generation cephalosporin) for the duration of chest tube placement. Eddy et al. (20a) found no occurrence of empyema in 105 patients with complete evacuation of the pleural space after thoracic trauma.

Often cited in support of prophylactic antibiotic use is a retrospective review of the experience at the Shock Trauma Center from 1982 to 1983 (21) that revealed a high incidence of empyema (16%) following chest tube placement. This high incidence occurred in a group of multiply traumatized patients, most of whom were mechanically ventilated and approximately one-half of whom received corticosteroids. In this study, the distribution of organisms differed substantially in patients having chest tubes placed for pneumothorax occurring after admission (unrelated to the original trauma). All "late" empyemas were caused by hospital-acquired Gram-negative bacteria as opposed to Gram-positive organisms predominating as the cause of empyema in thoracostomy tubes placed for hemopneumothorax at the time of admission. Organisms isolated in the former group were all resistant to commonly used "prophylactic" regimens. Continued infection surveillance at our institution has shown the occurrence of empyema to have decreased markedly since this previous study in the absence of any change in surgical procedure. This result has been attributed to a reduction in the incidence of barotrauma by a change from pressure- to volume-controlled mechanical ventilation during this period.

Based on our experience and in agreement with others (11, 20, 22), we do not believe that antibiotic coverage is indicated after chest tube placement for spontaneous pneumothorax. Although less generally accepted (16, 18, 20a), we similarly do not routinely advocate "prophylaxis" for chest tube placement after trauma in consideration of the necessity for prolonged antibiotic use, the risk of superinfection or adverse reactions, and the declining incidence of empyema at our center. If a patient is at greater risk of bacterial contamination or is immunocompromised, we agree with Eddy et al. (20a) that a short course of antibiotic "prophylaxis" may be used. In all cases, chest tubes should be removed as soon as possible.

Prophylaxis for Pneumonia

The use of antibiotics for the prevention of nosocomial pneumonia in intubated patients has generated far more controversy in the medical and surgical literature. Interest in prophylaxis against pneumonia has persisted after the realization that infection rates remained high even after great success in eliminating "exogenous" sources of infection from respiratory apparatus (23). Prophylaxis has been of particular concern for trauma patients due to the possibility of acute aspiration at the time of trauma or the presence of mechanical factors associated with injury that may increase the risk of nosocomial pneumonia. In a recent retrospective review from Parkland, Walker et al. (2) described a statistically significant benefit for prophylactic antibiotic use in preventing pneumonia and empyema following thoracic injury. The overall incidence of "major" infection in patients not receiving prophylaxis was 66% versus 21% in patients receiving prophylaxis (approximately one-fifth of infections were abdominal abscesses; the remainder were pneumonia or empyema). In this retrospective report, 16 different "prophylactic" regimens were used for varying periods of time. Pneumonia was also related to the duration of intubation, occurring in 50/65 (77%) patients intubated longer than 1 week. In the setting of a high incidence of nosocomial pneumonia despite prophylactic antibiotic use and the lack of activity of most commonly recommended prophylactic antibiotics against Gram-negative bacilli, any presumed statistical benefit for prophylactic antibiotics must be viewed with caution. The results of other studies have reached differing conclusions, with multiple studies both favoring and opposing routine antibiotic use to prevent pneumonia after thoracic intervention. Stone et al. (20), in trauma patients, and Kvale et al. (9), Cooper (24), and Ilves et al. (8), in elective pulmonary surgery, have found significant benefit for the use of antibiotics to prevent pneumonia in controlled studies; Mandal et al. (1), Truesdale et al. (6), Frimodt-Moller et al. (10), and Cameron et al. (7) found no advantage for prophylactic antibiotic use in preventing pneumonia after either thoracic trauma or elective pulmonary surgery.

Drawing a firm conclusion from these disparate studies is difficult due to the regimens that were used, the varying durations of coverage, and the different clinical settings (trauma versus elective surgery) in which the studies were performed. Of particular concern is the labeling of any regimen as "prophylactic"; a regimen of continuous antibiotic use during hospitalization to prevent pneumonia must be considered far different in both cost and potential adverse consequences than perioperative dosing to minimize wound infections. The strategy of continuous antibiotic use for prophylaxis of nosocomial pneumonia has been criticized by the infectious diseases community as ultimately increasing the incidence of infectious complications by selecting for resistant pathogens—a concern since early attempts to prevent pneumonia in all intubated patients. Nebulized polymyxin B therapy, despite initially showing a slight efficacy in the prevention of nosocomial pneumonia (25), has not been adopted for this reason. A more recent multicenter trial of nebulized gentamicin in intubated patients confirms the lack of clinical utility for this therapy while again selecting for resistant organisms (26). Similar arguments have been made against the use of systemic agents in all critically ill patients; there is no a priori reason to view thoracic trauma patients as different in this regard.

Reflecting the uncertainty in the multiple clinical studies that have been performed in patients after thoracic trauma, we do not currently recommend antibiotic use to prevent nosocomial pneumonia. We share the concern of selecting out resistant organisms that have been observed with indiscriminant antibiotic use (27). The cost and potential for significant morbidity from adverse drug reactions associated with uniform antibiotic use are significant. As in all decision analytic studies, the baseline incidence of disease (in this instance, infection) is a key variable in determining the potential benefit of intervention (i.e., prophylactic antibiotics). For pneumonia prophylaxis, as described below, we strongly favor an approach of aggressive diagnosis as the optimal method for both treating infection early and avoiding unnecessary antibiotic exposure. However, there have been reports from Europe of a more global, alternative approach to antibiotic prophylaxis in trauma. Following the trend of prophylactic antibiotic use in neutropenic patients, recent studies have described significant benefit for "selective decontamination" regimens in intubated patients (28–32). This approach combines systemic antibiotics, a topical antibiotic paste applied to the oropharynx, and instillation of nonabsorbable antibiotics (polymyxin/tobramycin/amphotericin) into the gastrointestinal tract through an orogastric tube. In addition, systemic prophylaxis with cefotaxime is given for the first 4–5 days of treatment. The regimen is predicated on the premise that most pneumonias result from oropharyngeal aspiration. Topical antibiotics "decontaminate" and sterilize the orophyarynx while gastric instillation of antibiotics prevents either primary colonization or recolonization of this area by endogenous gastrointestinal flora or nosocomial species. Early use of systemic antibiotics prevents infection prior to sterilization by this regimen. Results in intensive care unit patients from two centers have been extremely favorable (29, 30). Also observed was the prevention of early pneumonias (occurring in the first week of hospitalization), attributed to "treatment" of subclinical aspiration at the time of injury or intubation. Analysis by subgroup in the experience from Glasgow showed a statistically significant decrease in mortality in trauma patients treated with this regimen. Surprisingly, no emergence of resistant organisms was observed after 5 yr of this regimen at one center (32).

A theoretically similar approach to infection prophylaxis is found in the work of Craven (33) and Driks et al. (34), where the use of sucralfate is advocated to prevent stress ulceration and to maintain a lower pH environment. (The use of H2 antagonists to raise gastric pH has been previously associated with an increased gastric colonization by microorganisms (34) and a subsequent increased risk of nosocomial pneumonia by aspiration.) Although preliminary results are promising, large-scale confirmation that sucralfate is efficacious without increasing the risk of stress ulceration is pending. An interesting recent report compared these two potential therapies (sucralfate versus selective decontamination) in a cardiac surgery intensive care unit and found the decontamination regimen associated with a significantly lower postoperative infection rate (35).

Prophylaxis for Concurrent Abdominal Trauma or Esophageal Injury

Abdominal involvement in the patient with thoracic trauma is quite common, occurring in 25% of the patients in a series from Parkland (2). The use of prophylactic antibiotics both in elective abdominal surgery and after abdominal trauma has been well-studied. In the setting of blunt trauma where no laparotomy is planned, prophylaxis is not indicated. For patients undergoing elective laparotomy where a hollow viscus is to be violated, prophylaxis with either cefoxitin or an antibiotic combination containing aerobic Gram-negative bacilli and anaerobic coverage have been effective in preventing postoperative wound infections (36–38). These regimens have also been shown to prevent the later complication of intraabdominal abscess. In two large studies of patients undergoing posttraumatic laparotomy, Gentry et al. (39) and Oreskovich et al. (40) have shown antibiotic prophylaxis to be useful. There is consensus that, in the setting of penetrating abdominal injury, prophylactic antibiotics are indicated (perhaps better described as "anticipatory therapy") (3). Controversies have focused primarily on the specific therapy and the optimal duration of antibiotic treatment. Most of the recent studies addressing the former question have found single agents providing broad-spectrum anaerobic and aerobic coverage (e.g., cefoxitin, imipenem, and cefotetan (38, 41–43)) to be equivalent to antibiotic combinations that yield a similar spectrum of coverage. Other second-generation cephalosporins, e.g., cefamandole, have been shown to be less effective due to the lack of coverage of intestinal anaerobes, primarily *Bacteroides fragilis*. The appropriate duration of antibiotic coverage is less certain, although recent studies have steadily reduced the length of time that prophylaxis is felt necessary. A recent review of these studies (44) has led to the recommendation of 24–48 hr of antibiotic therapy for penetrating trauma. This guideline should be individualized by the degree of contamination in individual patients. In the absence of bowel injury, minimal risk of infection is anticipated; with bowel penetration, risk is far greater after colonic injury to the normally sterile stomach or duodenum in the setting of normal gastric acidity.

Esophageal injury is an uncommon but well-described complication of both penetrating and blunt trauma, although reports contain little data regarding infectious complications from this type of injury. The esophagus is colonized by oropharyngeal flora at the superior aspect and becomes progressively more sterile distally toward the gastric junction. Acute shock from abrupt rupture with accompanying acid-induced mediastinitis or pleuritis may overwhelm the clinical presentation and account for high mortality if this complication occurs; more commonly, perforation presents less dramatically and may be difficult to diagnose. Contamination of the mediastinum or thorax can occur with oral aerobic and anaerobic flora, leading to a severe secondary necrotizing infection. Although there are few formal studies, prophylaxis for complicated esophageal trauma is recommended and should include complete coverage for oral anaerobes. Clindamycin and ampicillin-sulbactam are acceptable agents; if indicated, broader coverage (i.e., addition of an agent with Gram-negative activity) may be appropriate. Instillation of topical neomycin or povidone-iodine solution into the esophagus has also been advocated prior to surgery. Increased aspiration of oropharyngeal flora is a known postoperative complication after esophageal injury and requires increased attention to pulmonary toilet.

Mediastinitis

Mediastinitis is a well-known and greatly feared complication of cardiothoracic surgery. Although estimated at an incidence of between 0.5 and 3.0% for elective procedures, the rate of this complication following trauma is unknown. The need for emergent surgery has been proposed as a risk factor for postoperative mediastinitis (45) and may be true following acute operative intervention for mediastinal or cardiac injury; other studies, however, have not found increased rates after emergency surgery (46). The high mortality of cardiac trauma limits the absolute incidence of this complication. However, even in emergency situations, risk may not be higher than in elective procedures; no mediastinal complications were seen in 25 patients surviving emergency room thoracotomy at the University of Maryland Hospital (47). Preoperative health status, chronic obstructive pulmonary disease (COPD), and a need for reexploration, in addition to the duration of surgery, have all been associated with an increased incidence of postoperative mediastinitis. Trauma patients would be expected to have a lower baseline incidence of these preoperative risk factors than patients undergoing elective cardiac surgery, perhaps decreasing infectious risk or compensating for increased risk in the emergent situation. "Classic" signs of mediastinitis (mediastinal widening, dysphagia, sternal tenderness) are uncommon and insensitive for diagnosis. Wound drainage or cellulitis was seen in the majority of patients with mediastinitis studied by Bor et al. (46). A "toxic" state was also seen in 38% of the patients in this series, although presentation ranged from occult fever to overwhelming sepsis. Findings from computed tomography (CT) scanning of the mediastinum have been of little aid in diagnosis (48).

Definitive diagnosis is by aspiration or apparent by findings at reexploration. Treatment requires immediate debridement, drainage, and broad-spectrum antibiotic coverage. In the study by Bor et al. (46), organisms isolated in the first week postoperatively were all Gram-negative; Gram-positive organisms were more common 1–2 weeks after surgery, although others have not found this pattern. Aggressive treatment combined with continuous mediastinal irrigation has been felt to account for improved outcomes in more recent series (48a). A recent report has also suggested that topical vancomycin may reduce the risk of postoperative sternal infection (48b).

Due to the morbidity associated with postoperative sternotomy infections or mediastinitis, antibiotic prophylaxis is strongly recommended for patients undergoing cardiothoracic surgery. The need to maintain adequate serum concentrations of antibiotic throughout surgery has been emphasized by some authorities (18). If mediastinal penetration has occurred with injury, antibiotic therapy with an agent active against *S. aureus* should be continued for a minimum of 2–3 days posttrauma.

GENERAL INFECTIOUS ISSUES IN THE TRAUMATIZED PATIENT
Diagnosis of Infection in the Posttraumatic Period

The diagnosis of infection in the posttraumatic period is often difficult. Fever, the most reliable marker of infection, is often caused by noninfectious mechanisms. Both penetrating and blunt thoracic trauma are commonly associated with lung parenchymal injury, manifested as pulmonary contusion and/or hemopneumothorax; fever in this situation is a common accompaniment of tissue trauma. If acute operative intervention is necessary, fever from tissue injury in surgery or from anesthesia may be present. Leukocytosis is often secondary to the traumatic event itself and is usually not contributory as a marker of infection. In the immediate posttraumatic period, especially in normally sterile injuries (e.g., limited to the thorax), infection is an unlikely cause of fever. Appropriate evaluation is necessary, but empiric antibiotics are indicated less often than during the later phase of hospitalization. Concern at this stage should be directed to associated factors or contamination at the time of injury (or perhaps during nonsterile aspects of resuscitation) that raise the likelihood of infection as a source of fever in this period.

Recognizing the morbidity and importance of infection in the postresuscitative phase of trauma, the infectious diseases service follows all patients admitted to the MIEMSS Shock Trauma Center. Surgical prophylaxis in the thoracic cavity is provided by the prompt drainage of hemothoraces and obliteration of potential spaces. Sputum Gram stains on each patient are examined by an infectious diseases staff member at least 3 times weekly to observe changes in the degree of sputum colonization. Knowledge of the changes in sputum colonization allows the clinician to better interpret both the results of concurrent sputum cultures and any changes observed on chest x-ray. All wounds are observed daily and cultures taken as necessary. Intravascular catheters are changed regularly after being in place a maximum of 4 days. After removal, catheter tips are sent for semiquantitative cultures (49, 50); we have not found alternative methods of evaluating line tips, e.g., Gram staining (51), to be practical or sensitive. We are currently evaluating the risk/benefit of line changes over wires and allow at most one change of a central catheter over a wire at a given site; therefore, the duration of a central line at any given site is restricted to no more than 8 days. Chest x-ray films are obtained daily on all intubated patients. If the source of infection is suspected to be of thoracic origin, CT has been shown to contribute to the interpretation of x-ray film abnormalties (52). Mirvis et al. (53) have also demonstrated the sensitivity of CT for the diagnosis of thoracic infections even in the absence of concomitant x-ray study changes. In the newly febrile patient, sputum Gram stain and culture, urinalysis, urine culture, blood cultures, and intravascular line changes are routine. It has been our experience that routine, careful attention to the "colonization" status of the patient allows us to anticipate the likely sites of infection if fever develops. This knowledge also serves to make a more appropriate choice for empiric therapy when indicated.

Although a strict definition of "sepsis" is somewhat controversial, this clinical entity is uniformly recognized. Despite the many noninfectious etiologies that can mimic a septic picture, most studies confirm infection as the primary cause of posttraumatic sepsis. Distinguishing between "infection" and "sepsis" is often difficult in the trauma patient where the early markers of sepsis (fever, leukocytosis, hyperdynamic state) are often present after severe injury; for this reason, we have focused on early detection of infection as the best "prophylaxis" against sepsis while minimizing the adverse effects of antibiotic use.

There have been many efforts to predict the risk of sepsis earlier and more specifically in critically ill populations by the use of indices of illness or by measurement of endogenous mediators, e.g., endotoxin assays (54). In the former case, although there has been success in identifying relative risk of infection in various groups, there is little reliability for predicting infectious risk on an individual basis (55). No measure of endogenous mediator activation has proven useful as a predictor of infection in the setting of acute trauma where such markers may be elevated due to the traumatic event itself; however, there may be a role for such measurements in the future (especially with blossoming research and application of various antiendotoxin mediators).

At the MIEMSS Shock Trauma Center, we attempt to minimize antibiotic use and, thereby, any associated adverse effects. Recently described toxicities, e.g., increased bleeding consequences from certain extended-spectrum penicillins (56), may alter the "risk/benefit" of certain antibiotics. It has been our clinical observation that the onset of fever temporally related to the initiation of certain medications is very common, although drug fever has received surprisingly little critical examination in the medical literature. Drug fever can also be delayed in onset, arising even as the fever from a true infection is replaced by one from antibiotic therapy.

Specific Infectious Etiologies
PNEUMONIA

Thoracic trauma predisposes the patient to pulmonary infection, the most common infectious cause of mortality following trauma. Walker et al. (2) noted a 33% incidence of major infection in patients with thoracic trauma (although 25% of the patients in this series underwent laparotomy for concurrent abdominal injury); in patients with major infections, pneumonia was diagnosed in 82 of 254 individuals. Occurrence of pneumonia was directly related to the duration of intubation: 50 of 65 patients (77%) intubated longer than 1 week developed pneumonia. The incidence of pneumonia was higher in blunt trauma patients, reflecting the usually more severe nature of the injury and more frequent multiple organ system involvement. This experience is similar to our observations.

The etiology of pneumonia in the injured patient follows a bimodal distribution. The overwhelming majority of all pneumonias are due to "aspiration" of oropharyngeal contents; in the early postinjury phase, this pneumonia usually reflects involvement by "community" oropharyngeal flora aspirated at the time of injury or shortly thereafter. *Hemophilus influenzae* has been increasingly recognized as a common cause of nosocomial pneumonia occurring early in the hospitalization course. Originally felt to be an uncommon pathogen, this organism has been increasingly recognized because of more widespread inclusion of bacteriologic media that support the growth of this organism from sputum specimens. Clinical evidence of pneumonia in the setting of a mixed Gram stain (i.e., one with various organisms but no predominant pathogen) increases the suspicion of anaerobic involvement. Other predominantly "early" pathogens include the pneumococcus and *S. aureus*. Later during hospitalization, nosocomial Gram-negative organisms (and *S. aureus*) replace the preexisting endogenous flora as both colonizers and the etiology of pneumonia.

Although the diagnosis of pneumonia is made by the criteria of fever and persistent pulmonary infiltrate (among others), in the early postinjury phase the majority of pulmonary infiltrates (even if accompanied by fever) can be resolved by aggressive physical therapy. This fact is especially important after thoracic trauma where pulmonary infiltrates are common, and it further underscores the importance of serial sputum examination. A recent study by Joshi et al. (57) have confirmed this principle by observing the resolution of x-ray changes by physical therapy in a cohort of intubated trauma patients who had early infiltrate and fever but who were not treated with antibiotics. This principle no doubt reflects the importance and frequency of atelectasis as a common source of early postinjury fever, often clinically indistinguishable from pneumonia. Other techniques of pulmonary mobilization (e.g., oscillating beds (57a)) may also reduce the incidence of infection.

Most seriously injured patients either arrive at our center intubated or are intubated shortly after admission. More than 90% of the more severely injured patients receive mechanical ventilation for some period during their hospital course. The common occurrence of pneumonia is associated with prolonged mechanical ventilation; the greatest risk factor for pneumonia in most studies is intubation (although the need for ventilation correlates directly with severity of injury). Following the early hospitalization phase, the cause of nosocomial pneumonia reflects the colonization by hospital-resident flora, most often Gram-negative bacilli. The almost 100% colonization of mechanically ventilated patients by these organisms (58–60) gives no utility to sputum culture as indicative of nosocomial infection; diagnosis of pneumonia is never made on the basis of sputum culture alone. Although the value of sputum Gram stain for diagnosing pneumonia has been questioned (61), we have had excellent success in using the combination of sputum examination and culture results to diagnose and treat pneumonia in the critically ill patient. We strongly believe this relates to the careful following of serial sputum specimens by the staff so that changes in character and type of organism are seen before infection becomes manifest. The Gram stain is often pathognomonic before culture results are available (e.g., *H. influenzae*) and the Gram stain may be more sensitive than culture for certain pathogens (e.g., pneumococcus). Sputum purulence is common in intubated patients from the irritation of endotracheal intubation, making gross examination of sputum nonspecific for the diagnosis of pneumonia. High-quality sputum specimens are readily obtainable by deep suctioning from trauma patients who are intubated or have undergone tracheostomy. The relationship of colonization of the oropharynx and trachea preceding infection in intubated patients has been well-recognized (60, 62), although "exogenous" lower respiratory tract infection is still occasionally seen, primarily as aerosolization of bacteria from contaminated ventilatory equipment. We believe that frequent suctioning and aggressive physical therapy have been major factors in the low incidence of nosocomial pneumonia at our center. The physical therapy service reviews x-ray films daily to plan intervention and maximize the benefits of percussion and drainage. Atelectasis can mimic pneumonia exactly with hypoxemia, fever, and x-ray examination changes, especially early in hospitalization; absence of pathogens on Gram stain supports this diagnosis.

If pneumonia is diagnosed, treatment is directed at the pathogen identified by Gram stain and subsequent culture results. We have rarely observed *Legionella* species in our center, although, in other areas, culture on buffered charcoal media and direct fluorescent antibody studies for *Legionella* species may be indicated. Nosocomial bronchitis is far less common than pneumonia; however, this entity has been described and in the appropriate clinical circumstances may warrant therapy. It is expected that many additional antibiotics will be available in the near future, especially a broader range of quinolones (e.g., ciprofloxacin) and carbapenems (e.g., Imipenem). The exact role of these agents in the critically ill patient remains to be established. Choice of a specific agent from a larger class of agents often reflects individual preference and cost considerations at a particular institution. In all cases, if a pathogen is documented, the choice of antibiotic should be predicated on in vitro sensitivities. For mixed Gram stains without a predominant organism, cefoxitin is a reasonable empiric choice. The dosage of antibiotic should be checked for adjustment in the setting of renal insufficiency; creatinine clearance is routinely monitored at our institute to anticipate the necessity for a change in antibiotic dose. The pharmacokinetics of many agents, e.g., aminoglycosides (63), are altered in patients with severe trauma and dosages must often be adjusted upwards due to greater drug clearance (64). Antibiotic levels should be carefully monitored in agents with well-known toxicities (e.g., renal and auditory effects of aminoglycosides and vancomycin). A clinical pharmacologist or infectious disease specialist should be consulted to suggest and adjust dosages in the critically ill patient. Consultation is also advisable when the indirect effects of certain antibiotics (e.g., the large volume of fluid necessary to administer trimethoprim sulfamethoxazole) may be more significant than the direct toxicity and in circumstances where there are imperfect correlations between in vitro and in vivo antibiotic sensitivities (e.g., enterococcal infections).

Duration of treatment depends on clinical response and infectious etiology. We favor 10–14 days of therapy for most pathogens. Certain pathogens, e.g., *Pseudomonas,* usually require the use of two drugs for synergistic therapy and to prevent the selection of resistant strains. When synergistic therapy is necessary, we use either an antipseudomonal penicillin or a cephalosporin, combined with an aminoglycoside; the poor lung penetration of aminoglycosides may make them less optimal for use as monotherapy for any form of Gram-negative pneumonia. Aerosolization of aminoglycosides for treatment of pneumonia in the mechanically ventilated patient is currently undergoing reexamination and may be a useful adjunctive therapy in the future (64), especially with resistant Gram-negative bacilli or where the systemic toxicity of aminoglycosides may be intolerable.

SINUSITIS

Sinusitis has been a common source of nosocomial infection at the MIEMSS Shock Trauma Center (65). Presentation is most notable for an absence of any physical signs of sinusitis (purulence and discharge) in a patient with occult fever. Infection usually involves the maxillary sinuses in a patient predisposed to infection by occlusion of the sinus ostia and lack of drainage; contributing factors include supine position, nasal and facial trauma (with intranasal packing often present), nasogastric tube placement, and nasotracheal intubation. These latter two manipulations have been seen with the majority of cases of nosocomial sinusitis and are avoided in favor of oral routes if at all possible; we attribute a steady decline in sinusitis to this practice. Other series have similarly described nasal intubation as a major cause of postoperative nosocomial sinusitis (66).

The presence of sinus opacification, even in the maxillary sinus, is often difficult to confirm by x-ray studies of the sinuses in the immobilized and intubated patient. If obtainable, CT is a more sensitive instrument for diagnosing sinus infiltrates. CT also has the advantage of better resolution of the sphenoid and ethmoid sinuses. If a maxillary sinus opacification or collection is seen, the involved sinus is aspirated at the bedside and the material is sent for Gram stain and culture (in our center, other causes, primarily hematoma from trauma, are more commonly responsible for sinus fluid). Because the aspiration is frequently contaminated by oral flora (usually Gram-negative organisms after hospitalization), review of the Gram-stained material for polymorphonuclear cells and organisms is necessary to make this diagnosis. Bacteremia or clinical deterioration from maxillary sinusitis is very unusual, although infection in other sinuses, particularly the sphenoid sinus, can be associated with high mortality (67). Many of our patients have head trauma and undergo frequent cranial CT scanning; it is common practice to obtain a few additional "cuts" through the sinuses to assess that they have remained clear during hospitalization. Doing so does not require a full sinus examination with narrow cuts and adds minimal time to the CT scan.

The majority of isolates obtained from sinus aspirates at our center are Gram-negative rods, reflecting primarily nosocomial acquisition. The primary treatment is removal of any possible osteal obstruction to allow drainage. Most cases are relieved by changing endotracheal and nasogastric tubes to the oral route (66). If no foreign body exists, our patients usually undergo irrigation and drainage, most commonly by antral window. Antibiotic choice for specific pathogens is dictated by in vitro sensitivity studies done on the material aspirated.

BACTEREMIA/LINE SEPSIS

Bacteremia is common in the traumatized patient as a direct consequence of the increasing need for (and bore of) sophisticated cardiovascular monitoring lines. Although any source of infection can lead to secondary bacteremia, intravascular catheter infection remains the primary source of bacteremia at our center. In an analysis of bacteremic episodes at the MIEMSS Shock Trauma Center by Stillwell and Caplan (68), *S. aureus* was the most common cause of bacteremia, with Gram-negative species (primarily *Klebsiella* and *Enterobacter*) less common.

Our practice is to send all intravascular lines for semiquantitative culture after removal, even in the absence of clinical signs of infection. Gram-negative rod phlebitis, common in intensive care units, is often without local signs of inflammation (50). The knowledge of potential pathogens isolated from catheter tips prior to the emergence of clinical signs of infection allows a more directed choice of empiric therapy.

Many controversies surround the use of central venous catheters. The most prominent has been the question of how long a catheter may safely remain in place. There have been varying recommendations from different authorities but near-uniform agreement that there has not been a definitive study or methodology to adequately resolve this issue (68a). Duration of catheter placement clearly correlates with incidence of infection (69) but the optimal duration where infectious risk outweighs other complications (and cost) and changes is uncertain. A major problem in arriving at a consensus is the difficulty in generalizing across the varied circumstances in which central monitoring lines are used. The use of large-bore triple-lumen catheters in trauma patients with frequent solution changes, blood sampling through the catheter, piggybacking of medications, and cardiac output measurements (through Swan-Ganz catheters) is far different than the insertion of a single-lumen, dedicated parental nutrition line. Each of these factors (bore size, type of line (Swan-Ganz versus triple-lumen), and frequency of manipulation) has been related to increased risk of catheter-related infection (70). As with other iatrogenic procedures, infection is only one of multiple complications that can occur with central monitoring (bleeding, tamponade, pneumothorax, nonbacterial endocarditis); as yet, there has been no large-scale controlled study of these complications. We are currently analyzing our experience with more than 2000 lines changed under different conditions. Other controversies exist regarding appropriate exit site covering (gauze versus clear dressings), with some studies clearly favoring the gauze dressing (71). Silver-impregnated catheter hubs have recently also been reported to decrease colonization and catheter infection (72). A dedicated, central-line-care nursing staff and the use of only experienced personnel to insert catheters have been cited as additional factors in decreasing infectious risk.

The current policy at our center is to change all intravascular lines (except single-lumen lines dedicated to parenteral nutrition) at 4-day intervals. Skin sites are prepared with povidone-iodine solution and dressings are changed each day. Although chlorhexidine has been associated with a decreased incidence of catheter-site colonization (70), we have observed frequent skin irritation with the use of this topical agent and prefer the povidone-iodine preparation. Increasing evidence suggests that at least one catheter change can be safely done over an intravascular guide wire (70a). If a line change is done over a wire, the subsequent change is to a new site. In a patient suspected to have bacteremia, lines are often changed over guide wires; if a catheter tip is then shown to be colonized with a potential pathogen, the replacement line is changed to a new site. If positive blood cultures are obtained with clinical signs of infection, all intravascular line sites are changed. The absence of inflammation at the catheter site should not lower the suspicion of catheter-related infection; inflammation at the site of catheter insertion is an insensitive sign of infection, especially for Gram-negative infection. Intraarterial catheters are changed at the same intervals as intravenous lines (72a) and can also be changed over guidelines.

Even with *S. aureus* as the most common etologic agent, most line-related bacteremias are treated as presumed hospital-acquired infections with a removable focus. Such an infection usually requires a 10–14-day course of antibiotics rather than a prolonged course of 4 weeks for presumed endocarditis. Previous studies have confirmed the low likelihood of native valve seeding in hospitalized patients with acute bacteremia (73). In patients with persistent bacteremia despite antibiotic therapy, relapse after completion of therapy, or mitigating factors (e.g., presence of a deep vein thrombus or preexisting valvular damage), antibiotics are continued for a full 4-week course. In any of these circumstances, thorough evaluation must be made for an intravascular source (e.g., septic thrombophlebitis) that may require surgical intervention.

URINARY TRACT INFECTION

Urinary tract infections are almost uniformly the most common nosocomial infections; in some centers, it is also the primary cause of nosocomial Gram-negative bacteremia. Bladder colonization by Gram-negative organisms is approximately 50% after 1 week of hospitalization in the catheterized patient and approaches 100% after 2 weeks (74). The incidence of true infection is, however, far lower. Nosocomial urinary tract infection is rarely due to organisms other than Gram-negative rods.

In male patients, we avoid the use of indwelling catheters if possible in favor of external condom catheterization. All urinary catheters are permanently joined to the collection urometer to avoid contamination by manipulation (75). Bladder irrigation with bactericidal solutions has not been shown to be of benefit (76) and is not used. The distinction between colonization and infection is based on a urinalysis sample obtained at the same time as urine culture; in most circumstances, the presence of more than 10 leukocytes in urine is felt to discriminate between infection and colonization. Two special circumstances are the presence of *S. aureus* or *Candida* species in the urine. The presence of *S. aureus* bacteriuria is of particular significance, as this commonly reflects bacteremia with secondary urinary tract seeding. In this situation, blood cultures should be obtained and possible intravascular foci carefully sought. Fungal colonization of the urine is commonly seen but, as with bacterial colonization, the incidence of true fungal cystitis is far lower. Complications of fungiuria have been described (e.g., ureteral obstruction), but in our experience these are exceptionally rare. Occasionally, local treatment is administered with amphotericin B intermittent irrigation, following the suggestions of Gantz (77), but there are few empirical data to support this practice.

The treatment of urinary tract infection should be approached as a clinical cure rather than a microbiologic eradication. In almost all cases, urine can be initially sterilized by an appropriate antibiotic. Even an "inappropriate" antibiotic can be useful; antibiotics that undergo renal excretion can reach supratherapeutic levels and become bactericidal even though they are "resistant" at the lower concentrations used by the microbiology laboratory to ascertain sensitivity. Although urine is easily sterilized, the focus of infection is rarely eradicated in the presence of a foreign body (the catheter) that harbors a persisting inoculum of organisms adherent to its surface. "Cure" is soon followed by the recurrence of bacteriuria after antibiotics are discontinued. Recent studies have used silver-impregnated catheters to reduce urinary tract colonization and infection (78), but it is uncertain if more widespread use is indicated.

Because many antibiotics are excreted in the urine, there are many choices for therapy for almost all pathogens. In the patient tolerating oral feeding by nasogastric tube, trimethoprim sulfamethoxazole, ampicillin, norfloxacin, and ciprofloxacin are useful agents. If intravenous therapy is necessary, antibiotics that undergo urinary excretion can usually be administered at doses lower than those required for systemic disease. Trimethoprim sulfamethoxazole, quinolones, and most β-lactam antibiotics undergo urinary excretion. Duration of treatment should be short (5–7 days) and any "cure" documented by urinalysis. Relapse of bacteriuria without pyuria is common and does not require therapy. Pyelonephritis may be suggested by symptoms, an increased severity of illness, the presence of white cell casts, or persistent pyuria. Similarly, perinephric abscess should be excluded by imaging studies if the clinical picture is suggestive of this diagnosis. In the uncommon situation where treatment is indicated for fungal cystitis, we administer amphotericin B by either intermittent instillation or continuous irrigation for 2–3 days to eliminate pyuria; gross clearing of the urine has been observed almost immediately, and microscopic clearing usually occurs by 2–3 days. Relapse is almost universal after cessation and requires treatment only if it is "symptomatic." Similar to bacterial urinary tract colonization, catheter removal is often the only way to definitively "cure" fungiuria.

Empiric Therapy

It is common to find fever, leukocytosis, and other signs of infection without an apparent source. In trauma patients, these are frequent accompaniments of acute injury; later during hospitalization, these manifestations are more likely due to infection or other complications of hospitalization (e.g., deep venous thrombosis). It cannot be overemphasized that subtle changes indicative of early infection are far more easily recognized when the patient has been followed continuously since admission. The initiation of antibiotics in this situation must be based on clinical suspicion and the risk/benefit of withholding therapy; withholding therapy while evaluation of potential sources of fever proceeds is the most prudent course in many situations. If used, empiric antibiotics should be chosen based on the "colonization" status of the patient, likely sources of infection, and experience at the unit where the patient is hospitalized. Any suspicion of infection mandates careful search for an infectious etiology. After complete physical examination (with attention to wounds and sites of previous intravascular lines), we have found CT scan of the thorax and abdomen particularly valuable for demonstrating undrained fluid collections or unsuspected lung disease. We have occasionally also found· unsuspected noninfectious sources of fever (e.g., acalculous cholecystitis) requiring emergency intervention. The record of all patient medications should be reviewed, as well as all blood products received. We have found "central" causes of fever uncommon, even in patients with severe head injury.

Although still uncommon, viral causes of fever are being increasingly recognized in critically ill patients. In patients with head injury, stomatitis due to reactivation of herpes simplex is well recognized (although infrequently a source of fever). Patients at risk for trauma are also at greater risk of human immunodeficiency virus-1 (HIV-1) infection than the general hospital admissions; in certain endemic areas, a substantial proportion of patients with penetrating trauma may harbor HIV. Although not a cause of fever per se, HIV infection should be considered in patients manifesting unusual complications after hospitalization.

CONCLUSION

Care of the patient with thoracic trauma is currently plagued by many controversies. The lack of a clear consensus in the medical literature has led to variable practices in different institutions based on individual interpretations of this literature. We have presented an overview of our approach to this problem, emphasizing that we view potential complications in these patients as similar to those in all critically ill patients. The cornerstone of this approach is careful monitoring and anticipatory care of every intubated patient; although labor intensive, we believe this practice has resulted in a low incidence of infection-related morbidity and deaths at our facility.

REFERENCES

1. Mandal AK, Montano J, Thadepalli H. Prophylactic and no antibiotic compared in penetrating chest trauma. J Trauma 1985;25:639–643.
2. Walker WE, Kapelanski DP, Weland AP, Stewart JD, Duke JH Jr. Patterns of infection and mortality in thoracic trauma. Ann Surg 1985;201:752–757.
3. Sacks T. Prophylactic antibiotics in traumatic wounds. J Hosp Infect 1988;11(suppl A):251–258.
4. Pollack AV. Surgical prophylaxis—the emerging picture. Lancet 1988;1:225–229.
5. Kaiser AB. Antimicrobial prophylaxis in surgery. N Engl J Med 1986;315:1125–1138.
6. Truesdale R, D'Alessandri R, Manuel V, Daicof G, Kluge RM. Antimicrobial vs. placebo prophylaxis in non-cardiac thoracic surgery. JAMA 1979;241:1254–1256.
7. Cameron JL, Imbembo A, Kieffer RF, Spray S, Baker RR. Prospective clinical trial of antibiotics for pulmonary resections. Surg Gynecol Obstet 1981;152:156–158.
8. Ilves R, Cooper JD, Todd TRJ, Pearson FG. Prospective, randomized, double-blind study using prophylactic cephalothin for major, elective, general thoracic operations. J Thorac Cardiovasc Surg 1981;81:813–817.
9. Kvale PA, Ranga V, Kopacz M, Cox F, Magilligan DJ, Davila JC. Pulmonary resection. South Med J 1977;70(suppl 1):64–68.
10. Frimodt-Moller N, Ostri P, Pederson IBK, Poulsen SR. Antibiotic prophylaxis in pulmonary surgery. Ann Surg 1982;195:444–450.
11. Bryant LR, Dillon ML, Mobin-Uddin K. Prophylactic antibiotics in noncardiac thoracic operations. Ann Thorac Surg 1975;19:670–676.
12. Tarkka M, Pokela R, Lepojarvi M, Nissinen J, Karkola P. Infection prophylaxis in pulmonary surgery: a randomized prospective study. Ann Thorac Surg 1987;44:508–513.
13. Walker WS, Faichney A, Raychaudhury T, et al. Wound prophylaxis in thoracic surgery: a new approach. Thorax 1984;39:121–124.
14. LeBlanc KA, Tucker WY. Prophylactic antibiotics and closed tube thoracostomy. Surg Gynecol Obstet 1985;160:259–263.
15. LoCurto JJ, Tischler CD, Swan KG. Tube thoracostomy and trauma—antibiotics or not? J Trauma 1986;26:1067–1072.
15a. Platt R, Zaleznik DF, Hopkins CC, Dellinger EP. Perioperative antibiotic prophylaxis for herniorrhaphy and breast surgery. N Engl J Med 1990;322:153–160.
16. Root RK, Trunkey DD, Sande MA. Contemporary issues in infectious diseases: new surgical and medical approaches in infectious diseases. New York: Churchill Livingstone, 1987.
17. Weigelt JA. Risk of wound infections in trauma patients. Am J Surg 1985;150:782–784.
18. Anonymous. Antimicrobial prophylaxis in surgery [Editorial]. Med Lett 1987;29:91–94.
18a. Kernodle DS, Classen DC, Burke JP, Kaiser AB. Failure of cephalosporins to prevent *Staphylococcus aureus* surgical wound infections. JAMA 1990;263:961–966.
18b. Scott SM, Sethi GK, Takaro T, Enright TJ. Thoracic surgical infections. In: Howard RJ, Simmons RL, eds. Surgical infectious diseases. Norwalk CT: Appleton & Lange, 1988:515–557.
19. Grover FL, Richardson J, Fewel JG, et al. Prophylactic antibiotics in the treatment of penetrating chest wounds: a prospective double blinded study. J Thorac Cardiovasc Surg 1977;74:528–536.

20. Stone HH, Symbas PN, Hooper CA. Cefamandole for prophylaxis against infection in closed tube thoracostomy. J Trauma 1981;21:975–977.

20a. Eddy AC, Luna GK, Copass M. Empyema thoracis in patients undergoing emergent closed tube thoracostomy for thoracic trauma. Am J Surg 1989;157:494–497.

21. Caplan ES, Hoyt NJ, Rodriguez A, Cowley RA. Empyema occurring in the multiply traumatized patient. J Trauma 1984;24:85–89.

22. Miller KS, Sahn SA. Chest tubes: indications, technique, management, and complications. Chest 1987;258–264.

23. Craven DE, Connolly MG Jr, Lichtenberg DA, et al. Contamination of mechanical ventilators with tubing changes every 24 or 48 hours. N Engl J Med 1982;306:1505–1509.

24. Cooper DKC. The incidence of postoperative infection and the role of antibiotic prophylaxis in pulmonary surgery. Br J Dis Chest 1981;75:154–160.

25. Feeley TW, DuMouln GC, Hedley-Whyte J, et al. Aerosol polymyxin and pneumonia in seriously ill patients. N Engl J Med 1975;293:471–475.

26. Lode H, Goecke J, Peg-endotracheal Gentamicin Study Group. Endotracheal application of gentamicin: randomized placebo-controlled-double-blind study in ventilated patients. Presented at the 28th Interscience Conference on Antimicrobial Agents and Chemotherapy, Los Angeles, 1988.

27. Sanders CC,Sanders WE Jr. Emergence of resistance during therapy with the newer beta-lactam antibiotics: role of inducible beta-lactamases and implications for the future. Rev Infect Dis 1983;5:639–648.

28. StoutenBeek CP, van Saene HKF, Miranda DR, Zandstra DF, Langrehr D. Nosocomial gram-negative pneumonia in critically ill patients: a 3-year experience with a novel therapeutic regimen. Intensive Care Med 1986;12:419–423.

29. Ledingham IM, Eastaway AT, McKay IC, Alcock Sr, McDonald JC, Ramsay G. Triple regimen of selective decontamination of the digestive tract, systemic cefotaxime, and microbiological surveillance for prevention of acquired infection in intensive care. Lancet 1988;1:785–790.

30. StoutenBeek CP, van Saene HKF, Miranda DR, Zandstra DF. The effect of selective decontamination of the digestive tract on colonization and infection rate in multiple trauma patients. Intensive Care Med 1984;10:185–192.

31. StoutenBeek CP, van Saene HKF, Miranda DR, Zandstra DF, Langrehr D. The effect of oropharyngeal decontamination using topical nonabsorable antibiotics on the incidence of nosocomial respiratory tract infections in multiple trauma patients. J Trauma 1987;27:357–364.

32. StoutenBeek CP, van Saene HKF, Zandstra DF. The effect of non-absorable antibiotics on the emergence of resistant bacteria in patients in an intensive care unit. J Antimicrob Chemother 1987;19:513–520.

33. Craven DE. Nosocomial pneumonia: new concepts on an old disease. Infect Control Hosp Epidemiol 1988;9:57–58.

34. Driks MR, Craven DE, Celli BA, et al. Nosocomial pneumonia in intubated patients randomized to sucralfate versus antacids and/or histamine type 2 blockers: the role of gastric colonization. N Engl J Med 1987;317:1376–1382.

35. Flaherty J, Nathan C, Kabins SA, Weinstein RA. Nonabsorbable antibiotics versus sucralfate in preventing colonization and infection in a cardiac surgery intensive-care unit [Abstract]. Presented at the 28th Interscience Conference on Antimicrobial Agents and Chemotherapy, Los Angeles, 1988.

36. Danziger L, Hassan E. Antimicrobial prophylaxis of gastrointestinal surgical procedures and treatment of intraabdominal infections. Drug Intell Clin Pharm 1987;21:415–416.

37. Bell G, Smith J, Murphy J. Prophylactic antibiotics in elective colon surgery. Surgery 1983;93:204–208.

38. Drusano GL, Warren JW, Saah AJ, et al. A prospective, randomized controlled trial of cefoxitin versus clindamycin-aminoglycoside in mixed anaerobic-aerobic infections. Surg Gynecol Obstet 1982;154:715–720.

39. Gentry LO, Feliciano DV, Lea AS, et al. Perioperative antibiotic therapy for penetrating injuries of the abdomen. Ann Surg 1984;200:561–566.

40. Oreskovich MR, Dellinger EP, Lennard ES, Wertz M, Carico CJ, Minshew BH. Duration of preventive antibiotic administration for penetrating abdominal trauma. Arch Surg 1982;117:200–205.

41. Hofstetter SR, Pachter HL, Bailey AA, Copa GF. A prospective comparison of two regimens of prophylactic antibiotics in abdominal trauma: cefoxitin versus triple drug. J Trauma 1984;24:307–310.

42. Mbawa NC, Rose RR, Schumer W. Evaluation of the efficacy of cefoxitin in the prevention of abdominal trauma infections. Am Surg 1983;49:582–585.

43. Rowlands BJ, Ericsson CD. Comparative studies of antibiotic therapy after penetrating abdominal trauma. Am J Surg 1984;148:791–795.

44. Falcone RE, Carey LC. Colorectal trauma. In: Ravo B, Khubchandani IT, eds. The surgical clinics of North America. Philadelphia: Saunders, 1988;68:1307–1318.

45. Sarr MG, Gott L, Townsend TR. Mediastinal infection after cardiac surgery. Ann Thorac Surg 1984;38:415–423.

46. Bor DH, Rose RM, Modlin JF, Weintraub R, Friedland GH. Mediastinitis after cardiovascular surgery. Rev Infect Dis 1983;5:885–896.

47. Tavares S, Hankins JR, Moulton AL, et al. Management of penetrating cardiac injuries: the role of emergency room thoracotomy. Ann Thorac Surg 1984;38:183–187.

48. Carroll CL, Jeffrey RB, Federle MP, Vernacchia FS. CT evaluation of mediastinal infections. J Comput Assist Tomogr 1987;11:449–454.

48a. Loop FD, Lytle BW, Cosgrove DM, et al. Sternal wound complications after isolated coronary artery bypass grafting: early and late mortality, morbidity, and cost of care. Ann Thorac Surg 1990;49:179–187.

48b. Vander Salm TJ, Okike ON, Pasque MK, et al. Reduction of sternal infection by application of topical vancomycin. J Thorac Cardiovasc Surg 1989;98:618–622.

49. Voiriot P, Marcoux JA, Duperval R, Teijera J. Staphylococcus aureus mediastinitis: prognostic usefulness of early medicosurgical therapy. Infect Control 1987;8:325–328.

50. Maki DG, Weise CE, Sarafin HW. A semiquantitative method for identifying intravenous-catheter-related infections. N Engl J Med 1977;296:1305–1309.

51. Cooper GL, Hopkins CC. Rapid diagnosis of intravascular catheter-associated infection by direct Gram staining of catheter segments. N Engl J Med 1985;312:1142–1147.

52. Roddy LH, Unger KM, Miller WC. Thoracic computed tomography in the critically ill patient. Crit Care Med 1981;9:515–518.

53. Mirvis SE, Rodriguez A, Whitley NO, Tarr RJ. CT evaluation of thoracic infections after major trauma. AJR 1985;144:1183–1187.

54. van-Deventer SJ, Buller HR, ten Cate JW, Sturk A, Pauw W. Endotoxemia: an early predictor of septicaemia in febrile patients. Lancet 1988;1:605–609.

55. Dellinger EP. Use of scoring systems to assess patients with surgical sepsis. Surg Clin North Am 1988;68:123–145.

56. Drusano GL, Schimpff SC, Hewitt WL. The acylampicillins: mezlocillin, piperacillin, and azlocillin. Rev Infect Dis 1984;6:13–32.

57. Joshi M, Cielsa E, Caplan ES. Diagnosis of pneumonia in the critically ill patient. American College of Chest Physicians. Anaheim, CA, 1988.

57a. Fink MP, Helsmoortel CM, Stein KL, Lee PC, Cohn SM. the efficacy of an oscillating bed in the prevention of lower respiratory tract infections in critically ill victims of blunt trauma: a prospective study. Chest 1990;97:132–137.

58. Kerver AJH, Rommes H, Mevissen-Verhage A, et al. Colonization and infection in surgical intensive care patients—a prospective study. Intensive Care Med 1987;13:347–351.

59. Johnason W, Pierce A, Sanford J. Changing pharyngeal bacterial flora of hospitalized patients: emergence of gram-negative bacilli [Study]. N Engl J Med 1969;281:1137–1140.

60. Johnason W, Pierce A, Sandord J, et al. Nosocomial respiratory infection with gram-negtive bacilli. Ann Intern Med 1972;77:701–706.

61. Berger K, Arango L. Etiologic diagnosis of bacterial nosocomial pneumonia in seriously ill patients. Crit Care Med 1985;13:833–836.

62. Schwartz SN, Dowling JN, Benkovic C, DeQuittner-Buchanan M, Protsko T, Yee RB. Sources of Gram-negative bacilli colonizing the tracheae of intubated patients. J Infect Dis 1978;158:227–231.

63. Dasta JF, Armstrong DK. Variability in aminoglycoside pharmacokinetics in critically ill surgical patients. Crit Care Med 1988;16:327–330.

64. Klastersky J, Thys JP. Local antibiotic therapy for bronchopneumonia. In: Pennington JE, ed. Respiratory infections: diagnosis and management. New York: Raven Press, 1983:481–489.

65. Caplan ES, Hoyt N. Nosocomial sinusitis. JAMA 1982;247:639–641.

66. Deutschman CS, Wilton PB, Sinow J, Thienprasit P, Konstantinides FN, Cerra FB. Paranasal sinusitis: a common complication of nasotracheal intubation in neurosurgical patients. Neurosurgery 1985;17:296–299.

67. Lew D, Southwick FS, Montgomery WW, et al. Sphenoid sinusitis. A review of 30 cases. N Engl J Med 1983;309:1149–1154.

68. Stillwell MS, Caplan ES. The septic multiple-trauma patient. Crit Care Clin 1988;4:345–373.

68a. Plit ML, Lipman J, Eidelman J, Gavoudan J. Catheter related infection: a plea for consensus with review and guidelines. Intensive Care Med 1988;14:503–509.

69. Sherertz RJ, Falk RJ, Huffman KA, et al. Infections associated with subclavian Udall catheters. Arch Intern Med 1983;143:52–56.

70. Hampton AA, Sherertz RJ. Vascular access infections in hospitalized patients. Surg Clin North Am 1988;68:57–71.
70a. Snyder RH, Archer EJ, Endy T, et al. Catheter infection: a comparison of two catheter maintenance techniques. Ann Surg 1988;208:651–653.
71. Maki DG, Ringer M. Evaluation of dressing regimens for prevention with peripheral intravenous catheters. Gauze, a transparent polyurethane dressing, and an indoor-transparent dressing. JAMA 1987;258:2396–2403.
72. Maki DG, Cobb L, Garman JK, et al. An attachable silver-impregnated cuff for prevention of infection with central venous catheters: a prospective randomized multicenter trial. Am J Med 1988;85:307–314.
72a. Norwood SH, Cormier B, McMahon NG, Moss A, Moore V. Prospective study of catheter-related infection during prolonged arterial catheterization. Crit Care Med 1988;16:836–839.
73. Ehni WF, Reller LB. Short-course therapy for catheter-associated Staphylococcus aureus bacteremia. Arch Intern Med 1989;149:533–536.
74. Warren JW. Catheter-associated urinary tract infections. In: Moellering R, ed. Infectious disease clinics of North America. Philadelphia: Saunders, 1987;1:823–854.
75. Kunin CM, McCormack RC. Prevention of catheter-induced urinary-tract infections by sterile closed drainage. N Engl J Med 1986;274:1155.
76. Clark LW. Neomycin in the prevention of postcatheterizatin bacteriuria. Med J Aust 1973;1:1034–1036.
77. Gantz NM. Urinary catheter-related infections. In: Gantz NM, Gleckman RA, Brown RB, Esposito AL, eds. Manual of clinical problems in infectious disease. Boston: Little, Brown, 1986:237–244.
78. Akiyama H, Okamoto S. Prophylaxis of indwelling urethral catheter infection: clinical experience with a modified Foley catheter and drainage system. J Urol 1979;121:40–42.

8 Heart Assist Devices in Cardiothoracic Trauma

Safuh Attar, MD
John R. Hankins, MD

Heart assist devices have become useful adjuncts to the management of the postcardiotomy syndrome in patients who cannot be weaned from the heart lung machine following open heart surgery, in transplant patients awaiting a suitable heart donor, in babies with respiratory distress syndrome, and in patients with acute cardiogenic shock complicating myocardial infarction. The use of ventricular assist devices in cardiothoracic injuries is still in its infancy, requiring definition of the indications and contraindications for its application.

Ventricular heart assist devices provide circulatory support for normal life to patients with severe cardiothoracic trauma. They are intended to "buy time" while a definitive diagnosis and/or treatment is being established. For this purpose, only temporary heart assist devices are used.

A large number of cardiac assist devices have been developed. Although quite varied in approach, they all have one basic objective: to assist the heart in maintaining the circulation. Essential prerequisites for such a system are simplicity, ease of connection with the circulation, and initiation of mechanical support; thus, complicated intracorporeal systems are excluded.

An extracorporeal pump that can be connected rapidly to the circulatory system without the need for anticoagulation would be ideal. Rose et al. (1) utilized veno-arterial bypass using the roller pump to support patients who could not be weaned from cardiopulmonary bypass. Another system that has been used extensively in the clinical setting is the centrifugal pump (Bio-pump, Biomedicus) (Fig. 8.1) (2). In the Bio-pump, the blood passes through a vortex created by the spinning motion of smooth rotator cones, which are made of nonthrombogenic acrylics. They impart a circular motion to the blood, generating centrifugal force, pressure, and flow. The hydrodynamically designed flow path of the pump eliminates turbulence, cavitation, and resulting damage to the blood elements. A magnetic drive and solid-housing design prohibit air and contaminant induction.

Other pump systems that have been used for temporary ventricular assistance include the Pierce-Donachy Pennsylvania blood pump (Fig. 8.2) (3). It is an extracorporeally placed pneumatic pump. A flexible segmental polyurethane blood sac with a seam-free, highly smooth internal surface is enclosed within a rigid polysulfone

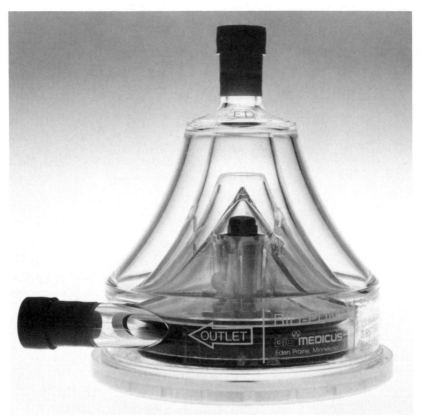

Figure 8.1.   The Biomedicus centrifugal pump.

case. The inner chamber of the case is in the shape of an oblate spheroid. A flexible diaphragm transects the frontal plane of the outer case, separating the air inlet port from the thin-walled blood sac. Bjork-Shiley disc valves are used to provide unidirectional flow. The pump is run in a full-to-empty mode, since this provides maximum washout of the blood sac, thus decreasing the possibility of thrombus formation. The stroke volume is 65 ml.

A new miniature cable-driven axial flow pump, the Hemo-pump (Fig. 8.3) (Nimbus Medical, Rancho Cordova, CA) has been developed to provide active left ventricular assistance (4). Dr. Richard K. Wampler invented this pump after watching water pumps in Africa that used the Archimedes principle. First described by Archimedes as a means of pumping water, a practical application of this principle employs a screw turning in a cylinder, which causes water to rise from a lower level to a higher one. This concept was applied by Wampler to develop a rotational pump using axial flow technology (4).

The Hemo-pump system consists of disposable elements and a control console. The disposable pumping system comprises an inlet cannula, an axial flow blood pump, a drive cable contained in a polymeric sheath, and a motor rotor and bearing set (Fig. 8.4). The inlet cannula, blood pump, and a portion of the sheath are inserted in the femoral artery and advanced through the aorta until the cannula has passed retrograde through the aortic valve, with the tip positioned within the left ventricle (Fig. 8.5). The Hemo-pump blood pump is a size 21 French axial flow device with a 20-cm inlet

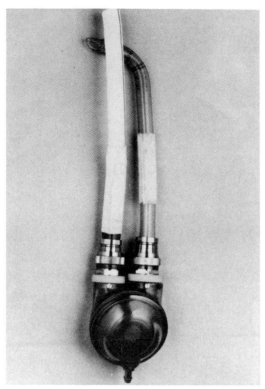

Figure 8.2.   The Pierce-Donachy pump.

cannula (Fig. 8.6). The blood flow through the pump is illustrated in Figure 8.5. Blood is withdrawn from the left ventricle and discharged from the pump into the descending aorta. The pump is driven by a flexible cable that is enclosed in a size 9 French sheath. The sheath also serves as a conduit for a 40% dextrose purge fluid. The fluid lubricates the drive cable and hydrodynamic bearings, which support the rotating elements of the device. The Hemo-pump control console (Fig. 8.3) is a 25-pound unit that contains the roller pump that is responsible for the delivery and collection of the 40% dextrose solution, motor control electronics, monitor alarm, and replaceable rechargeable batteries for back-up. The pump is capable of generating 0.5–3.0 liters/min of nonpulsatile, continuous blood flow at up to 25,000 rpm. Use of the Hemo-pump is contraindicated in patients with significant blood dyscrasias, patients with known dissecting thoracic and abdominal aortic aneurysms, patients with severe disease of the aortic wall, patients with severe aortic valve stenosis and/or insufficiency, and patients in whom the femoral artery cannot be dilated for insertion of the size 21 French cannula. The latter contraindication does not apply when smaller cannulas (which are being developed) become available.

INDICATIONS

Indications for the use of heart assist devices in cardiothoracic trauma are not yet well-defined. Mattox and Beall (5) reported the use of portable cardiopulmonary bypass in 10 patients with massive thoracic trauma: two had extensive tracheobronchial injury, two had extensive injury to the pulmonary veins or arteries, and five had cardiac

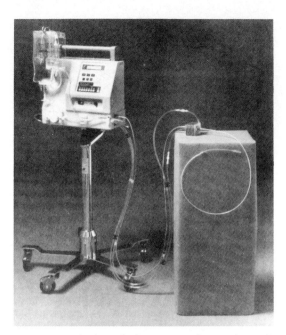

Figure 8.3. The Hemo-pump, which includes a control console, a disposable pump, and a disposable purge assembly. (Courtesy of Richard K. Wampler and the American Society for Artificial Internal Organs.) (From Wampler RK, Moise JC, Frazier H, Olsen DB. In vivo evaluation of peripheral vascular access axial flow blood pump. Trans Am Soc Artif Intern Organs 1988;34:450–454).

injuries. None of these patients could be resuscitated by routine measures. Phillips et al. (6, 7) reported on four patients with massive trauma in whom resuscitation was attempted via percutaneous cardiopulmonary bypass. All four died of uncontrollable hemorrhage during the resuscitation attempts.

In defining the indications for ventricular assist devices, several patient groups can be identified. Candidates for this support include patients sustaining massive cardiothoracic trauma and presenting in critical condition, such as in shock, and not responding to standard resuscitative measures; those in cardiac arrest with cerebral function, in whom the diagnosis is not clear; and victims of accidental hypothermia. The contraindication to cardiopulmonary resuscitation and ventricular assistance in trauma is the presence of significant bleeding. Intracranial hemorrhage, gastrointestinal hemorrhage, as well as active bleeding from other organs constitute absolute contraindications to the use of heart assist devices. This contraindication is not related to the use of heparin (since some pumps such as the Biomedicus pump do not require heparinization) but to the advisability of controlling the bleeding prior to the consideration of the use of the assist device.

TECHNIQUE

Percutaneous cannulation of the femoral artery and vein is carried out with the patient under local anesthesia, using the Seldinger technique (Fig. 8.7). If the femoral pulse cannot be palpated because of shock or cardiac arrest, the femoral vessels are exposed by a cutdown. A guide wire is introduced through an angiographic needle into the

Hemo-pump assembly

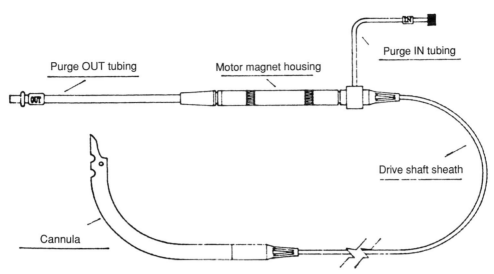

Figure 8.4. The disposable pumping system. (Courtesy of Richard K. Wampler and the American Society for Artificial Internal Organs.) (From Wampler RK, Moise JC, Frazier H, Olsen DB. In vivo evaluation of peripheral vascular access axial flow blood pump. Trans Am Soc Artif Intern Organs 1988;34:450–454.)

femoral vessel. A size 20 French multihole catheter is passed over the guide wire into the inferior vena cava and then to the right atrium. A size 18–20 French catheter is next inserted over a guide wire placed in the right femoral artery and advanced to the distal aorta. Both cannulas are then connected to the ventricular assist system, which consists of a pump and oxygenator.

The Biomedicus pump has the advantage of simplicity, availability, relatively low cost, less blood trauma, and little or no need for systemic heparinization. Flow rates of 3.0–5.0 liters/min can be achieved with this device. Pump flow rates through a flow meter are displayed digitally on the Bio console and are determined by the venous return. A compact cardiopulmonary support system is commercially available through Bard. Such a system has been used successfully at the University of Maryland Hospital for short-term support while performing percutaneous angioplasty and aortic valvuloplasty in 15 patients with poor ventricular function (8).

The use of the ventricular assist device system can be extended up to 2 weeks, as shown in the postcardiotomy support group, with a survival rate of 48%. The most frequent complication is bleeding. Pennington (9) reported that half of his patients supported with the Biomedicus pump had thrombi in the vortex pump system. Other complications include hemolysis and infection.

DISCUSSION

Ventricular assist devices have proven to be very useful in postcardiotomy ventricular failure, as a bridge to heart transplantation, and in respiratory distress syndrome. In the absence of myocardial ischemia, left ventricular assist results in significant reduction in systolic fractional shortening, reflecting systolic unloading; significant reduction in left ventricular end diastolic pressure; maintenance of aortic pressure while cardiac work is

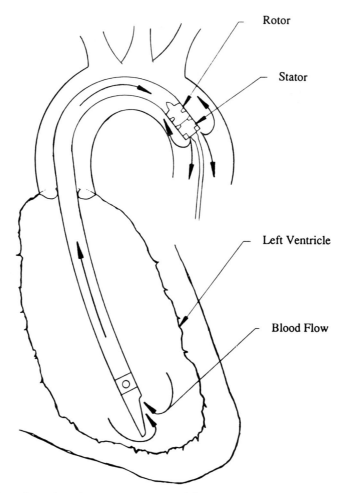

Rotor

Stator

Left Ventricle

Blood Flow

Figure 8.5. Pumping principle: Hemo-pump axial flow pump. The pump's position in the left ventricle. (Courtesy of Richard K. Wampler and the American Society for Artificial Internal Organs.) (From Wampler RK, Moise JC, Frazier H, Olsen DB. In vivo evaluation of peripheral vascular access axial flow blood pump. Trans Am Soc Artif Intern Organs 1988;34:450–454.)

decreased; and significant reduction in myocardial perfusion, which is secondary to decreased metabolic demands of the unloaded heart. In the presence of myocardial ischemia, there is a favorable distribution of blood flow in the heart; reduced cardiac work; diastolic unloading of the heart, manifested by reduced left ventricular end diastolic pressure; and maintenance of aortic pressure (10). The value of the ventricular assist system in cardiothoracic trauma is still to be determined. So far it has had limited application. Mattox (5) reported the use of portable cardiopulmonary bypass in 10 patients with massive cardiothoracic trauma. Eight of the 10 had control of hemorrhage and repair, allowing bypass to be discontinued. Two of these patients had sustained transection of the proximal left anterior descending artery. Phillips (7) reported the use of percutaneous cardiopulmonary bypass in four patients with massive trauma. All four died of uncontrollable hemorrhage during the resuscitation attempts.

The largest application of this modality of therapy has been in the resuscitation of

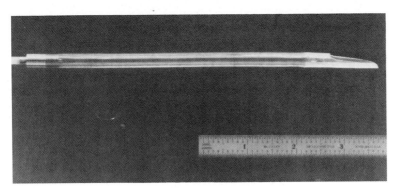

Figure 8.6. The Hemo-pump blood pump. (Courtesy of Richard K. Wampler and the American Society for Artificial Internal Organs.) (From Wampler RK, Moise JC, Frazier H, Olsen DB. In vivo evaluation of peripheral vascular access axial flow blood pump. Trans Am Soc Artif Intern Organs 1988;34:450–454.)

accidental hypothermia victims. At the present time, over 40 patients with profound hypothermia who were resuscitated with cardiopulmonary bypass have been reported in the literature (11). The survival rate in this collection of independent reports is 55%. The largest reported series resulted from the Mt. Hood disaster of 1986, when 10 patients were treated by cardiopulmonary bypass, with a survival rate of 20% (11). This contradicts the earlier studies that demonstrated nearly complete success with

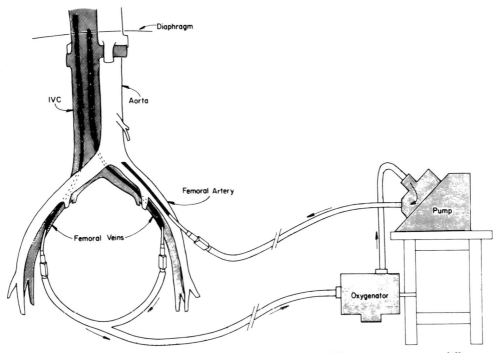

Figure 8.7. Perfusion system for percutaneous femoral-femoral bypass. At present, a different kind of oxygenator located at a different position is an option. (Courtesy of Steven J. Phillips, B. Ballantine and D. Slonine.) (Reprinted with permission from The Society of Thoracic Surgeons, THE ANNALS OF THORACIC SURGERY, Vol. 36, 1983, pp 223–225.)

cardiopulmonary bypass in hypothermia. The patients at Mt. Hood had the lowest core temperatures (mean, 17.8°C) of any group in the literature.

The Hemo-pump is still in the investigative stage. Its use has been limited to patients with cardiogenic shock secondary to myocardial infarction. Rutan et al. have accomplished six successful insertions (12). Sixty-seven percent of the patients were weaned from the device, with a survival rate of 50%. When compared with a mortality rate of more than 80% in patients with cardiogenic shock, it appears that the Hemo-pump is a very promising tool in the treatment of patients requiring ventricular assistance.

REFERENCES

1. Rose DM, Colvin SB, Culliford AT, et al. Long term survival with partial left heart bypass following perioperative myocardial infarction and shock. J Thorac Cardiovasc Surg 1982;83:483–492.
2. Olivier HF Jr, Maher TD, Liebler GA, Park SB, Burkholder JA, Magovern GJ. Use of the Biomedicus centrifugal pump in traumatic tears of the thoracic aorta. Ann Thorac Surg 1984;38:586–591.
3. Gaines WE, Pierce WS. Left and right ventricular assistance for postoperative cardiogenic shock. In: Attar S, ed. New developments in cardiac assist devices. New York: Praeger, 1985.
4. Wampler RK, Moise JC, Frazier OH, Olson DB. In vitro evaluation of a peripheral vascular access axial flow blood pump. Trans Am Soc Artif Intern Organs 1988;34:450–454.
5. Mattox KL, Beall AC Jr. Resuscitation of the moribund patients using portable cardiopulmonary bypass. Ann Thorac Surg 1976;22:436–442.
6. Phillips SJ, Ballantine B, Slonine D, et al. Percutaneous initation of cardiopulmonary bypass. Ann Thorac Surg 1983;36:223–225.
7. Phillips SJ, Zeff RH, Kongtahworn C, et al. Percutaneous cardiopulmonary bypass: application and indication for use. Ann Thorac Surg 1989;47:121–123.
8. Vogel RA. The Maryland experience: angioplasty and valvuloplasty using percutaneous cardiopulmonary support. Am J Cardiol 1988;62:11K–14K.
9. Pennington DG, Joyce LD, Pae WE Jr, Burkholder JA. Patient selection (for ventricular assist devices). Ann Thorac Surg 1989;47:77–81.
10. Merhige ME, Smalling RW, Cassidy D, Barrett R, Wise G, Short J, Wampler RK. Effect of the Hemo-pump left ventricular assist device on regional myocardial perfusion and function. Circulation Suppl. Part 2, 1989;80:III-158–III-160.
11. Hauty MG, Esrig BC, Hill JG, Long WB. Prognostic factors in severe accidental hypothermia: experience from the Mt. Hood tragedy. J Trauma 1987;27:1107–1112.
12. Rutan PM, Rountree WD, Myers KK, Barker LE. Initial experience with the Hemo-pump. Crit Care Nursing Clin North Am 1989;1:527–534.

9 Injuries of the Chest Wall, the Lungs, and the Pleura

Aurelio Rodriguez, MD

INJURIES OF THE CHEST WALL

Chest wall injuries are one of the most common thoracic injuries seen in trauma care, representing 50–70% of them (1). Their magnitude and severity vary greatly. Kemmerer et al. (2) evaluated 585 patients who died as a result of thoracic trauma and found that 35% of them had relevant rib fractures and 5% had sternal fractures. The correlation between the number of rib fractures and the intrathoracic and intraabdominal pathology has been emphasized by several authors (3–5).

Pathophysiology

Penetrating trauma is inflicted by assaults with knives and guns. Stab wounds usually are not so severe unless the intercostal or internal mammary arteries are lacerated. The morbidity and mortality associated with gunshot wounds and shotgun blasts depend on the velocity of the missile and the distance between the muzzle and the victim.

The main mechanisms of blunt injury to the chest wall are direct impact and shearing forces. Other less common forces are deceleration and rotation. A combination of the above can be seen in the so-called crushing injury with its consequent great increase in morbidity and mortality. Several studies (5, 6) have shown that the severity of chest wall injury correlates very well with the characteristics and intensity of the impact, with the use of restraining devices, and last, but not least, with the age of the patient.

Rib Injuries

Rib injuries are the most common of all chest injuries (5–7). Fractures of the ribs occur more frequently in adults than in children, due to differences in anatomic structures. Children's ribs have a resilient cartilaginous nature and are less likely to break; older individuals have more brittle and breakable ribs. The weakest point on impact is the posterior angle, while the 5th to the 9th ribs are the most commonly broken. Fracture of the 10th to the 12th ribs should raise the possibility of liver or spleen injuries (5, 6).

DIAGNOSIS

The diagnosis of rib fractures is mostly clinical, since approximately 50% of them cannot be visualized in the initial chest roentgenogram (8) without often bulky techniques (Figs. 9.1 and 9.2). Pain and localized tenderness are usually severe during the first 3

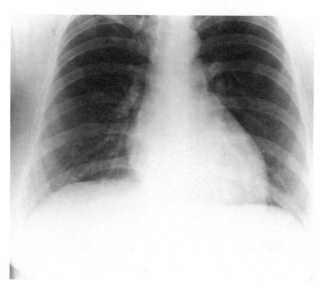

Figure 9.1.   Chest x-ray film of a blunt trauma patient. Fractured ribs are not visible.

days and subside almost completely in 3–4 weeks. The presence of subcutaneous emphysema is generally accompanied by a pneumothorax. However, in some cases, due to the symphysis of the parietal to the visceral pleura caused by a previous inflammatory process, a pneumothorax is not apparent in the initial chest roentgenogram and sequential series are required for its visualization.

TREATMENT

The treatment of rib fractures depends upon the number involved and the underlying pathology. A single rib fracture is more likely to be managed by oral analgesics. However, the presence of multiple injured ribs usually mandates the use of intercostal nerve blocks, transcutaneous nerve stimulators, and the recently demonstrated advantage of epidural and/or intrapleural analgesics. The techniques and indications are discussed in Chapter 5. Coughing, nasotracheal suction, physiotherapy (including fiberoptic bronchoscopy) should be included as part of the management of rib fractures in order to prevent atelectasis and pneumonia.

The morbidity and mortality are usually related to inherent anatomic and physiologic complications. Atelectasis, pneumonia, hemopneumothorax, massive hemothorax, and intraabdominal injuries may complicate the clinical picture. Hypoventilation may occur secondary to decreased residual capacity and respiratory failure.

FIRST AND SECOND RIB FRACTURES

Because of the remarkable protection of these two ribs by the clavicle, scapula, humerus, and soft tissue, the kinetic force capable of disrupting their anatomy is thought to be tremendous. Some authors (9–13) have found a significant association of that pathology with injuries of the subclavian artery and vein and of the brachial plexus and thoracic aortic rupture. We have been unable to find this correlation (5). However, we

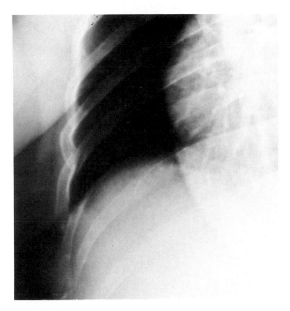

Figure 9.2.   Fractured ribs: special x-ray view.

emphasize the importance of the alertness of the physician who encounters those injuries and the need for a systematic examination for vascular or neurologic injuries.

Costochondral Injuries

Separation or fractures of the costochondral junction are not rare. The diagnosis is made by pain that is usually more severe and persistent than that associated with regular rib fractures. An elicited clicking sensation during respiration helps to corroborate the diagnosis, since these injuries cannot be visualized on the chest roentgenogram. The treatment is the same as for rib fractures, except, when the pain is chronic and incapacitating, part of the cartilage may be removed surgically.

Fractures of the Sternum

Fractures of the sternum are being reported with increasing frequency, particularly since the most common cause of this injury is the impact of the victim's chest with a steering wheel. As is the case with rib fractures, sternum fractures are more common in the elderly and usually are transverse. An increase in the incidence of associated injuries (e.g., pulmonary contusion, tracheobronchial tree disruption, and myocardial contusion) is appearing in the literature (14–18).

DIAGNOSIS

The clinical diagnosis is based on pain and localized tenderness. Lateral or oblique sternal radiographic views are necessary most of the time (Fig. 9.3).

TREATMENT

The treatment varies depending on the degree of deformity and cardioventilatory impairment. The only indication for surgical correction is severe deformation or

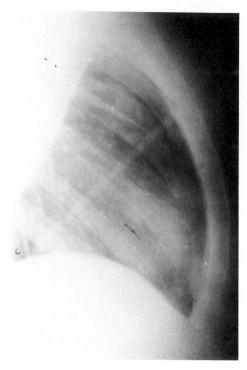

Figure 9.3. Lateral chest roentgenogram reveals fractured sternum.

intolerable pain. The procedure is done through a vertical incision, with horizontal wiring of the fracture and attention being given to the protection of the heart (Fig. 9.4).

Scapular Fracture

This is an uncommon fracture that implies a massive energetic impact. Other associated injuries should be sought (8), particularly injuries of the ipsilateral lung, shoulder girdle, subclavian and axillary artery, and brachial plexus. Young adults are more often the victim of this pathology. The most common mechanisms of injury are motor vehicle accidents, motorcycle accidents, and falls (19). The body of the scapula is the most frequent site of fracture, followed by the neck and glenoid; the spine, coracoid, and acromion are less frequently involved.

The diagnosis is often overlooked: 20–30% of these injuries are not diagnosed at the time of admission (8). Radiologic diagnosis of scapular fracture requires the proper views: a true anteroposterior view of the scapula (Fig. 9.5), followed by a true lateral view (Y view), having the coracoid process and the spine-acromion process as the upper limbs and the body of the scapula as the vertical limb. Occasionally, the need to visualize the coracoid process requires projection of the beam 60° cephalad in the infraclavicular area (20).

The treatment is usually conservative. The patient should be started on early passive range-of-motion exercises with a progression to active range-of-motion exercises. Excellent results have been reported with this method (19). Unless there is significant involvement of the glenoid fossa or acromion, open reduction and internal fixation is recommended (21). Even patients with isolated scapular fractures should be admitted

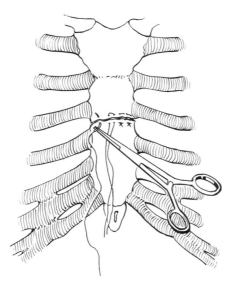

Figure 9.4. Surgical repair of fractured sternum.

to the hospital in order to monitor them for late presentation of pneumothorax or hemothorax.

Flail Chest

Flail chest is one of the most potentially fatal injuries in trauma. Its incidence has increased markedly in the past 20 years and is related to the overwhelming increase of automobile accidents, its major cause. The flail chest segment most commonly found is the lateral, but anterior or posterior sections can also be involved.

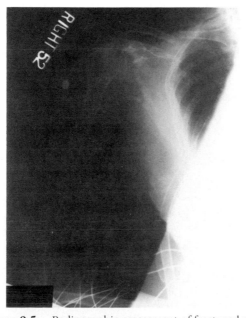

Figure 9.5. Radiographic assessment of fractured scapula.

PATHOPHYSIOLOGY

The disruption of more than three ribs with or without costochondral junction involvement, the presence of pain, and, particularly, an underlying lung contusion are responsible for the severe derangements of respiratory physiology found in the clinical manifestations of flail chest.

The "pendelluft" or pendulum-like movements have long been disregarded as the mechanism causing these alterations (22, 23). However, during inspiration, the flailing portion of the chest wall fails to expand, and this part subsequently is driven inward into the chest by atmospheric pressure and increased intranegative pressure. On expiration, an opposite mechanism causes outward projection of the flailing segment due to a change in the ratio of intrathoracic pressure and atmospheric pressure.

Lung parenchymal injuries (lung contusion) produce alterations in the alveolar ventilation:perfusion ratios.

As a consequence of the pain associated with flail chest, the patient exhibits shallow inspiratory efforts and is unable to clear secretions (23, 24).

All of the physiologic alterations produced by the above mechanisms are manifested by

Decreased vital capacity
Decreased tidal volume
Decreased functional residual capacity
Decreased lung compliance
Increased shunting

These may lead to respiratory insufficiency, atelectasis, and pneumonia.

DIAGNOSIS

Several factors determine the clinical presentation of flail chest: the magnitude of the chest wall injury and the lung contusion as well as the premorbid status and pain tolerance of the patient. Chest wall pain, dyspnea, tachypnea, tachycardia, and even hypotension and cyanosis are the main clinical pictures. Good lighting and a tangential plane examination will allow the discovery of any paradoxic movement of the chest wall, even though this can be less apparent in posterior wall and upper anterior wall fractures. The chest roentgenogram usually reveals the associated injuries (lung contusion, pneumothorax, or hemothorax) but sometimes fails to demonstrate the flail segment (Fig. 9.6). Arterial blood gas evaluation is important to determine the magnitude of the physiologic respiratory alterations.

TREATMENT

The treatment of flail chest depends upon the degree of chest instability, the quantity of pain, the magnitude of lung contusions, and the extent of impairment of oxygenation and ventilation. Consequently, the goals in management of flail chest should be (*a*) stabilization of the chest wall, (*b*) control of pain, and (*c*) optimization of oxygenation. To accomplish all of these, the surgeon has to decide first if the patient needs mechanical ventilatory support. The combination of a respiratory rate > 35, a $PaCO_2$ > 50 mm Hg, and a PaO_2 < 60 mm Hg with supplemental oxygenation should be an indication for assisted mechanical ventilation (25–30), particularly if the patient has increased work of breathing. Since it usually takes 2–3 weeks for the flailing segment to stabilize, the patient should probably be on a respirator for this period of time, depending also

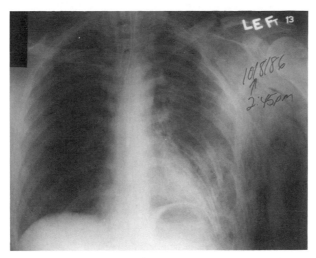

Figure 9.6.   Flail chest.

on the degree of lung contusion and presence of complications related to the respiratory support (e.g., barotrauma, respiratory sepsis). Also, at this initial point, the decision regarding the modality of pain control is imperative because, in some cases, a good pain management plan can avoid even mechanical ventilatory support if the patient does not exhibit the above criteria. Oral or intravenous analgesics (Chapter 5), transcutaneous nerve stimulator, and intercostal blocks have been used with variable results in the management of pain in patients with flail chest. However, epidural and intrapleural analgesics recently have had a tremendous impact and, at this point, are considered the most effective (31, 32).

Occasionally, internal stabilization of the chest wall disruption has been done, especially when the patient needs a thoracotomy for another reason. This has been accomplished with wires, plates, or staples (Fig. 9.7). Some European groups have shown significant patient improvement following the placement of fixator devices; this technique also avoids the complications of mechanical ventilatory support (33, 34).

The judicious use of fluids should be emphasized as part of the pulmonary contusion treatment. Steroid and diuretic administration still remains controversial. Continuous respiratory toilet is imperative. Sterile nasotracheal suctioning, fiberoptic bronchoscopy, and appropriate chest physiotherapy are invaluable in the total care of these patients.

INJURIES OF THE LUNG

The anatomic configuration of the lungs, with a broad area of contact with the anterior, lateral, and posterior chest wall, makes them frequently vulnerable to penetrating and blunt trauma of the thorax, the upper part of the abdomen, and even the lower portion of the neck. The evidence of lung injuries varies with the etiology. Gunshot and stab wounds are more preponderant in certain geographic areas, but, in general, the incidence is reported to be 60–80% among patients with penetrating thoracic wounds (35–37). In blunt trauma, 80% of the lesions are caused by motor vehicle accidents (5), 17% by falls, and 17% by cardipulmonary resuscitation and other events (5, 38). The

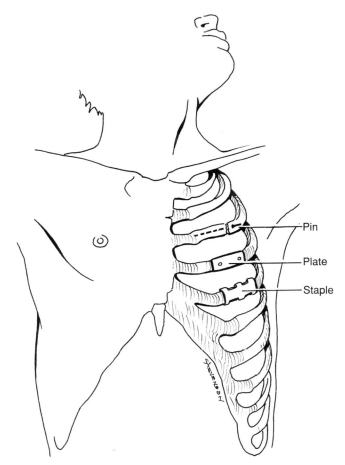

Figure 9.7. Techniques of internal fixation of flail chest.

mortality when there is an association between pulmonary contusion and flail chest is 40% (37).

Lung Contusion
PATHOPHYSIOLOGY

The high-energy dissipation produced by motor vehicle accidents, falls, or the secondary missiles in gunshot wounds is responsible for disruption of the microvasculature, interstitial extravasation, and alveolar flooding with red cells, plasma, and proteins. These derangements result in severe physiologic changes such as intrapulmonary shunting, which is partially compensated by hypoxic vasoconstriction. The decrease in compliance leads to hypoventilation and increased work of breathing. All of these have a major impact on gas exchange (39).

DIAGNOSIS

Lung contusion should be entertained in any patient with penetrating, blast, or blunt thoracic trauma, the latter usually being produced by a high-speed motor vehicle crash or a fall. Respiratory insufficiency and hemoptysis are not found as frequently as hemothorax or pneumothorax secondary to lung lacerations or pleural injuries.

Radiologic findings are directly related to the severity of the pulmonary contusion, although in the initial roentgenogram, this correlation may not exist. The radiologic findings vary tremendously in extension and appearance and occur abruptly—70% within 1 hr after injury and 30% with a lag time of 4–6 hr (8, 37). The subsequent presence of infiltrates despite an initial clear chest roentgenogram indicates that other pathology may be more likely: aspiration pneumonia or atelectasis (Fig. 9.8).

Recently, some authors (40) have suggested computed tomographic scanning as the most accurate available method for assessment of pulmonary contusions. They have elaborated a method of quantitating the degree of lung contusion and using that information to plan treatment and to predict outcome (Fig. 9.9).

One of the most important parameters in the clinical assessment and diagnosis of lung contusion is evaluation of arterial blood gases. Oxygenation usually is decreased and the $PaCO_2$ varies according to the degree of ventilatory impairment.

TREATMENT

The majority of lung contusions, when properly treated, show signs of resolution within 48–72 hr (39, 41). However, complete resolution could take 2–3 weeks.

The treatment and prognosis of patients with pulmonary contusion parallel the severity of lung injury. Unfortunately, many aspects of therapy are controversial and are discussed separately here.

Ventilatory Support and Monitoring

In the majority of cases, conservative management with supplemental oxygenation is all that is necessary. Several authors (27, 28, 42) have championed the selective management of patients with lung contusion and flail chest. Furthermore, they established criteria for ventilatory support in patients with lung contusions:

1. Ventilatory impairment—patient unable to maintain a vital capacity greater than 12 or 14 ml/kg, with difficulty in breathing, coughing, and clearing secretions.
2. Hypoxemia—patient unable to maintain a PaO_2/FIO_2 ratio greater than 300 or 350 without ventilatory support

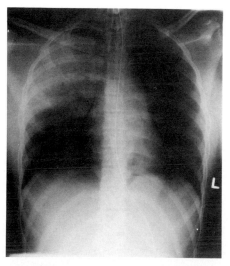

Figure 9.8.   Lung contusion.

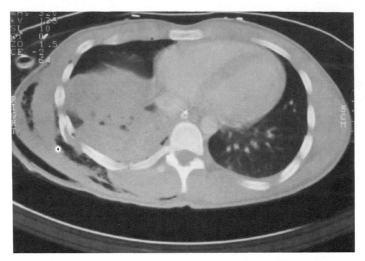

Figure 9.9. CT scans allow accurate assessments of lung contusion.

3. Head injuries
4. Shock
5. Major surgical procedures

However, for this subset of patients, ventilatory therapy can be challenging, particularly if the patient has extensive lung contusions. Because of the localized nature of the injury, the indiscriminate application of positive end expiratory pressure (PEEP) and continuous positive airway pressure (CPAP) could be harmful; this is a result of diffuse pressure in the entire lung with subsequent decrease of blood flow in ventilated alveoli, diversion of blood to less compliant alveoli, and increase of intrapulmonary shunt (43). These side effects can be avoided with continuous monitoring of ventilatory pressures and use of intermittent mandatory ventilation (IMV) with low PEEP.

Another important aspect in the management of patients with lung contusion is the need for close monitoring, particularly if they do not have ventilatory support. This should be done in an intensive care unit, with careful administration of fluid with the assistance of a Swan-Ganz catheter and active blood gas surveillance (43).

Fluid Administration

Recently, some authors, based on their own experiences and review of the experimental and clinical literature (43–45), have concluded that there is no evidence that administration of crystalloids, given in adequate volume to restore normal perfusion, is harmful to patients with pulmonary contusion. After all, the contusion should start clearing clinically and radiologically in 72 hr; if it does not, another complication—pneumonia or aspiration—should be suspected.

Steroids

Despite some experimental evidence of its benefits, no clinical justification for the routine use of steroids has been demonstrated (46, 47).

PROGNOSIS

The final outcome is more commonly related to associated injuries. Some determinants of outcome have been implicated: Injury Severity Score (ISS) > 25, Glasgow Coma Scale (GCS) score < 7, transfusion > 3 units, and PaO_2/FIO_2 ratio < 300.

No significant relationship has been found between outcome and shock, excess fluid administration, or extended ventilatory support (48). Furthermore, initial hypoxemia has not correlated with the final outcome.

Regression analysis of data from our facility showed that the overall mortality rate of 13% (49) is, in our view, not directly related to pulmonary contusion per se. It is more likely related to the adult respiratory distress syndrome, the volume of blood products received in 24 hr, the admission GCS score, and the age of the patient.

Traumatic Lung Pseudocyst (Traumatic Pneumatocele)

PATHOPHYSIOLOGY

Despite the varied terminology, the etiology is the same: penetrating or blunt trauma. The characteristic histopathology of this injury-induced cavity is the lack of bronchial wall elements, particularly epithelium. The frequency is variable; we have found 35 cases among patients admitted to our facility between 1975 and 1983 (50).

The pathophysiology is different in penetrating and blunt trauma. In the former, the path of the missile and the associated infection create the cavity. In blunt trauma, the increase of intrapulmonary pressure with an intact pleura and a closed glottis disrupts the pulmonary parenchyma. Whatever the mechanism of parenchymal disruption, small capillaries, vessels, and arteries are torn (50, 51). The blood accumulated in the site of the tear takes a rounded shape due to the elasticity of the lung parenchyma surrounding the lesion. When the air leaks into the tear, an air/fluid level cavity is found.

The lesions are usually located in the periphery of the lungs (50–52). It appears that children are particularly prone to develop pseudocysts (53). These lesions are single or unilocular but occasionally are multiple and multilocular.

DIAGNOSIS

The physical symptoms of chest pain, cough, hemoptysis, and mild fever can be elusive. Chest roentgenograms continue to be the cornerstone of diagnosis. However, it is necessary to emphasize the need for serial chest films daily, since the traumatic pseudocyst could appear several hours or days after injury. It is also advisable to obtain an erect x-ray film in blunt-injured patients to demonstrate the air/fluid level (see Chapter 4). The time span of radiographic appearance is from 7 days to 3 months.

CT scans are very helpful in identifying traumatic pseudocysts at a very early stage and in following their progression very closely (Fig. 9.10) (40).

The differential diagnosis should include congenital cyst, tuberculosis, fungal cavities, emphysematous blebs, necrotic neoplasms, and lung abscess. Some authors (50) make a distinction between pulmonary hematoma and lung pseudocyst. Hematomas usually persist longer (50).

TREATMENT

The treatment is conservative: postural drainage and chest physiotherapy. Antibiotics are not used routinely since only 15% of pseudocysts become infected.

The indications for surgery are (*a*) progressive pseudocyst enlargement with

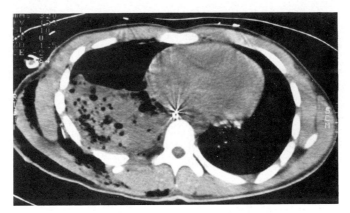

Figure 9.10. CT scan: contusion with traumatic lung cyst.

impairment of hemodynamic or ventilatory function and (*b*) an unresolved infected cyst with generalized sepsis.

OUTCOME

Most pseudocysts subside completely in 2 weeks. A small percentage may remain, and they need to be differentiated from coin lesions.

Pulmonary Lacerations

Despite the fact that pulmonary lacerations are not nearly as common as pulmonary contusions and are usually unrecognized (particularly in patients with blunt trauma), they could be a threat to life. The diagnosis should be entertained in any patient with penetrating or blunt trauma who presents with a varying degree of hemoptysis, air leak in the chest tube, and/or the characteristic radiologic picture of an ill-defined shadow with an upward convexity (Fig. 9.11).

PATHOPHYSIOLOGY

In blunt trauma, there appear to be two mechanisms: (*a*) direct piercing or tear of the lung parenchyma by fractured ribs and (*b*) indirect mechanism without rib fractures (usually the same sequence of events that produces lung contusion).

TREATMENT

Most of these lacerations, especially those due to penetrating trauma, are treated satisfactorily with the placement of a chest thoracostomy tube. In blunt trauma, however, in addition to the need to evacuate a pneumohemothorax and monitor arterial blood gases, continuous bleeding and massive air leak could be the most common indications for thoracotomy. At surgery, a major laceration can be controlled by sutures only, and, in 40% of cases, with formal lung resections. If air embolism is suspected, expeditious clamping of the hilum will prevent further entrance of air into the vascular system. Then the leak should be controlled and the anesthesiologist asked to use vasopressors, if possible, to flush the air out of the coronaries. Some authors have suggested the use of temporal systemic anticoagulation (8, 37, 38).

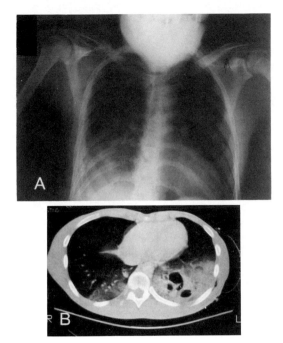

Figure 9.11.   A, the radiographic presentation of a pulmonary laceration is characteristic: an ill-defined shadow with an upward convexity. **B,** CT scan: lung contusion with laceration.

Pulmonary Hematoma

When blood accumulates in a lung laceration, a space-occupying lesion—a pulmonary hematoma—is created. It can manifest clinically with chest pain, hemoptysis, and/or low-grade fever. The differential diagnosis with lung contusion can be difficult; however, the radiographic appearance of pulmonary hematoma is more uncertain. These lesions are more dense; more centrally located, preferentially in the lower areas; and circumscribed, despite the fact that they can take any shape and be of any size (from 1–10 cm). Their radiographic resolution is usually more prolonged (2 weeks and occasionally even months). A CT scan is an excellent means of differentiating them (46). The treatment, in the absence of pulmonary complications, is conservative.

INJURIES OF THE PLEURAL CAVITY
Pneumothorax

Undoubtedly, pneumothorax is one of the most common lesions secondary to thoracic trauma. It could result from nonpenetrating or penetrating mechanisms and is not infrequently associated with a hemothorax. Despite being a common consequence of a lung injury, it could result from injuries to the esophagus or the tracheobronchial tree.

Air can gain entry to the pleural space by several mechanisms. If there is communication with the atmosphere, the disorder is called an open or communicating pneumothorax or a sucking chest wound. When there is no continuity between the pleural space and the skin or chest wall, a closed or noncommunicating pneumothorax exists. A closed pneumothorax can be further defined as a simple pneumothorax if the lung parenchymal, esophageal, or tracheal injury is self-limited or as a tension pneumothorax if there is no sealing effect, causing escape of air during inspiration, a continuous increase of intrapleural pressure, and significant hemodynamic and respiratory embarrassment.

OPEN OR COMMUNICATING PNEUMOTHORAX (SUCKING CHEST WOUND)

An open pneumothorax can result from penetrating injuries, usually those caused by small weapons/implements, or from blunt chest trauma, usually associated with a large defect. The pathophysiologic changes result in ventilatory impairment of both lungs in both the inspiratory and the expiratory phases. Consequently, the functional dead space increases, with marked accumulation of carbon dioxide in arterial blood.

Diagnosis

The most prevalent symptom is respiratory distress. A sucking wound carries the possibility of lung herniation through the defect. Subcutaneous emphysema is invariably present, the extent of which is usually generalized not only to the thorax but also to the anterior abdominal wall and even to the neck.

Treatment

The wound should be covered temporarily with a nonocculusive dressing. The patient should be intubated endotrachcally and expeditiously, and a chest tube thoracostomy should be placed in the anterolateral thorax in an area removed from the original wound. After initial stabilization of the patient, the wound should be explored with the patient under general anesthesia. Subsequent primary closure of the defect should be attempted.

SIMPLE PNEUMOTHORAX

Simple pneumothoraces are most frequently found in patients with thoracic trauma. The etiology is similar to that previously mentioned.

Diagnosis

The clinical presentation of a simple pneumothorax depends upon the lung volume loss produced by pulmonary collapse and the degree of air occupying the pleural space. A small pneumothorax, affecting 10–15% of the pleural cavity, usually manifests radiologically by a 1-cm rim of air and is usually asymptomatic. It sometimes is found incidentally on a CT scan of the chest (Fig. 9.12**A**). A moderate pneumothorax, occupying 15–50% of the volume of the pleural cavity, is manifested radiographically by a rim of air larger than 2 cm and is always symptomatic (Fig. 9.12**B**). Finally, a pneumothorax involving more than 60% of lung volume is manifested radiographically by a unilateral or bilateral lung collapse and is invariably symptomatic (Fig. 9.12**C**).

Respiratory embarrassment, chest pain, discomfort, and even cyanosis may be present. Decreased breath sounds on auscultation and hyperresonance to percussion may be detected. Ultimately, the diagnosis can be confirmed by chest roentgenograms, with disclosure of a radiolucency around the pulmonary parenchyma. However, a small pneumothorax may not be obvious in the initial roentgenograms, especially on inspiration, requiring additional roentgenograms at the end of expiration or repeated serially during the first 48 hr. Lateral decubitus views with the suspected affected side uppermost have been useful in questionable cases. If the hemodynamic status of the

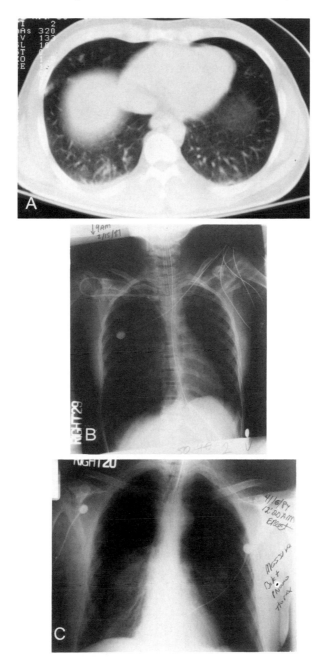

Figure 9.12.   Presentations of pneumothoraces. **A,** minimal. **B,** moderate. **C,** massive.

patient is not stable and there is a suspicion of a pneumothorax, diagnosis may be elicited by the exit of air or hemodynamic improvement of the patient when the chest tube is placed.

Treatment

Several factors determine the mode of therapy: the clinical stability of the patient, the volume of air in the pleural cavity, the need for general anesthesia and surgical intervention, and the time from the occurrence of injury. In fact, if the patient has a very small pneumothorax, is not experiencing respiratory distress, and does not need further surgical intervention, he or she can be monitored with serial chest x-ray films for 48 hr. The chances of the pneumothorax disappearing in that period are very high. Otherwise, the patient will require a chest tube insertion. For technique details, see Chapter 3.

Several factors may account for incomplete evacuation of a pneumothorax following chest tube insertion: improper positioning of the chest tube, the need for more chest tubes, mucous plugs, or associated tracheobronchial, esophageal, or pulmonary ruptures. In this circumstance, it will be necessary to take diagnostic measures such as checking the position and functionality of the chest tubes and employing fiberoptic bronchoscopy. The chest tube should be left in place until there is no evidence of air leak and less than 100 ml of chest tube drainage is obtained in 24 hr, on water seal only. This usually occurs 48 hr after insertion.

TENSION PNEUMOTHORAX

The etiology of tension pneumothorax can be the same as for the previously described pneumothoraces: blunt or penetrating mechanisms. The threat to life posed by this entity necessitates expeditious diagnosis and treatment.

Pathophysiology

The progressive increase of the intrapleural pressure with compression of the ipsilateral lung, vena cava, and mediastinum and the displacement to the contralateral side, causing mechanical impairment of the opposite lung, produce hypoxia, decreased cardiac output, and acidosis. All of these events are lethal unless corrected rapidly.

Diagnosis

The clinical diagnosis is based on marked respiratory embarrassment, restlessness, cyanosis, hypotension, tachycardia, nasal flaring, and intercostal retention. Breath sounds are absent over the involved hemithorax and hyperresonance is detected in the same area. Furthermore, there is classic displacement of the trachea and apical impulse toward the side opposite the lesion. A chest roentgenogram will confirm the diagnosis, disclosing a collapsed lung, flattening of the diaphragm, and mediastinal shift (see Chapter 4.)

Treatment

Immediate decompression of the pleural cavity is mandatory. The treatment should precede radiologic confirmation, particularly if the patient is in respiratory distress. Temporary relief of the tension pneumothorax can be obtained with a 14-gauge needle placed in the second intercostal space, midclavicular line (54). A gush of air is commonly heard; however, many times, even if exiting air is not heard, the hemodynamic status of the patient improves, suggesting relief of the tension pneumothorax.

Definite treatment is accomplished subsequently with the placement of a chest tube thoracostomy in the fourth interstitial space, midaxillary line (we prefer this level for pneumothoraces and/or hemothoraces). The care of the chest tube and its removal time follow the same criteria as for a simple pneumothorax.

Hemothorax

A common sequela of penetrating and blunt trauma, hemothorax usually develops secondary to injuries of systemic vessels (such as intercostal vessels, internal mammary artery, the aorta, and pulmonary vessels) and to lung lacerations. Injuries of the aorta and great vessels usually produce a massive hemothorax and are associated with great mortality. Because of the lungs' great resilience capability, injuries to them are usually self-limited.

PATHOPHYSIOLOGY

Depending upon the magnitude of the traumatic hemothorax, several immediate adverse effects can be produced. As a consequence of hypovolemia and, less likely, mediastinal displacement, the patient can become hypotensive with all the associated consequences of shock. Mechanical displacement of the lungs, however, can contribute to hypoxia and carbon dioxide retention. Adverse effects also may be delayed and are mainly secondary to the presence of blood and clots in the pleural cavity. Several therapeutic modalities based on the volume and degree of loculation have been elaborated. Many controversies have been generated regarding the treatment of retained clot hemothorax because of its potential for empyema and fibrothorax (37, 55). Studies of these clots have shown that they are invaded by fibroblasts and angioblasts by the fourth week, with subsequent formation of a peel by this time.

DIAGNOSIS

The diagnosis of traumatic hemothorax is based on its clinical manifestation, the consequences of the rate and source of bleeding, as well as the involvement of other thoracic organs. The diagnosis is usually confirmed by chest roentgenography. Diffuse radiodensity is apparent in the entire hemithorax on films taken with the patient in a supine position, and a definite radiodensity in the lower hemithorax, with even displacement of the diaphragm and mediastinum, can be seen on films taken in the upright position. Minimal amounts of blood, less than 200 ml, more than likely will not show in regular chest roentgenograms. On the other hand, an air/fluid level will be apparent in the presence of hemopneumothorax (Fig. 9.13).

TREATMENT

The treatment of traumatic hemothorax should be individualized. A conservative approach with close monitoring is warranted for a patient with a minimal hemothorax without clinical manifestations of cardiorespiratory insufficiency. A moderate or massive hemothorax should receive a more aggressive approach: restoration of volemia, correction of hypoxemia, and immediate drainage of the hemothorax with large chest tubes, preferably no. 40, placed in the fifth intercostal space, midaxillary or anterior axillary lines (the technique is described in Chapter 3). The most important parameter in the decision for an urgent thoracotomy is the bleeding trend, which should be monitored every 15 min for the first 2 hr. The indications for urgent thoracotomy in the presence of a traumatic hemothorax are

1. Evacuation of more than 1500 ml at the time of chest tube placement
2. Thoracic bleeding—more than 300 ml/hr for 3 consecutive hours
3. Bleeding more than 150 ml/hr for 3 consecutive hours in the elderly patient
4. All of the above plus hemodynamic instability

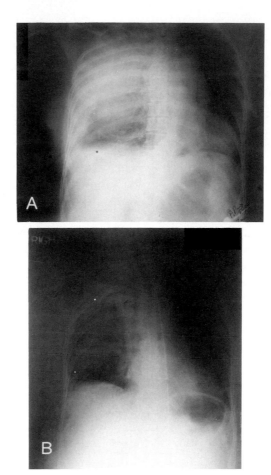

Figure 9.13.   A, hemothorax: pleural and extrapleural components. **B,** hemothorax following evacuation.

Only 10% of patients with traumatic hemothorax require thoracotomy (54, 56). However, there are controversial issues regarding the management of the delayed or retained clotted hemothorax: the indications for thoracotomy and evacuation of these clots should be

1. Residual clotted hemothorax occupying more than half the hemithorax
2. Septic course in the presence of the above
3. Multiloculated hemothoraces
4. Respiratory and cardiovascular embarrassment due to mechanical progression in the size of the hemothorax

Small retained hemothoraces (less than one-third of the hemithorax) will reabsorb in 3–4 weeks, provided the pleura is not infected (56).

If a hemothorax is associated with a pneumothorax, additional chest tubes should be inserted. If air leak persists despite that maneuver and the amount of suction increases, fiberoptic bronchoscopy should be performed to rule out bronchial tear. Small air leaks can be treated conservatively for 2 weeks, provided no clinical derangements are produced. Persistent (lasting more than 2 weeks) moderate to large leaks should be evaluated for possible thoracotomy and definite surgical control, according to the patient's clinical condition.

Thoracic Empyema

Infected pleural fluid with or without purulent appearance could be a definition of thoracic empyema (54). This can be secondary to blunt or penetrating trauma and its incidence is variable: 15–60% in injured civilian populations (57–59).

The etiology of thoracic empyema is multifactorial. The most common cause continues to be contiguous pneumonia; however, empyema could be the consequence of distal seeding of the pleural cavity from a subphrenic abscess or other infected source. We propose the theory that patients with lung contusions and associated small lacerations of the lung could develop empyema secondary to seeding of the pleural space with bacteria of the oropharynx blown off distally into the lacerated lung by the respirator (60).

DIAGNOSIS

The clinical manifestations are malaise, fever, chills, and weight loss. If the patient is being ventilated, it is very difficult to differentiate this entity from other clinical septic etiologies. Therefore, the diagnosis needs to be confirmed by chest roentgenogram (Fig. 9.14) and thoracentesis or chest tube thoracostomy. An immediate Gram stain of the thoracostomy drainage may disclose many bacteria, usually *Streptococcus* and *Staphylococcus* species; 20% of fluid cultures from patients with empyema can be negative (58, 59) because many patients are usually placed on prophylactic antibiotics. As stated earlier, a purulent appearance is not mandatory in this diagnosis (58, 59). The CT scan also has contributed to the diagnosis and decision process regarding the need for thoracotomy (61).

TREATMENT

The treatment of traumatic thoracic empyema has not changed since Burford, Parker, and Samson established basic therapeutic criteria in 1944 (62):

1. Proper antibiotic therapy (Fig. 9.15)
2. Expansion of the lung and obliteration of the pleural cavity (Fig. 9.15)
3. Proper drainage of the empyema (Fig. 9.16) via one of the following modalities:
    a. Thoracentesis—effective only in small children
    b. Chest tube thoracostomy—no. 40 midaxillary line
    c. Rib resection—rarely used in trauma
    d. Decortication—thoracotomy is indicated for patients with thoracic empyema with the following characteristics:
        1. Multiple loculated empyema collections
        2. Marked enlargement of the fluid collection, with impairment of oxygenation and ventilation
        3. Septic course, not explainable from any other cause except the clotted hemothorax

Normally, after thoracotomy, defervescence requires several weeks. A mild degree of fever and cardiorespiratory instabilities continues but is followed by complete normalization of respiratory and cardiac function.

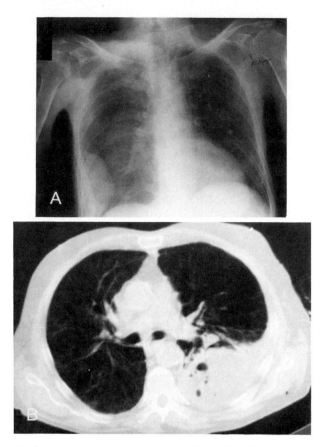

Figure 9.14.   A, right loculated empyema shown on chest film. **B,** loculated empyema on CT scan.

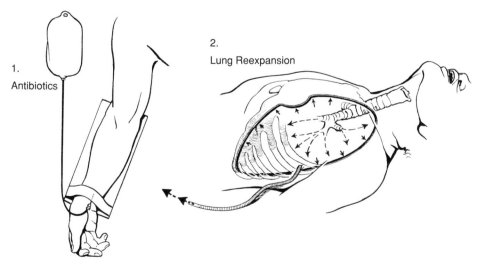

Figure 9.15.   The treatment of thoracic empyema includes antibiotic therapy and reexpansion of the lung.

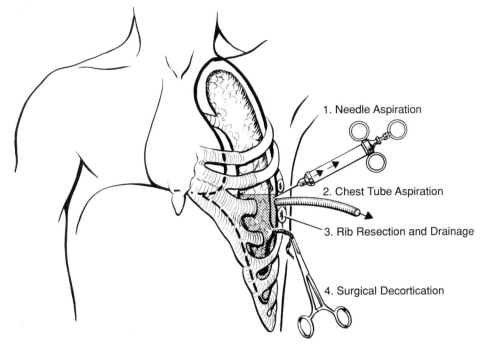

1. Needle Aspiration

2. Chest Tube Aspiration

3. Rib Resection and Drainage

4. Surgical Decortication

Figure 9.16. Techniques for drainage of empyema.

REFERENCES

1. Besson A, Saegesser F. Color atlas of chest trauma and associated injuries, vol 1. Oradell, NJ: Medical Economics, 1983.
2. Kemmerer WT, Eckert WG, Gathright JB, Reemtsma K, Creech O Jr. Patterns of thoracic injuries in fatal traffic accidents. J Trauma 1961;1:595–599.
3. Wilson RF, Murray C, Antonenko DR. Nonpenetrating thoracic injuries. Surg Clin North Am 1977; 57:17–36.
4. Schaal MA, Fischer RP, Perry JF. The unchanged mortality of flail chest injuries. J Trauma 1979;19:492–496.
5. Shorr RM, Crittenden M, Indeck M, Hartunian SL, Rodriguez A. Blunt thoracic trauma: analysis of 515 patients. Ann Surg 1987;206:200–205.
6. Conn JH, Hardy JD, Fain WR, Netterville RE. Thoracic trauma: analysis of 1022 cases. J Trauma 1963;3:22–40.
7. Rasmussen OV, Brynitz S, Struve-Christensen E. Thoracic injuries: a review of 93 cases. Scand J Thorac Cardiovasc Surg 1986;20:71–74.
8. Blaisdell FW, Trunkey DD. Trauma management. New York: Georg Thieme, 1986; 140–142.
9. Richardson JD, McElvein RB, Trinkle JK. First rib fracture: a hallmark of severe trauma. Ann Surg 1975;181:251–254.
10. Wilson JM, Thomas AN, Goodman PC, Lewis FR. Severe chest trauma: morbidity implications of first and second rib fracture in 120 patients. Arch Surg 1978;113:846–849.
11. Phillips EH, Rogers WF, Gaspin MR. First rib fractures: incidence of vascular injury and indications for angiography. Surgery 1981;89:42–47.
12. Pierce GE, Maxwell JA, Boggan MD. Special hazards of first rib fractures. J Trauma 1975;15:264–267.
13. Leguerrier A, Rosat P, Lebeau G, et al. Multiple lesions from closed chest injury: right bronchus rupture, right subclavian artery rupture, and bilateral fracture of first rib. J Chir (Paris) 1985;122:561–565.
14. O'Malley MK, Duignan JP, Lavelle JS. Fractured sternum associated with the use of seat belts. Ir Med J 1983;76:131–132.
15. Gibson LD, Carter R, Hinshaw DB. Surgical significance of sternal fractures. Surg Gynecol Obstet 1962;114:443–448.

16. Richardson JD, Grover FL, Trinkle JK. Early operative management of isolated sternal fractures. J Trauma 1975;15:156–158.

17. Kurzweg FT, Danna SJ, Lolley RT. Open reduction and fixation of a commuted fracture of the sternum. J Thorac Cardiovasc Surg 1972;63:424–426.

18. Harley DP, Mena I. Cardiac and vascular sequelae of sternal fractures.. J Trauma 1986;26:553–555.

19. McGinnis M, Denton J. Fractures of the scapula: a retrospective study of 40 fractured scapulae. J Trauma 1989;29:1488–1493.

20. Neer CS, Rockwood CA Jr. Fractures and dislocation of the shoulder. In: Rockwood CA Jr, ed. Fractures in adults. 2nd ed. Philadelphia: Lippincott, 1984:675–721.

21. Hardegger FH, Simpson LA, Weber BG. The operative treatment of scapular fractures. J Bone Joint Surg (Br) 1984;66:725–731.

22. Brauer L. Erfahrungen und Uberlengun ger zur Lungenkollapstherapuie. Beitr Klin Tuberk Spezif Tuberk Forsch 1909;12:49.

23. Duff JH, Goldstein M. McLean APH, et al. Flail chest: a clinical review and physiological study. J Trauma 1968;8:63–74.

24. Parham AM, Yarbrough DR III, Redding JS. Flail chest syndrome and pulmonary contusion. Arch Surg 1978;113:900–903.

25. Blair E, Mills E. Rationale of stabilization of the flail chest with intermittent positive pressure breathing. Am Surg 1968;34:860–868.

26. Cullen P, Modell JH, Kirby RR, et al. Treatment of flail chest: use of intermittent mandatory ventilation and positive end-expiratory pressure. Arch Surg 1975; 110:1099–1103.

27. Richardson JD, Adams L, Flint LM. Selective management of flail chest and pulmonary contusion. Ann Surg 1982;196:481–487.

28. Shackford SR, Smith DE, Zarins CK, et al. The management of flail chest: a comparison of ventilatory and nonventilatory treatment. Am J Surg 1976;132:759–762.

29. Glinz W. Problems caused by the unstable trauma wall and by cardiac injury due to blunt trauma. Injury 1986;17:322–326.

30. Barone JE, Pizzi WF, Nealor TF Jr, Richman H. Indications for intubation in blunt chest trauma. J Trauma 1986;26:334–338.

31. Mackensie RC, Shaekford SR, Hoyt DB, Karajiens TG. Continuous epidural fentanyl analgesic: ventilatory function improvement with routine use in treatment of blunt chest trauma. J Trauma 1987;27:1207–1212.

32. Cullen M, Staren E, Ganzouri AE, Logus W, et al. Continuous epidural infusion for analgesic after major abdominal operations: a randomized, prospective double blind study. Surgery 1985;98:718–728.

33. Sanchez-Lloret J, Letang E, Mateau M, et al. Indications and surgical treatment of the traumatic flail chest syndrome: an original technique. Thorac Cardiovasc Surg 1982;30:294–297.

34. Thomas AN, Blaisdell FW, Lewis FR Jr, Schlobohm RM. Operative stabilization for flail chest after blunt trauma. J Thorac Cardiovasc Surg 1978;75:793–801.

35. Graham JM, Mattox KL, Beall AC Jr. Penetrating trauma of the lung. J Trauma 1979;19:665–669.

36. Boland FK. Traumatic surgery of the lungs and pleura: analysis of 1009 cases of penetrating wounds. Ann Surg 1936;104:572–579.

37. Symbas P. Cardiothoracic trauma. Philadelphia: Saunders, 1989:232–259.

38. Hankins JR, McAslan TC, Shin B, Ayella RJ, Cowley RA, McLaughlin JS. Extensive pulmonary laceration caused by blunt trauma. J Thorac Cardiovasc Surg 1977;74:519–527.

39. Trinkle JK, Furman RW, Hinshaw MA, et al. Pulmonary contusion: pathogenesis and effect of various resuscitative measures. Ann Thorac Surg 1973;16:568–573.

40. Wagner RB, Jamieson P. Pulmonary contusion: evaluation and classification by computed tomography. Surg Clin North Am 1985;69:31–40.

41. Hankins JR, Attar S, Turney SZ, et al. Differential diagnosis of pulmonary parenchymal changes in thoracic trauma. Am Surg 1973;39:309–318.

42. Richardson JD, Adams L, Flint LM. Selective management of flail chest and pulmonary contusion. Ann Surg 1982;196:481–487.

43. Carrico J. Lung contusion. In : Mattox KL, Moore EE, Feliciano DV, eds. Trauma. East Norwalk, CT: Appleton & Lange, 1988.

44. Fulton RL, Peter ET. Physiological effects of fluid therapy after pulmonary contusion. Am J Surg 1973;126:773–777.

45. Fulton RL, Peter ET. Compositional and histologic effects of fluid therapy following pulmonary contusion. J Trauma 1974;14:783–790.

46. Franz JL, Richardson JD, Grover FL, et al. Effect of methylprednisolone sodium succinate on experimental pulmonary contusion. J Thorac Cardiovasc Surg 1974;68:842–844.

47. Svennevig JL, Bugge-Asperheim B, Bjorgo S, Kleppe H, Birkeland S. Methylprednisolone in the treatment of lung contusion following blunt chest trauma. Scand J Thorac Cardiovac Surg 1980;14:301–305.

48. Johnson JA, Cogbill TH, Winga ER. Determinants of outcome after pulmonary contusion. J Trauma 1986;26:695–697.

49. Dunham CM, Gbaanador G. Factors influencing outcome in lung contusion, personal communication, 1989.

50. Dunn MG, Rodriguez A, Brotman S. Traumatic pseudocyst of the lung. Contemp Surg 1983;23:51–54.

51. Nielsen GD, Grønmark T. Traumatic cyst of the lung. Injury 1975;6:241–243.

52. Ellis R. Traumatic lung cyst. JAMA 1976;236:1976–1977.

53. Sorsdahl OA, Powell JW. Cavitary pulmonary lesions following nonpenetrating chest trauma in children. AJR 1965;95:118–124.

54. Trunkey D. Torso trauma. Curr Probl Surg 1987;24:234–235.

55. Langston HT, Tuttle WM. Pathology of chronic traumatic hemothorax. J Thorac Surg 1947;16:99–116.

56. Kirsh M, Sloan H. Hemothorax: blunt chest trauma. Boston: Little, Brown, 1977.

57. Caplan ES, Hoyt NJ, Rodriguez A, Cowley RA. Empyema occurring in the multiply traumatized patient. J Trauma 1984;24:785–789.

58. Caplan ES, Hoyt NJ. Infection surveillance and control in the severely traumatized patient. Am J Med 1981;70:638–640.

59. Coon JL, Shuck JM. Failure of tube thoracostomy for post-traumatic empyema: an indication for early decortication. J Trauma 1975;15:588–594.

60. Rodriguez A. Empyema in the multiple trauma patient, personal communication, 1989.

61. Mirvis SE, Rodriguez A, Whitley NO, Tarr RJ. CT evaluation of thoracic infections after major trauma. AJR 1985;144:1181–1187.

62. Samson PC. Empyema thoracis. Ann Thorac Surg 1971;11:210–221.

10 Tracheobronchial Injuries

Larry R. Kaiser, MD
Joel D. Cooper, MD

Injuries to the trachea or major bronchi comprise only a small percentage of those occurring in the spectrum of thoracic trauma. The incidence of tracheobronchial rupture resulting from blunt chest trauma has been reported to range from a high of 2.8% (1) to 0.85% (2). Bertelsen and Howitz (1) reviewed autopsy reports on 1178 patients who died following an injury and found 33 cases (2.8%) of tracheobronchial injuries, with all but five accompanied by other injuries. When Kemmerer et al. (2) looked at 585 deaths from traffic accidents in general, they found five (0.85%) tracheobronchial transections. The higher incidence of tracheobronchial trauma noted by Bertelsen and Howitz probably results from the fact that all individuals dying from trauma were included in their review, including those who suffered penetrating injuries. Even in a busy trauma center, no more than a handful of patients with injuries to the upper airway would be expected to be seen in a given year. One only needs to review recent reports detailing experience in thoracic trauma from Houston and New Orleans to underscore this fact (3, 4).

As with other organ systems, it is convenient to classify airway trauma based on the mechanism of injury: penetrating or nonpenetrating. We consider iatrogenic injury, particularly that which may occur during or because of endotracheal intubation, under the heading of penetrating injuries. Inhalation injuries form a separate and distinct group, though their management involves techniques remarkably similar to those used for other types of airway trauma.

Isolated injury to the tracheobronchial tree is distinctly unusual. This is especially true following penetrating trauma. There are, however, occasional patients who, having sustained blunt chest trauma, present with an isolated bronchial rupture. Ironically, this type of injury frequently may be overlooked because of the subtlety of the clinical signs and symptoms and a lack of suspicion on the part of the treating physician. Truly, this must be one of the few instances where a major injury may go unrecognized, and it is a testament to the stout nature of the connective tissue that ensheathes the upper airway, allowing maintenance of air flow despite occasional complete bronchial rupture. The elasticity of the thorax tends to dissipate an applied force and thus plays a role in allowing this type of injury to occur. Significant airway trauma may be seen frequently even in the absence of rib fractures.

PENETRATING TRAUMA

In a review of trauma victims admitted to the University of Texas Medical Center in Houston during the 5-year period July 1980 to June 1985, Thompson et al. (3) found that

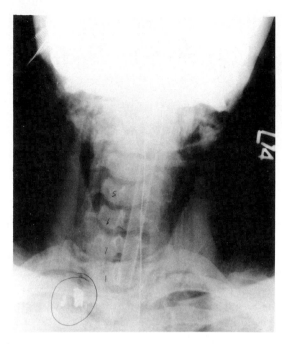

Figure 10.1.   Gunshot wound to the neck. Massive subcutaneous emphysema caused by a single hole in the anterior trachea is seen. This injury was also associated with a small right pneumothorax. Aortogram with selective injection of brachiocephalic vessels demonstrated no vascular injury.

36% of all injured patients (2608/7283) had injuries that included the chest. Of those sustaining penetrating trauma, 41% (945/2302) involved thoracic structures. Only 28% of patients underwent emergent or urgent thoracotomy as compared with 7.5% of those with blunt trauma. Only five patients (1.2%) had isolated tracheobronchial disruption. Overall, patients with lung injuries who required pulmonary resection did poorly and, of note, all nine patients who required pneumonectomy for hemorrhage died.

Findings on presentation vary according to both location and severity of the penetrating injury. Often, the manifestations of an associated injury, particularly a vascular injury, may obscure those clinical findings expected with an airway injury. Patients with penetrating injuries to the cervical trachea commonly present with dyspnea, usually accompanied by subcutaneous emphysema of the neck (Fig. 10.1). Mild hemoptysis is seen relatively frequently, but massive hemoptysis would be distinctly unusual with an isolated injury to the tracheobronchial tree; its presence usually indicates an associated vascular injury. Patients sustaining a thoracic tracheal injury may have a pneumothorax, depending upon the site of the wound and whether or not there is communication with the free pleural space. It is common for patients with penetrating injuries to present with a pneumothorax, though this finding is not specific for an airway injury. Conversely, an airway injury may present with findings as subtle as pneumomediastinum and subcutaneous emphysema seen only on close inspection of the chest radiograph.

Bronchoscopy and esophagoscopy should be carried out as a matter of routine in patients with penetrating injuries. Obviously, if the clinical condition of the patient mandates emergent exploration to control bleeding, endoscopy is delayed until the patient's clinical condition stabilizes. A chest radiograph should be obtained rapidly as initial resuscitative measures begin. Immediate control of the airway is mandatory. The need for further diagnostic studies, such as angiography, must be balanced against the lability of the patient's condition.

In what is perhaps the largest series of patients with penetrating chest trauma, Kelly et al. (4) from Tulane reported on 100 patients with injuries to the trachea and major bronchi. The cervical trachea was injured in 78 patients whereas the other 22 injuries involved the intrathoracic trachea or major bronchi. The highest mortality rate (50%) occurred in patients sustaining intrathoracic tracheal injuries; those with injuries to the cervical trachea had a mortality rate of 14%, underscoring the increased severity of the injuries associated with intrathoracic trauma. It is illustrative to examine the causes of death in this series to determine what measures, if any, may prevent similar occurrences. The fate of six patients seemingly was determined prior to arrival: three presented with irreversible shock and required thoracotomy in the emergency room, and three others had associated massive carotid artery injuries. Among those who arrived in the emergency room alive and in whom death may have been preventable, four patients died because of problems secondary to airway management. Two of them, who had combined laryngeal and cervical tracheal trauma, died because of inability to establish an airway. In one patient, inability to control a thoracic tracheal injury resulted in intraoperative death, and in the fourth, who had multiple gunshot wounds, the diagnosis of tracheal laceration was made only at autopsy.

Principles of management revolve around immediate control of the airway for any injured patient, but the patient with a primary airway injury presents some unique problems. Most patients, even those with injury to the trachea, may be managed with nasotracheal or orotracheal intubation. Occasionally, however, intubation with the aid of a flexible bronchoscope may be required, especially in a situation where there may be disruption of the cervical trachea. Tracheostomy, though rarely required, may be necessary in the presence of the combined laryngeal and tracheal injury, or in the individual with concomitant massive facial trauma. Since primary airway repair is the treatment of choice, we prefer to avoid tracheostomy whenever possible, as it may affect the outcome of the definitive repair.

Three additional patients in Kelly et al.'s series died due to massive aspiration of blood following an injury to the trachea and a nearby vascular structure. With a large amount of blood in the airway, rigid bronchoscopy may be required, as it allows for ventilation as well as provides a large channel through which to suction; therefore, a surgeon facile in insertion of the necessary instrument should be available.

Two patients died because of missed esophageal injuries, both of whom had normal contrast esophagrams in the emergency room. In Kelly et al.'s series (5), 21 patients were seen with combined airway and esophageal injuries resulting from penetrating trauma. Mortality in this group was 20.8% (5). Essentially all patients had cervical esophageal injuries. Missing an esophageal injury is a disaster and must not be allowed to occur. The result of delayed recognition is markedly increased mortality. Definitive treatment mandates primary repair of the airway injury and the esophageal injury, but the key remains making the diagnosis.

With any significant penetrating neck injury, we perform esophagoscopy along with bronchoscopy, as long as the hemodynamic status of the patient permits. If endoscopy is not performed prior to neck exploration, the esophagus must be explored thoroughly as the consequences of missing an esophageal injury cannot be overestimated. Rarely, if ever, is it necessary to divert the esophagus if an injury is recognized early and, even if discovered late, primary repair usually suffices.

Symbas et al. (6) also noted the high frequency of associated major injury with penetrating wounds to the trachea. They treated 20 patients at Grady Memorial Hospital in Atlanta from 1966 to 1975, half of whom had other major injuries. Fifteen of the 20 airway injuries involved the cervical trachea and five, the thoracic trachea. The most frequent site of injury was the anterior lateral wall of the cervical trachea.

The approach to the airway in order to effect primary repair is mandated both by the location of the airway injury as well as by associated vascular or other injuries. For cervical trauma, a transverse neck incision that can be extended to either side, if vascular injuries are present, is preferred. A right thoracotomy is the approach of choice for the intrathoracic trachea and carina, while major bronchial injuries are dealt with on the appropriate side. If the vascular injury mandates sternotomy, the airway injury is readily approached through this exposure, whether it be the right or left main bronchus.

Despite all of this, one would do well to keep in mind how infrequently these injuries are seen. As Kelly et al. (4) point out in the review from Charity Hospital in New Orleans, one of the busiest trauma centers in the United States, they see on average only five such injuries each year. Thus, the average surgeon must maintain a high level of suspicion regarding these injuries, despite their rarity, if a diagnosis is to be made in a timely fashion and primary repair carried out.

A discussion of penetrating wounds of the trachea and bronchi would be incomplete without including iatrogenic injuries. These injuries most commonly occur during or following endotracheal intubation and usually involve double-lumen endobronchial tubes, with either the membranous trachea or membranous bronchus sustaining the injury. The instrument of injury may be the tip of the endotracheal tube, the stylet used to facilitate passage of the tube, or the tracheal or bronchial cuff (7). The wire stylet should be removed immediately after the tip of the tube passes through the vocal cords. Interestingly, nitrous oxide absorption by the permeable cuffs, causing overinflation, has been implicated in a number of anecdotal reports of tracheal or bronchial rupture (8).

Despite the fact that these tubes have soft, low-pressure tracheal and bronchial cuffs, injuries can and do occur. No more than 2–2.5 ml of air should be placed in the bronchial cuff of the polyvinyl chloride double-lumen tubes. Of note, after 3 ml of air are placed in the bronchial cuff, the cuff behaves like a high-pressure cuff (8). If more than 3 ml of air is required, it is likely that the cuff is not in an optimal location. Tube position should be reevaluated if the bronchial cuff fails to seal after inflation with 2–3 ml of air. Because of diffusion of nitrous oxide across the plastic, the bronchial cuff should be kept deflated and inflated only when one-lung anesthesia is being employed; optimally, nitrous oxide should not be administered when an endobronchial tube is in use. If nitrous oxide is being used, the cuff should be deflated periodically. To determine tube position accurately, a pediatric bronchoscope may be passed down both the tracheal and bronchial limbs of the tube so that the bronchial cuff may be positioned in the optimal location relative to the carina. The bronchial cuff should be situated just distal to the carina, but the cuff should not be able to herniate out of the appropriate main bronchus.

Rollins and Tocino described early radiographic signs of tracheal rupture related to intubation (9). All ruptures occurred in the membranous trachea. The distal portion of the endotracheal tube was seen radiographically to be displaced toward the right side and was accompanied by an overdistended balloon in all seven cases. These findings preceded the development of subcutaneous and mediastinal emphysema in four cases. The authors identified a markedly decreased distance between the cuff and tip of the tube (<1.2 cm) in six of the cases, due to eccentric inflation allowed by the tracheal rupture (Fig. 10.2).

Wagner et al. (10) postulated that changes in the membranous trachea in the patient with emphysema may allow tracheal rupture to occur more readily. Perhaps the membranous trachea becomes thin and inelastic, as well as stretched, due to the emphysematous changes in the lung parenchyma. A partial-thickness tracheal wall laceration may allow air to dissect insidiously into the adventitia, thereby expanding it and producing aneurysmal dilatation of the membranous tracheal wall. The dilatation may take several hours to form and signs of injury may not occur until rupture into the mediastinum or pleural space occurs. Anytime there has been difficulty in passing the endotracheal tube prior to thoracotomy, bronchoscopy should be performed and full mediastinal inspection, with both lungs ventilated, should be carried out by the operating surgeon. Primary repair should be performed if any laceration is identified.

NONPENETRATING TRACHEOBRONCHIAL TRAUMA

Nonpenetrating injuries, most commonly resulting from motor vehicle accidents, account for the majority of injuries to the tracheobronchial tree. The true incidence of these injuries is also difficult to assess because many of the patients have associated

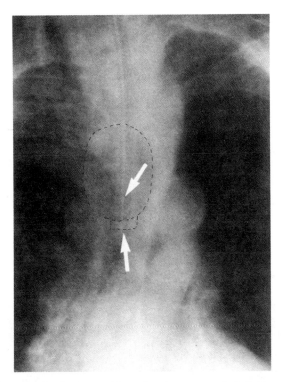

Figure 10.2.   Endotracheal tube in position showing eccentric inflation of the cuff causing a decrease in the distance between the cuff and the tip of the tube. This finding is highly suggestive of tracheal rupture. (From Rollins JR, Tocino I. Early radiographic signs of tracheal rupture. AJR 1987;148:695–698.)

lethal injuries and never make it to the hospital; a second group have airway injuries that go unrecognized at the time of initial presentation and subsequently present with complications resulting from the misdiagnosis. The difficulty in trying to ascertain a true incidence is further compounded by the propensity of authors to look at either hospital admissions following trauma (3, 4) or autopsies on those dying from their injuries (2). The former overlook a potentially large group with other associated lethal injuries, while the latter fail to account for those with isolated tracheobronchial injuries, many of whom survive. Bertelsen and Howitz (1) identified 33 airway injuries at autopsy following death caused by trauma over a 5-year period and treated an additional 11 patients with tracheobronchial injuries over a 14-year period. Alyono and Perry (11) noted only seven cases of tracheobronchial rupture among 966 patients seen with chest injuries resulting from motor vehicle accidents over a 12-year period. All of these occurred before 1974, when the speed limit was reduced, and the authors point out that morbidity, mortality, and severity of chest injury were lower after this reduction from 70 to 55 mph. Similarly, in a series of 353 patients treated with major chest injuries over a 10-year period, Dougall et al. (12) treated only eight (2.2%) tracheobronchial ruptures.

The historical aspects leading to the recognition and management of tracheobronchial rupture provide some fascinating insights. Webb, in 1848, reported finding a ruptured left main bronchus at autopsy in a patient who died following a massive liver injury (13). Winslow (14), in 1871, added significantly to knowledge of airway injury and reported the first survival from a bronchial injury. Unfortunately, the "patient" was a wild canvasback duck that, while being prepared for the oven, was incidentally found to have a fibrous pouch that had presumably developed in response to a rupture of the left main bronchus. Krinitzki (15) found a completely occluded right mainstem bronchus at autopsy in a patient who had sustained a severe blunt injury to the right chest some 20 years earlier.

Initial surgical attempts at treating airway rupture were aimed at relieving mediastinal shift and pulmonary sepsis (16, 17). Griffith (18), in 1949, reported the first successful management of a posttraumatic bronchial stricture, the result of a bronchial disruption occurring 6 months previously. The stricture was resected and an end-to-end anastomosis performed using interrupted wire sutures. Three years later, Scannell (19) reported the first successful case of a bronchial laceration treated by immediate thoracotomy and repair. The patient was a 10-yr-old boy struck by a car, who presented with a complete pneumothorax that failed to respond to chest tube placement. When he continued to have signs and symptoms of a tension pneumothorax with continued clinical deterioration, thoracotomy was performed. Primary repair of a cervical tracheal disruption was first reported by Beskin (20) in 1956, in a patient who sustained a "steering post" injury and presented with severe respiratory distress. Emergency tracheostomy was attempted only to find that the trachea was absent in the region above the suprasternal notch. The distal trachea was retrieved after incising the still-intact deep cervical fascia, and after debridement, the ends were sutured together with interrupted wire sutures. The patient had no further difficulty and the trachea healed without stricture formation.

MECHANISM OF INJURY

Isolated blunt injury to the cervical trachea tends to be unusual, accounting for only 10–15% of cases, mainly because of the protection afforded by the mandible and the cervical spine. Identifying the mechanism of injury that produces cervical tracheal trauma is fairly easy. With the neck hyperextended, a direct blow to the trachea may result in rupture with only minimal external evidence of trauma (21). This injury most commonly results from motor vehicle trauma when the neck strikes the edge of the dashboard, which is soft enough to preclude laceration but firm enough to cause tracheal rupture. Theoretically, this injury should be nonexistent if all car occupants wore shoulder retrains. Similarly, tracheal rupture or laceration may result from a so-called clothesline injury, in which the neck strikes a tethered line.

Over 80% of blunt tracheobronchial injuries occur within 2.5 cm of the carina (22). In order to injure the intrathoracic trachea, carina, or mainstem bronchi, sudden forceful compression of the thoracic cage is required. The anteroposterior force from rapid deceleration applied to the tracheobronchial tree, which is fixed at the level of the cricoid and at the carina, may easily result in disruption. Also, sudden chest compression occurring in the presence of a closed glottis may result in an increase in the intratracheal and intrabronchial pressure, which may be greater than the elasticity of the trachea or bronchi, and thereby result in rupture. Acute blunt chest compression in an anteroposterior direction forces the trachea and carina against the vertebral bodies, causing lateral shearing forces that may also result in tearing. Probably, a combination of these factors accounts for most blunt tracheobronchial injuries. In younger patients, in whom the chest wall is elastic and therefore more compressible, these types of injuries seem to be more common. Nahum et al. (23) demonstrated significant variation in chest wall damage sustained by cadavers subjected to blunt sternal impact based on age. Younger cadavers suffered essentially no rib fractures while older ones sustained multiple rib fractures, sternal fractures, and damage to the heart and lungs. This compressibility of the younger chest wall may partly explain why many of these injuries are not associated with a parenchymal or significant vascular injury. Less than one-half of blunt chest injuries have associated injuries more severe than rib fractures (24).

The absolute force of the injury may not be as important a factor as the way in which the force is applied to the chest wall. Both the magnitude of skeletal deflection and the time required to develop such deflections seem to be more closely correlated (25). Alyono and Perry (11) noted a statistically significant decrease in four categories of thoracic injury when they compared incidence, morbidity, and mortality of blunt chest injuries occurring before and after the reduction in speed limit from 70 to 55 mph. Hemothorax occurred in 42% of patients sustaining chest trauma before the reduction in the speed limit versus 29% after. Sternal fractures and flail chest injuries also significantly decreased, but, of note, no (0/503) tracheobronchial ruptures were seen after the speed limit reduction as compared to 1.5% (7/463) before the reduction was instituted. They concluded that speed limit reduction was, at least in part, responsible for less severe chest injuries in victims of motor vehicle accidents. This, along with the relative compliance of the pulmonary vessels, may account for the low incidence of accompanying pulmonary vascular injuries. The only exception to this may be injury to the middle lobe bronchus, which may be more readily associated with pulmonary artery injury, perhaps because of the anatomic relationship of the middle lobe bronchus to the middle lobe pulmonary arterial branch. Zapolanski (26) reported three cases of injury to the middle lobe bronchus associated with pulmonary artery injury.

CLINICAL PRESENTATION

The diagnosis of blunt tracheobronchial injury may be difficult, as the severity of symptoms and signs may be quite variable. Most patients complain of dyspnea and some degree of respiratory distress, which varies with the rate and amount of air loss. This, of course, depends upon the degree to which the airway is disrupted and whether or not there is free communication with the pleural space. Depending upon whether there is free communication between the site of the disruption and the pleural space determines the findings at presentation. Without free communication, there tends to be little or no pneumothorax (Fig. 10.3). Despite the fact that the bronchus may be totally transsected, the patient may have only a minimal amount of air in the mediastinum, which may be easily missed on the first chest x-ray film. Deep cervical emphysema and subcutaneous emphysema of the chest may also be present. The pretracheal fascia and peribronchial tissue may be stout enough to maintain an airway and the patient may be only minimally symptomatic, with reasonable oxygenation and ventilation. Minimal hemoptysis may also accompany this injury. Rarely is there massive hemoptysis. Occasionally, a patient may present with signs and symptoms of a tension pnuemothorax, which mandates rapid tube thoracostomy. When there is communication between the airway disruption and the pleura, a complete pneumothorax usually occurs (Fig. 10.4). Further confirmation of the severity of injury usually is obtained at time of placement of the chest tube, when a massive air leak is demonstrated, and incomplete expansion of the lung results, despite suction. The patient may, in fact, experience more respiratory difficulty when the chest tube is placed to suction, and this finding is almost invariably associated with bronchial disruption, as pointed out by Deslauriers et al. (27). The presence of rib fractures should not be the basis for deciding that "significant" chest trauma has occurred.

Injuries to the cervical trachea lend themselves more readily to early diagnosis. Respiratory distress may be a more frequent accompaniment, and significant deep cervical emphysema usually results. Severe cyanosis and evidence of a tension pneumothorax occasionally may be present. Computed tomographic scans of the neck may prove useful in the patient suspected of having a tracheal injury but in whom the classic findings of pneumomediastinum, subcutaneous emphysema, or pneumothorax

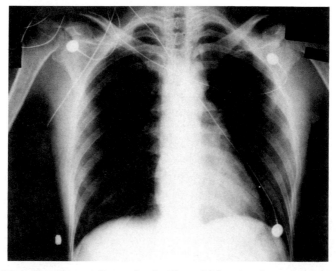

Figure 10.3.   Presenting chest radiograph of a 32-yr-old female who was involved in a head-on collision. Her chest struck the steering wheel. Note the lack of significant findings on the x-ray film. The patient was experiencing no respiratory distress. Her only other significant injuries were several long bone fractures.

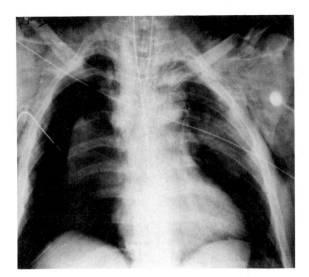

Figure 10.4.   Presenting chest radiograph of a 27-yr-old male struck by a truck. Note the large right pneumothorax persisting after placement of a chest tube. Note also the large amount of subcutaneous emphysema. Bronchoscopy demonstrated complete disruption of the right main bronchus, and he underwent thoracotomy and reanastomosis of the bronchus.

are absent (28) (Fig. 10.5). Findings on plain film such as overdistension of the balloon cuff of the endotracheal tube, oblique orientation of the endotracheal tube, or caudal displacement of the balloon over the shaft of the tube may also be helpful (8) (Fig. 10.6). Despite complete transection, the pretracheal fascia may temporarily serve to maintain airway patency. It is probably safest to intubate these patients with the use of a flexible bronchoscope in order to maintain airway patency prior to going to the operating room for urgent airway repair. If the airway is unable to be secured with endotracheal intubation, emergent neck exploration with retrieval of the distal end of the severed trachea and placement of a tracheostomy tube may be required prior to definitive repair. One should be aware of the possibility of concomitant esophageal injury that may not become apparent until several days following repair of the tracheal injury (29).

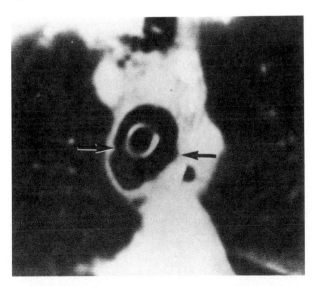

Figure 10.5.   Computerized tomographic scan demonstrating the presence of an overdistended balloon cuff of an endotracheal tube. *Arrows* point to the junction of the cartilaginous and membranous trachea. (From Rollins JR, Tocino I. Early radiographic signs of tracheal rupture. AJR 1987;148:695–698.)

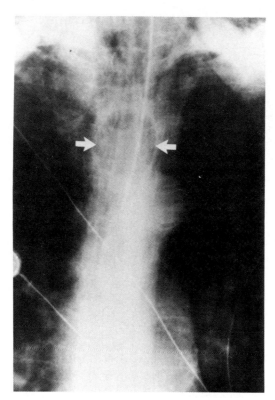

Figure 10.6.   Chest radiograph demonstrating abnormalities in the endotracheal tube positioning with the presence of a tracheal rupture. Note the oblique orientation of the endotracheal tube and overdistention of the cuff. (From Tocino I, Miller MH. Computer tomography in blunt chest trauma. J Thorac Imaging 1987;2:45–59.)

MANAGEMENT

Once the diagnosis is established, a tracheal or bronchial injury should be repaired urgently. Bronchoscopy is mandatory to determine the location as well as extent of the injury in order to allow for planning of the operative approach. The presence of co-existing injuries sometimes mandates a change in the operative strategy. As pointed out by Ramzy et al. (30), a group with extensive experience with motor vehicle trauma, at times it may be necessary to proceed first with laparotomy in patients with significant abdominal trauma who have ongoing intraperitoneal blood loss. This requires that an airway be established, almost always possible with either an endobronchial tube or a bronchoscopically positioned endotracheal tube in the uninjured side, and that adequate oxygenation be maintained. The operative plan must be individualized for each patient with an airway injury and injury to other organ systems, despite the intuitive desire to deal with the airway first. Repair involves direct reanastomosis of the trachea or disrupted bronchus or primary suture repair of a membranous wall tear. Pulmonary resection is rarely required and should be reserved for extraordinary circumstances. If there is massive parenchymal injury accompanying an airway injury, pulmonary resection may be the preferred procedure. An injury to a lobar bronchus may also be an indication for pulmonary resection. Rarely is pneumonectomy indicated.

Exposure of the cervical trachea is readily accomplished via a neck incision. It may occasionally be necessary to do a partial sternotomy in order to facilitate repair of distal tracheal injuries. With a known intrathoracic tracheal injury, exposure is probably best achieved via a right thoracotomy. Mainstem bronchus disruptions are readily approached via thoracotomy on the appropriate side of the injury. Placement of an endobronchial tube with one-lung ventilation may be required for optimal anesthetic management. Occasionally, airway injuries are amenable to nonoperative management, especially if, at bronchoscopy, one finds only a small laceration in the membranous trachea or bronchus or less than one-third of the cartilaginous arch involved. A course of nonoperative management of a bronchial tear may be pursued if the lung fully expands, after chest tube placement, and the air leak is of a manageable size and seals within several days. If the lung is unable to be maintained fully expanded with chest tube drainage, operative intervention should be pursued. Many trivial tracheal injuries may never even be clinically apparent, except for minimal subcutaneous emphysema, because they may seal off so quickly. Any nonoperative course depends on finding minimal injury at bronchoscopy and probably is applicable only for the minority of cases that are clinically apparent.

Depending upon the extent of accompanying injuries, one should strive to extubate patients with airway injuries as soon as possible following definitive repair. There are few indications for performing a prophylactic tracheostomy following repair of a cervical tracheal injury. Ideally, the endotracheal tube should be removed immediately following the operative procedure.

Repair of the trachea or bronchi is usually accomplished by debriding the disrupted edges and then using interrupted, monofilament sutures to complete an anastomosis. We prefer to use a monofilament absorbable suture. Bronchial suture lines should be wrapped with either a pleural flap or intercostal muscle bundle to separate the suture line from the pulmonary artery. Cervical tracheal suture lines ideally should be wrapped with strap muscle. A thorough inspection of the esophagus should accompany repair of any cervical tracheal injury, as missed esophageal injuries may result in significant morbidity and mortality (5). Though rare, tracheoesophageal fistula may occur following blunt trauma. The classic sign of coughing immediately upon swallowing may not manifest itself until several days following the initial injury. This may be due to segmental ischemia of the esophagus at the level of the tracheal injury due to the initial insult (29). Necrosis with resultant fistula formation requires several days to develop. Reconstruction of these injuries may be complex but primary repair is preferred, if possible. Occasionally, blunt airway injury may be accompanied by injury to the aorta or brachiocephalic vessels (31). If a sternotomy is performed to repair the vascular injuries, the airway injury may also be repaired through this approach. Exposure of the distal trachea, carina, and both main bronchi is easily accomplished via median sternotomy.

Shorr et al. (32) reviewed the records of 515 patients who sustained blunt thoracic trauma over a 3-year period, looking for injury patterns, complications, and mortality. Not surprisingly, most patients were young (mean, 37 years), and most injuries occurred as a result of motor vehicle accidents. Eighty-four patients (16.3%) had isolated thoracic injuries and only four had thoracic tracheal or bronchial injuries; three of the four had injury to two or more extrathoracic systems.

Deslauriers et al. (27) reported on 13 patients treated for major bronchial tears over a 12-year period. Bronchoscopy confirmed the diagnosis and localized the tear in every case. All patients with rupture of a main bronchus had radiographic evidence of pneumomediastinum. Primary bronchial repair was the procedure of choice, but lobectomy was performed when a lobar bronchus was involved.

That these injuries occur rarely hardly needs to be restated. Bates (33), reporting on the experience of 25 British thoracic surgeons, estimated that a thoracic surgeon in the United Kingdom would see approximately two cases, only one of which would be acute, over a career of 30 years.

Smoke inhalation injury represents an entirely distinct class of airway trauma. The major pathophysiology involves edema to the soft tissues of the oropharynx, apparently resulting from the release of both oxygen-free radicals and thromboxane A2 from the injured tissues (34). With the increasing capillary and microvascular pressure and permeability, mucosal edema is noted. The tracheobronchial injury results mainly from the chemicals in smoke.

The inhalation injury produces an exudative response accompanied by dissolution of the epithelium. This is followed by a period of cast formation, which occurs in association with increased respiratory resistance. Usually, a major inhalation injury is accompanied by significant parenchymal injury, usually manifest by pulmonary edema (34).

Initial management following a significant inhalation injury usually requires endotracheal intubation for a variable period of time. Formerly, tracheostomy was performed readily in burn patients, but now it is reserved for specific indications, rather than as prophylactic airway management. In a recent study from the New York Hospital Burn Center, a review of 5 years' experience showed 99 tracheostomies performed in 3246 patients who had either acute loss of the airway or prolonged ventilator dependence (35). Twenty-eight patients developed late upper-airway sequelae, including tracheal stenosis, tracheoesophageal fistula, or tracheal arterial fistula. These complications were associated with a particularly high mortality. Seventy-four of the 99 patients who underwent tracheostomies died, with 54% of the deaths related to respiratory complications. Interestingly, there was a significantly higher mortality in patients with less than 30% total body surface area burned who underwent tracheostomy, while no difference in mortality was seen in patients with larger body surface area burns who required tracheostomy versus those who did not.

Despite the use of high-volume low-pressure cuff tracheostomy tubes, the development of major, late, upper-airway sequelae remains a significant problem following tracheostomy. This may also occur following endotracheal intubation, as illustrated by Figure 10.7. This 20-yr-old male sustained an inhalation injury in a mobile-home fire and required two separate episodes of endotracheal intubation, one for 3 days and one for 7 days. Approximately 6 weeks following his initial injury, he noted the increasing onset of respiratory distress manifest by stridor. Tracheal tomograms (Fig. 10.8) demonstrated tracheal stenosis beginning immediately distal to the glottis and extending for 6 cm. Because of increasing respiratory difficulties, a tracheostomy was performed through the strictured area. Subsequently a Montgomery T-tube (Hood Laboratories, Pembrook, MA) was placed to stent the airway.

It has been noted by Jones that younger patients tend to respond in a hypertrophic fashion to the effects of inhalation injury, resulting in the development of tracheal granulation tissue and stenosis (35). He feels that the insult of an inhalation injury with subsequent infection combined with intubation produces this response. Older patients are more likely to respond in a degenerative fashion, with necrosis of the tracheal wall leading to either tracheoesophageal fistula or tracheal arterial fistula. With more

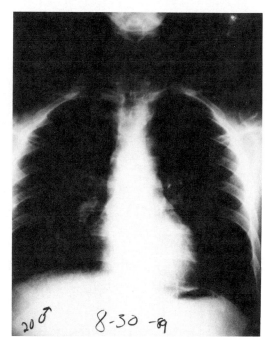

Figure 10.7. Chest radiograph 1 month following inhalation injury sustained in a mobile-home fire by a 20-yr-old male. Note the narrowing of the tracheal air column seen even on this plain film.

patients surviving significant burn injury, we expect to see greater numbers of patients with upper-airway sequelae who will require definitive treatment.

Many of these airway problems may not be amenable to immediate resection and reanastomosis. The use of an airway stent, such as the Montgomery silicone tracheal T-tube, then assumes greater importance (Fig. 10.9). Cooper et al. (36) described the use of this tube for the management of complex tracheal injuries and noted four categories of problems that may require its use. These included the use of the tube prior to definitive resection, as an adjunct at the time of resection, following resection for anastomotic problems, or as definitive treatment in cases deemed unsuitable for resection. They described the use of this tube in 18 patients who presented with a variety of problems, but included three patients with inhalation injury and nine patients with postintubation injuries. Five patients underwent placement of a T-tube for definitive management. The tube is positioned with the use of a rigid bronchoscope and is surprisingly well-tolerated for long periods of time, even when the proximal limb is placed between the vocal cords. The T-tube has been used for lesions in all locations of the upper airway and custom tubes have been designed for use at the carina or at either mainstem bronchus (Fig. 10.10). Warming and humidification of inspired air occurs in a normal fashion, since airflow occurs along the usual route, as the horizontal limb of the tube usually is kept corked. Speech is maintained, though at decreased amplitude, even when the proximal limb passes through the vocal cords. The availability of these

Figure 10.8. Tracheal tomograms showing the subglottic stricture resulting from inhalation injury and endotracheal intubation. Note the onset of the stenosis just distal to the vocal cords and extending for approximately 6 cm.

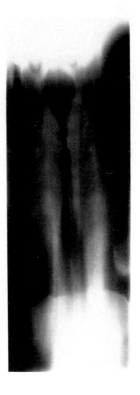

tubes, however, should not detract from the fact that, whenever possible, resection with reanastomosis remains the definitive treatment for these injuries and should be performed whenever feasible.

CHRONIC SEQUELAE OF BRONCHIAL DISRUPTION

At times, the initial presentation of bronchial disruption resulting from nonpenetrating trauma may be subtle enough that the injury is missed. Clinical findings referable to the airway may be absent and the radiologic findings may be subtle, demonstrating nothing more than a minimal pneumomediastinum, which may be visible only in retrospect.

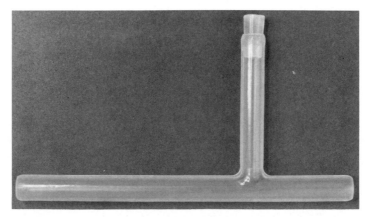

Figure 10.9. The standard Montgomery silicone T-tube (Hood Laboratories, Pembrook, MA). This tube comes in several sizes and is usually placed with the aid of a rigid bronchoscope.

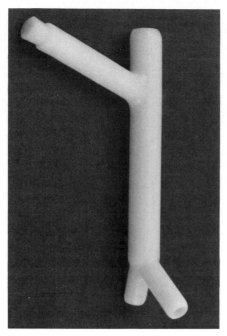

Figure 10.10.   A Y-bifurcation silicone stent (Hood Laboratories, Pembrook, MA) designed for lesions involving the carina and both proximal mainstem bronchi.

Follow-up chest x-ray studies to look for evidence of airway trauma or pulmonary contusion should be obtained in anyone suspected of having sustained significant blunt chest trauma. If an airway injury is missed, signs and symptoms develop within several weeks. Figure 10.11 is the chest radiograph of a young female taken 3 weeks following a motor vehicle accident, when she sought medical attention because of the insidious onset of an audible wheeze, which could be heard even by others around her. Bronchoscopy showed a narrowing of the left main bronchus resulting from the formation of granulation tissue and fibrosis. Bronchography, which may be an extremely useful imaging study if a bronchial stricture is suspected, demonstrated a marked narrowing in the left main bronchus (Fig. 10.12).

This illustrates the sequelae of a tracheobronchial rupture that is missed and not repaired acutely. The airway, at the time of the initial injury, may be completely disrupted yet held together by the strong connective tissue present, especially in young people. Likewise, an airway may be only partially disrupted, but in either case ventilation may be maintained. The disruption heals with the formation of granulation tissue and subsequent stricture formation usually within 3–4 weeks.

A critical factor is whether or not the stenosis causes complete obstruction or only partial obstruction. With partial obstruction, infection distal to the stenosis, that is, in the lung itself, commonly results, often causing a necrotizing process that destroys lung tissue. However, paradoxically, if the obstruction is complete, infection is unlikely; numerous reports have detailed late resection of a stricture, bronchial reconstruction, and restoration of lung function to almost normal (37, 38). The critical factor for determining whether resection of the stricture and primary reanastomosis will result in return of functioning lung parenchyma is the presence or absence of necrotizing infection. The presence of chronic infection often results in bronchiectatic or fibrous

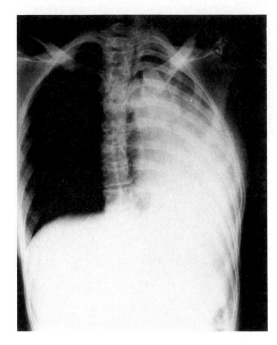

Figure 10.11.   Complete opacification of the left hemithorax occurring 3 weeks following blunt chest trauma, when the patient presented with an audible wheeze. Only minimal breath sounds could be heard on auscultation of the left chest.

changes that may, in some instances, mandate pulmonary resection. Nonoyama et al. (38) reported successful repair of a left main bronchus 9 years following injury in a 26-year-old patient. Improving pulmonary function in the left lung was documented over the first 9 weeks after operation, and by the 60th postoperative day the vital capacity in the left lung was 41% of the total. Unless there is definite evidence of infection, an attempt should be made to resect the strictured area of the bronchus, reserving pulmonary resection only for those cases where lung parenchyma has been destroyed.

SUMMARY
Injuries to the trachea or main bronchi require prompt recognition and early definitive primary repair of the airway. Occasionally, a trivial airway injury may be managed expectantly. The major morbidity and mortality following these injuries usually depend more on the associated injuries, mainly to the major vascular structures. Bronchoscopy remains the definitive diagnostic procedure, though suspicion of an airway injury should be high in the patient sustaining chest trauma who presents with a pneumothorax that fails to completely resolve following chest tube insertion. Often, these patients become symptomatically worse when the chest tube is connected to suction, and this finding is almost pathognomonic of airway disruption. Failure to recognize a disrupted airway often leads to stricture formation with the possibility of obstructive necrotizing pneumonia and potential destruction of lung parenchyma. Injury to the airway, especially as an isolated finding, is a rare occurrence and, if not suspected in certain circumstances, is easily missed. The true incidence of these injuries remains unknown, since many individuals sustaining them die of associated injuries prior to reaching the hospital.

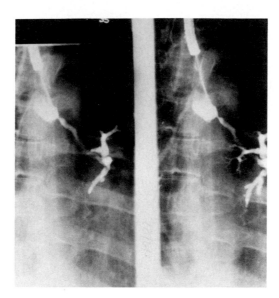

Figure 10.12. Bronchogram of the same patient depicted in Figure 10.11, showing the significant bronchial stenosis. Note the pooling of contrast proximal to the stricture and then the short segment of stricture with contrast flowing into segmental bronchi.

REFERENCES

1. Bertelsen S, Howitz P. Injuries to the trachea and bronchi. Thorax 1972;27:188–194.
2. Kemmerer WT, Eckert WG, Gathright JB, Reemtsma K, Creech O Jr. Patterns of thoracic injuries in fatal traffic accidents. J Trauma 1961;1:595–599.
3. Thompson DA, Rowlands BJ, Walker WE, Kuykendal RC, Miller PW, Fischer RP. Urgent thoracotomy for pulmonary or tracheobronchial injury. J Trauma 1988;28:276–280.
4. Kelly JP, Webb WR, Moulder PV, Everson C, Burch BH, Lindsey ES. Management of airway trauma. I. Tracheobronchial injuries. Ann Thorac Surg 1985;40:551–555.
5. Kelly JP, Webb WR, Moulder PV, Moustoukas NM, Lirtzman M. Management of airway trauma. II. Combined injuries to the trachea and esophagus. Ann Thorac Surg 1987;43:160–163.
6. Symbas PN, Hatcher CR, Boehm GAW. Acute penetrating tracheal trauma. Ann Thorac Surg 1976;5:473–477.
7. Brodsky JB, Shulman MS, Mark JBD. Airway rupture with a disposable double lumen tube (letter). Anesthesiology 1986;64:415.
8. Burton NA, Fall SM, Lyons T, Graeber GM. Rupture of the left main bronchus with a polyvinyl chloride double lumen tube. Chest 1983;83:928–929.
9. Rollins JR, Tocino I. Early radiographic signs of tracheal rupture. AJR 1987;148:695–698.
10. Wagner DL, Gammage GW, Wong ML. Tracheal rupture following insertion of a disposable double lumen tube. Anesthesiology 1985;63:698–700.
11. Alyono D, Perry JF. Impact of speed limit. I. Chest injuries, review of 966 cases. J Thorac Cardiovasc Surg 1982;83:519–522.
12. Dougall AM, Paul ME, Finley RJ, Holliday RL, Coles JC, Duff JH. Chest trauma: current morbidity and mortality. J Trauma 1977;17:547–553.
13. Webb A (cited in Roxburg JC). Rupture of the tracheobronchial tree. Thorax 1987;42:681–688.
14. Winslow WH. Rupture of bronchus of wild duck. Phila Med Times 1871;1:255.
15. Krinitzki SI. Zur Kasuistik einer vollstandigen Zerreibung des rechten Luftrohrenastes. Virchows Arch Pathol Anat Physiol Klin Med 1928;266:815–819.
16. Clerf LH. Rupture of main bronchus from external injury. Surgery 1940;7:276–279.
17. Kinsella TJ, Johnsrud LW. Traumatic rupture of the bronchus. J Thorac Surg 1947;16:571–583.
18. Griffith JL. Fracture of the bronchus. Thorax 1949;4:105–109.
19. Scannell JG. Rupture of the bronchus following closed injury to the chest. Ann Surg 1951;133:127–130.

20. Beskin CA. Rupture-separation of the cervical trachea following a closed chest injury: report of a case successfully treated by primary anastomosis. J Thorac Surg 1957;34:392–394.

21. Butler RM, Moser F. The padded dash syndrome: blunt trauma to the larynx and trachea. Laryngoscope 1968;78:1172–1182.

22. Payne WS, DeRemu R. Injuries of the trachea and major bronchi. Postgrad Med J 1971;49:152–157.

23. Nahum AM, Kroell CK, Schneider DC. The biochemical basis of chest impact protection. II. Effects of cardiovascular pressurization. J Trauma 1973;13:443–459.

24. Chesterman JT, Satsangi PN. Rupture of the trachea and bronchi by closed injury. Thorax 1966;21:21–27.

25. Attar S, Kirby WH Jr. The forces producing certain types of thoracic trauma. In: Daughtry DC, ed. Thoracic trauma. Boston: Little, Brown, 1980:1–10.

26. Zapolanski A, Ilvis R, Todd TRJ. Injury to the middle lobe bronchus and pulmonary artery: an unusual pattern. Ann Thorac Surg 1983;35:156–158.

27. Deslauriers J, Beaulieu M, Archambault G, LaForge J, Bernier R. Diagnosis of long term follow up of major bronchial disruptions due to non-penetrating trauma. Ann Thorac Surg 1982;33:32–39.

28. Tocino I, Miller MH. Computer tomography in blunt chest trauma. J Thorac Imaging 1987;2:45–59.

29. Braun RA, Goldware RR, Flores LM. Cervical tracheal transection with esophageal fistula. Arch Otolaryngol 1972;96:67–71.

30. Ramzy AI, Rodriguez A, Turney SZ. Management of major tracheobronchial ruptures in patients with multiple system trauma. J Trauma 1988;28:1353–1357.

31. Sadow SH, Murray CA, Wilson RF, Mansoori S, Harrington SD. Traumatic rupture of ascending aorta and left main bronchus. Ann Thorac Surg 1988;45:682–683.

32. Shorr RM, Crittenden N, Indeck M, Hartunian SL, Rodriguez A. Blunt thoracic trauma: analysis of 515 patients. Ann Surg 1987;206:200–205.

33. Bates N. Rupture of the bronchus. In: Williams WG, Smith RE, eds. Trauma of the chest (the Coventry conference). Bristol: John Wright and Sons, 1977:142–150.

34. Haponik EF. Smoke inhalation. Am Rev Respir Dis 1988;138:1060–1063.

35. Jones WG, Madden M, Finkelstein J, Yurt RW, Goodwin CW. Tracheostomies in burn patients. Ann Surg 1989;209:471–474.

36. Cooper JD, Todd TRJ, Ilvis R, Pearson FG. Use of the silicone tracheal T-tube for the management of complex tracheal injuries. J Thorac Cardiovasc Surg 1981;82:559–568.

37. Logeais Y, Florent D, Danrigal A, et al. Traumatic rupture of the right main bronchus in an eight year old child successfully repaired eight years after injury. Ann Surg 1970;172:1039–1047.

38. Nonoyama M, Masuda A, Kasahara K, Mogi T, Kagawa T. Total rupture of the left main bronchus successfully repaired nine years after injury. Ann Thorac Surg 1976;21:445–448.

11 Esophageal Injuries

John R. Hankins, MD
Safuh Attar, MD

Full-thickness injury of the esophagus, i.e. laceration, perforation, or rupture, usually has disastrous consequences because of the aggressive infection that rapidly occurs in the mediastinal tissues. Prompt diagnosis and early institution of effective treatment may obviate not only a fatal outcome but also a protracted convalescence.

CLASSIFICATION ACCORDING TO ETIOLOGY

It is helpful to classify esophageal injuries according to etiology or causative mechanism, since this may affect the patient's symptomatology or clinical presentation (Table 11.1). This classification is a modification of the one proposed by Seiler and Brooks (1). The intraluminal agents and extraluminal forces that can cause esophageal injuries are well-defined. The former are listed first in the classification since they are far more common. So-called "spontaneous" rupture has a less well-defined cause and is listed as a separate entity. It does not properly fit either within the intraluminal agent

Table 11.1.
Classification of Esophageal Injuries According to Etiology

A. Injury from intraluminal agents or forces
    1. Instrumentation- and manipulation-associated injuries
        a. Diagnostic endoscopy
        b. Dilatation
        c. Esophageal intubation with/without balloon tamponade
        d. Attempted endotracheal intubation
        e. Sclerotherapy
    2. Foreign bodies
    3. Pneumatic or blast injury
    4. Caustic or corrosive agent ingestion
B. Injury from extraluminal agents or forces
    1. Penetrating wounds (gunshot wounds, stab wounds)
    2. Blunt trauma
    3. Injury during thoracic surgical procedures
C. Spontaneous rupture
    1. Barogenic (Boerhaave's syndrome)
    2. Nonbarogenic (secondary to esophageal ulceration or other disease)
D. Perforations occurring on the basis of preexisting disease of the esophagus
    1. Neoplasms
    2. Esophagitis with ulceration

nor the extraluminal force category. Last, perforations occurring on the basis of preexisting disease are listed as a separate heading because they usually are more complicated and more difficult to manage than those in the three preceding categories.

Injury from Intraluminal Agents or Forces
INSTRUMENTATION- AND MANIPULATION-ASSOCIATED INJURIES

Instrumentation is the most common cause of esophageal perforation. A 1974 survey by the American Society of Gastrointestinal Endoscopy (2) found that perforations occurred in 0.03% of esophagogastroduodenoscopies and in 0.25% of esophageal dilation procedures, for an overall rate of 0.13%. Although many authors have considered the flexible, fiberoptic endoscopes safer than the rigid instruments, Katz (3) reported similar perforation rates for the two types of instruments: 0.74% for the rigid and 0.93% for the fiberoptic esophagoscope. Michel et al. (4) noted an incidence of perforation of 0.15% for elective esophageal instrumentation during a 20-yr period.

Of the three anatomic areas of narrowing of the esophagus, the pharyngoesophageal junction is the narrowest and is the area most often perforated during instrumentation (1). The second narrowing, where the esophagus curves around the aortic arch, is much less commonly perforated. The third narrow segment, and the second most common site of perforation, is at the lower end of the esophagus, where it curves to the left just before passing through the diaphragm. This segment is also a common site of esophageal disease, such as esophagitis, stricture, or achalasia, and this factor further increases the risk, particularly for dilation.

The addition of biopsy or dilation to esophagoscopy increases the possibility of perforation. The esophagus in older patients is more friable and is easily perforated by biopsy forceps. The flexible, tapered, mercury-filled rubber bougies (such as, for example, the Maloney bougies), although they are supposedly safer than the rigid, woven variety, are not free of hazard if too large a size or too much force is used in dilating a stricture. The same is true of dilations performed with direct vision using a rigid esophagoscope. Last, the incidence of perforation with pneumatic or hydrostatic dilation for achalasia is four times greater than the incidence of esophageal leak after esophagomyotomy (5).

The various types of indwelling esophageal tubes that are inserted for therapeutic purposes have all been associated with perforations. The Sengstaken-Blakemore tube, which is utilized to provide balloon tamponade of bleeding varices, can produce perforation through pressure necrosis or erosion. The funnel-shaped intraluminal or endoesophageal tubes that are placed through unresectable neoplasms to provide a channel for alimentation can lead to perforation, either during the process of insertion or through erosion of the esophageal wall by the tip or the unyielding flange of the tube. The risk exists with both types of placement of these tubes—"traction" and "pulsion"—but has lessened somewhat in recent years by the inauguration of the softer silicone rubber tubes (6). Perforations also have been produced by simple nasogastric (Levin) tubes (7).

Attempted endotracheal intubation can cause perforation of the hypopharynx or cervical esophagus. These injuries are more likely to occur when the intubation is performed blindly, with inadequate exposure, under urgent conditions, or by an inadequately trained or inexperienced physician (8, 9). Another type of airway, the esophageal obturator airway employed by emergency medical technicians for resuscitation, also has been reported to have produced esophageal disruption (10). A patient with a perforation caused by the insertion of this type of airway has been treated recently in the Shock Trauma Center of the Maryland Institute for Emergency Medical Services Systems.

Sclerotherapy for esophageal varices is an uncommon cause of esophageal perforation. It was responsible for only 1 of the 115 perforations reported by Nesbitt and Sawyers (11). This complication of sclerotherapy has been described by Soderlund and Wiechel (12) and by Huizinga et al. (13). Postlethwait (14) surveyed the literature and found 977 bleeding episodes that were treated by sclerotherapy. Perforations occurred in 3.8%. Perforation after sclerotherapy probably results from injection of too large an amount of sclerosing material outside the varix, with resultant necrosis and sloughing of the esophageal wall.

FOREIGN BODIES

Foreign bodies are a common cause of perforation. A wide variety of objects have been described as having caused perforation. Perforations may be produced by a sharp object penetrating the wall of the esophagus, by a smooth foreign body producing pressure necrosis, or by instrumental laceration of the esophagus during endoscopic removal. The foreign body may be organic rather than metallic. We have seen two instances of perforation following endoscopic removal of meat impacted in the lower esophagus. At thoracotomy, it was impossible to tell whether the perforation had been caused by pressure necrosis from the impacted meat or by the instrumental manipulation. The endoscopic removal of foreign bodies, particularly of sharp objects, may be quite difficult. The procedure usually should be done under general anesthesia. Exact localization of the foreign body in the esophagus by radiographic studies, usually with contrast, should be obtained beforehand. A contrast esophagogram should be performed immediately afterward to rule out a perforation. If the foreign body proves difficult to retrieve, the clinician should not persist in attempts at endoscopic removal but, rather, should use an open thoracotomy approach.

PNEUMATIC OR BLAST INJURY

Pneumatic or blast injury is listed under external blunt trauma in some classifications of esophageal injuries. However, we think this injury is more properly classified with those due to intraluminal agents. This unusual injury occurs when there is a sudden accidental release of gas under high pressure near the face or into the oral cavity of the victim. Another reported variant of pneumatic injury occurs in children who bite into an exposed inner tube bulging through a defect in a tractor tire (15, 16). Michel et al. in their collective review (17) found only 13 reported cases of blast or pneumatic injuries of the esophagus.

CAUSTIC OR CORROSIVE AGENT INGESTION

Damage to the esophagus from ingestion of caustic or corrosive agents is not an "injury" in the usual sense of the word. However, we believe the chemical "burn" of the esophageal wall produced by these agents, which is often full-thickness, should be included in any discussion of esophageal injuries. These corrosive chemical agents may lead directly to perforation through full-thickness necrosis of the esophageal wall, or perforation of the inflamed, scarred esophagus may occur when dilation is attempted during the healing phase. In recent years, we have seen three patients with perforation of the esophagus due to the direct necrotizing effect of the caustic material and one with perforation secondary to attempted dilation of the scarred, inflamed esophagus.

Injury from Extraluminal Agents or Forces
PENETRATING WOUNDS (GUNSHOT WOUNDS, STAB WOUNDS)

Penetrating wounds are a relatively uncommon cause of injury to the thoracic esophagus, doubtless because of its small diameter in relation to the dimensions of the surrounding vital organs. In the neck, penetrating wounds are a somewhat more common cause of esophageal injury. Thus, among the 115 patients with esophageal perforation reported by Nesbitt and Sawyers (11), penetrating wounds were the cause in only 14 patients (gunshot, 13; stab, 1). These penetrating types of wounds were responsible in 11 of the 27 patients with cervical esophageal perforations, but in only 3 of the 69 patients with perforations of the thoracic esophagus, and in none of the 19 patients with abdominal esophageal perforations. These penetrating injuries, particularly if they involve the intrathoracic esophagus, are associated with a high mortality rate, principally because of problems with exposure and complex associated injuries. Thus, Defore et al. (18) had 18 deaths (23%) among 77 patients with penetrating injuries of the esophagus. Four of the deaths were attributed to missed injury, five to anastomotic breakdown, and six to associated injuries. Symbas et al. (19) had 10 deaths (21%) among 48 patients with gunshot wounds of the esophagus. They stressed that the physical and radiographic findings of esophageal injury in such patients often are nondiagnostic, being masked by associated injuries to other vital structures. A high index of suspicion is needed for diagnosis in such patients. Glatterer et al. (20) reported 22 patients with penetrating esophageal trauma and 4 with blunt esophageal trauma. Seventeen of the penetrating wounds involved the cervical esophagus and five, the thoracic esophagus. Four patients (15%) died early, and there was one late death. Six patients with penetrating injuries of the cervical esophagus underwent contrast esophagograms; two were false-negative studies. Of the three contrast studies that were performed in patients with injuries of the thoracic esophagus, one was falsely negative. Six patients underwent esophagoscopies; one, in a patient with a thoracic esophageal injury, was falsely negative. Therefore, the authors (20) recommended that any patient with penetrating trauma whose physical findings suggest esophageal injury should undergo a contrast esophagogram and, if that is negative, an esophagoscopy.

BLUNT TRAUMA

Perforation or rupture of the esophagus from blunt trauma is quite uncommon. In the reported cases, the blunt force usually has been applied to the abdomen rather than the chest, although Lundberg et al. (21) reported lacerations of the gastroesophageal junction following closed-chest cardiac massage. The 1982 collective review by Michel et al. (17) included 31 cases of solitary esophageal rupture or perforation from blunt trauma that had been reported up to that time. The pathogenesis of these injuries was thought by Michel et al. (17) to be similar to that of postemetic rupture. Among the instances of perforation or rupture analyzed in the collective review, 90% occurred in the thoracic esophagus and only 10% in the cervical esophagus. Only one of the cervical esophageal ruptures was caused by trauma from a steering wheel. However, Hagan (22) reported four cases of pharyngoesophageal perforations or lacerations due to blunt trauma to the neck, to which he added nine others found in a review of the literature. Of those 13 pharyngoesophageal injuries, 4 were due to steering wheel impact. Hagan postulated a "barometric" mechanism for these perforations and thought they resulted from the combined effect of three factors: the natural anatomic weakness at the junction of hypopharynx and cervical esophagus caused by a lack of supporting longitudinal muscle fibers in this region; and closure of the upper airway by blunt impact at the hyoid bone level that, combined with an upper chest impact that forcibly empties air out of the lungs into the upper airway, may exceed its bursting pressure. An independent or associated factor might be hyperextension of the neck due to an impact on the head, with resultant shearing of the hypopharynx and larynx against the extended cervical vertebral bodies.

INJURY DURING THORACIC SURGICAL PROCEDURES

Esophageal perforation can occur during several different types of paraesophageal operations, including antireflux procedures (17), vagotomy (23), and pneumonectomy for cancer (17). The sutures placed through the esophageal muscle layer during various antireflux operations can tear the wall and result in a perforation. We have observed such an occurrence in connection with a Belsey Mark IV antireflux operation. Perforations also have been noted in connection with the Hill median arcuate ligament hiatal hernia repair and with the Nissen fundoplication (17). The incidence of esophageal perforation following abdominal vagotomy is approximately 0.5%. (23.)

Esophageal myotomy also should be included with hiatal hernia repair and vagotomy as one of the operations involving the external aspect of the esophagus that most frequently results in leakage or perforation (24, 25). A tiny opening made inadvertently in the mucosa during the myotomy may not be recognized, or if recognized, it may not be repaired adequately. Also, we have seen instances in which the delicate, unsupported mucosa at the site of the myotomy has been perforated by the blind passage of a nasogastric tube.

Spontaneous Rupture

Since Boerhaave (26, 27) originally described a case of transmural postemetic rupture of the esophagus in 1724, the terms "spontaneous perforation" or "spontaneous rupture" have generally been used to encompass all full-thickness perforations associated with prolonged or forceful vomiting. This clinical entity also may occur with weight lifting, defecation, childbirth, and seizures.

Abbott et al. (28) proposed a classification of this entity based on three postulated etiologic factors: (*a*) increased intraesophageal pressure, (*b*) preexisting disease of the esophagus, and (*c*) neurogenic causes. A marked and precipitous increase in pressure within an apparently normal esophagus is the most common cause of "spontaneous" rupture. The usual mechanism is a vomiting episode in which the sudden increment in intraabdominal pressure is transmitted to an esophagus which is relaxed but obstructed at its upper end by spasm, or a failure to relax, of the esophageal musculature (17). In more than 90% of patients, the rupture occurs in the left lateral aspect of the distal esophagus, where the esophagus deviates to the left and anteriorly before passing through the diaphragm (11).

Preexisting disease of the esophagus has been postulated as the etiologic factor in those patients who develop "spontaneous" perforation without having experienced prior vomiting or other events that produce increased intraesophageal pressure. The preexisting disease in these patients usually is one that causes obstruction of the distal esophagus, such as a web, a stricture, or a carcinoma. If an associated abnormal motility is present with the resulting weak peristalsis, a voluntary swallowing effort may occur to supplement the weak peristalsis. As a meal bolus being thus propelled meets the obstructing lesion, a rise in intraesophageal pressure occurs which, if rapid and severe enough, can result in esophageal rupture (17).

Several reports have documented rupture or perforation of the esophagus in connection with intracranial diseases or after intracranial operations (17). Cushing (29) postulated that stimulation of the vagi could lead to vasospasm with consequent ischemia in the wall of the upper gastrointestinal tract. The resultant area of softening or ulceration in the esophagus could rupture with any elevation of intraluminal pressure.

We, with some other authors, such as Nesbitt and Sawyers (11), prefer simply dividing spontaneous perforations into just two categories: *barogenic* and *nonbarogenic.* The barogenic category would include the classic Boerhaave type of perforation occurring in an esophagus, which may have been previously normal, in response to emesis or other barogenic events such as defecation. Also included in the barogenic category are patients with preexisting esophageal disease producing partial distal obstruction but in whom the perforation would not have occurred without the added factor of a sudden increase in intraluminal pressure. This increase in pressure may be caused by a forceful voluntary swallowing effort intended to supplement a disordered, weak motility rather than by emesis or defecation. The nonbarogenic category is comprised principally of those ruptures due to neurogenic factors, such as those associated with the softening and ulceration of the esophageal wall that Cushing (29) postulated to be due to vagal stimulation leading to vasospasm, with resultant local ischemia.

Because spontaneous perforation or rupture is relatively uncommon, and because the symptoms and signs often simulate those of other diseases such as perforated peptic ulcer, pancreatitis, myocardial infarction, or dissecting aneurysm, the diagnosis is frequently delayed (11). In the series of Nesbitt and Sawyers (11), the diagnosis was delayed in 58% of the patients. Chest pain and fever were the two most frequent clinical findings, occurring in 86.4 and 63.6% of the patients, respectively. However, *abdominal* pain occurred in 45% of the patients and was thought possibly to have confused the diagnosis in several. Walker et al. (30) reported that the "classic" triad of symptoms and signs (emesis, chest pain, and subcutaneous emphysema) occurred in only 1 of their 14 patients.

Perforations Occurring on the Basis of Preexisting Disease of the Esophagus

Perforations that are actually caused by a preexisting esophageal disease itself, rather than by endoscopic or other interventions performed for such disease, are relatively uncommon. The two disease categories that have been identified most frequently as causing perforations are neoplasms and esophagitis with ulceration. The perforations caused by neoplasms are seldom free perforations, but more often lead to a mediastinal abscess or an esophagorespiratory fistula. In the series of Skinner et al. (24) that comprised 48 perforations in 47 patients, there were 13 patients with perforations due to neoplasm. In five of these, the tumors perforated into the pleura or mediastinum: two spontaneously and three during a course of radiation therapy. The remaining eight patients had malignant tracheoesophageal fistulae. Our series includes only one patient with spontaneous free perforation of a carcinoma into the pleura; it also includes one patient whose tumor spontaneously perforated into the lung parenchyma.

Perforation caused by peptic esophagitis with ulceration is even less common than malignant perforation. The series of Skinner et al. (24) included two such patients, one of whom had the Zollinger-Ellison syndrome. In the other, peptic ulceration of the esophagus developed cephalad to an esophagogastric anastomosis after a resection for carcinoma and led to a tracheoesophageal fistula with, ultimately, a fatal outcome.

The part that a usually unrecognized, preexisting, distally obstructing disease may play in producing one type of so-called spontaneous perforation has been discussed above (see "Spontaneous Rupture").

DIAGNOSIS
Symptoms and Physical Examination Findings

The diagnosis of esophageal perforation is facilitated if the physician has a high index of suspicion. The index of suspicion is likely to be higher in the case of instrumental perforations and, therefore, such perforations are generally diagnosed fairly early. The diagnosis of perforations caused by blunt trauma, and of spontaneous perforations, is more likely to be delayed.

The presenting symptoms and signs and the initial roentgenographic findings differ according to the location of the perforation. By far, the most common symptom is pain, which is present in 70–90% of patients, although it is acute in onset in only 30% (3). But the pain with cervical esophageal perforations is more often located in the chest, whereas with thoracic esophageal perforations, it more likely occurs in the abdomen or back (31). Considering perforations at all locations, dyspnea is the second most common symptom but, although it occurs in 41% of those with thoracic perforations, it is seen relatively uncommonly with cervical or abdominal perforations (11). The third most common symptom, dysphagia, was found in only 4% of the patients in the overall series of Bladergroen et al. (32).

Fever and subcutaneous emphysema are the two most common physical signs; the latter finding is present in about 60% or more of cervical perforations but occurs in less than 20% of thoracic perforations (3, 11, 32, 33). Abdominal tenderness and cyanosis are less common physical findings, the latter being found principally in patients with delayed diagnosis.

Michel et al. (3) made a point of comparing the clinical manifestations of cervical and thoracic esophageal perforations. They found that, in cervical perforations, subcutaneous emphysema was the most frequent finding, occurring in nearly 60% of the patients, followed (in order) by pneumomediastinum and hydrothorax. Dyspnea was noted in less than 30%, and pneumothorax and shock were each observed in only about 20%, or less, of the patients. Among the thoracic perforations, on the other hand, hydrothorax was the most common manifestation, followed by dyspnea and then by shock. Less common were pneumomediastinum, occurring in slightly less than 40% of the patients, pneumothorax (30%), and subcutaneous emphysema (less than 20%).

Radiographic Studies
PLAIN CHEST ROENTGENOGRAMS

In addition to chest roentgenograms, soft-tissue posteroanterior and lateral films of the neck should be obtained in suspected perforations of the cervical esophagus. In some cases with perforation, the films will show dissection of air in the periesophageal region, retropharyngeal swelling, or an increased diameter of the retrotracheal space.

As pointed out by DeMeester (34), the finding of abnormalities on chest roentgenography depends on three factors: the time elapsed since perforation, the site of the perforation, and the integrity of the mediastinal pleura. First, mediastinal emphysema, or pneumomediastinum, is present in only about 40% of patients with thoracic perforations and, even then, it takes at least 1 hr to appear; mediastinal widening due to edema may take several hours to develop. Second, the site of the perforation affects the chest roentgenographic findings. As mentioned earlier, cervical (subcutaneous) emphysema is quite common in cervical esophageal perforations, but the less common pneumomediastinum tends to develop late. In thoracic esophageal perforations, pneumomediastinum tends to occur earlier, but it may be missed if the radiograph is underexposed. Frequently, a roentgenogram of the neck, if it is obtained along with the chest roentgenogram, will demonstrate air in the vicinity of the deep cervical (erector spinae) muscles before it can be clearly identified in the intrathoracic mediastinum. Third, the integrity of the mediastinal pleura will affect the radiographic findings: if the integrity is preserved, mediastinal emphysema (pneumomediastinum) occurs early; hydrothorax, on the other hand, develops slowly and a pneumothorax does not occur. The appearance of a pneumothorax means that a breach has occurred in the mediastinal pleura. In DeMeester's experience (34), a pneumothorax occurs in approximately 77% of the patients with esophageal perforation (left-sided in 67%, right-sided in 20%, and bilateral in 10%).

CONTRAST ESOPHAGOGRAPHY

Even if roentgenograms of the neck and chest provide evidence that an esophageal perforation has occurred, a contrast esophagogram is ordinarily indicated for the following purposes: to confirm the diagnosis, to demonstrate the location and size of the perforation and to show whether it is contained or free, and to elucidate the relationship of the perforation to any preexisting disease that may be present.

Controversy exists regarding the type of contrast medium that should be used in a patient with a suspected esophageal perforation. Barium sulfate normally is the contrast material of choice for radiographic visualization of the gastrointestinal tract because of its high density, superior mucosal coating, isoosmolarity, and relatively inert nature. However, the instillation of barium, with or without an accompanying inoculum of oral bacteria, into the mediastinum in cats has been shown to cause granuloma formation and, in some instances, extensive pleural adhesions (35). To our knowledge, there have been no studies in humans bearing out the clinical significance, if any, of this mediastinal reaction. Nor are we aware of any documented evidence that the entry of barium into the mediastinum or pleural cavity is innocuous (36). There is cause for concern that, if the granulomatous mediastinitis and fibrosis shown to develop in cats occurred to a sufficient degree in humans clinically significant complications could result. Another lesser disadvantage of barium is that the material, by its long-term persistence in the tissues, may obscure or confuse certain details on subsequent chest roentgenograms.

Water-soluble iodinated contrast agents, such as diatrizoate methylglucamine (Gastrografin), when instilled into the mediastinum of cats by James et al. (35), did not cause a significant inflammatory reaction. However, water-soluble contrast medium does have certain disadvantages in comparison to barium. Its inferior radiographic density and mucosal coating ability can result in missing or inadequately demonstrating 25–50% of esophageal perforations (37). It has a high osmolality—about 6 times that of normal human serum if undiluted (36). Therefore, if it is aspirated or in some other way gains entry into the tracheobronchial tree, it causes, at the very least, irritation and respiratory distress and, in larger amounts, life-threatening pulmonary edema or pneumonitis. Water-soluble medium may draw fluid from the intravascular space into the bowel lumen, with resultant hypovolemia and electrolyte derangement (36).

Generally speaking, a careful review of the patient's history, physical findings, and chest roentgenogram will be a useful guide as to which type of contrast medium should be used. If there is a suspicion that an esophagorespiratory fistula is present, barium sulfate should be the medium used. If, however, one suspects an esophageal perforation into the mediastinum or the pleural or peritoneal cavities, the initial contrast material should be a water-soluble one. If the patient's swallowing mechanism is impaired or he/she is unconscious or has an endotracheal tube in place, the contrast medium can be instilled through a nasogastric tube. If the esophagogram using the water-soluble agent shows no perforation, it should *not* be construed as ruling out a perforation but, rather, it should be followed immediately by an esophagogram using barium.

We have found that, in the great majority of patients, the perforation can be demonstrated adequately by the use of water-soluble contrast medium alone (Fig. 11.1).

With the use of proper radiographic techniques and the appropriate contrast medium, the incidence of false-negative esophagograms should not exceed 10% (32, 34). The positioning of the patient during the study is important. If the examination is performed with the patient only in the erect position, the contrast medium may pass through the esophagus too rapidly to demonstrate a small perforation. Prone oblique projection views and cross-table left or right lateral decubitus views should also be obtained (34, 37).

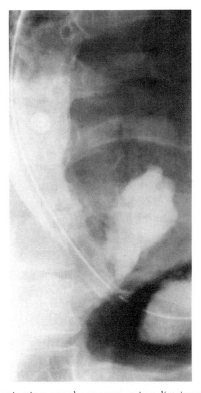

Figure 11.1.   An oblique-projection esophagogram using diatrizoate methylglucamine (Gastrografin) clearly demonstrates a perforation (endoscopic) of a narrowing at the esophagogastric junction, which proved to be a carcinoma. A nasogastric tube is in place in the esophagus and stomach.

COMPUTED TOMOGRAPHY

Computed tomography is not recommended as a routine diagnostic measure in a patient with a suspected esophageal perforation, but it has on occasion proved helpful in diagnosing a perforation that was unsuspected because of an atypical presentation (38) and in detecting the late complications of an anastomotic leak after esophago-gastrectomy (39).

Diagnostic Esophagoscopy

This procedure ordinarily does not help in the diagnosis of esophageal perforation. The one outstanding exception is in patients who have sustained external penetrating trauma with suspected esophageal involvement. In such patients, because of the presence of associated injuries to other organs, the contrast esophagography frequently is performed under less than ideal conditions and, therefore, the false-negative rate is high (20). If the contrast esophagogram is negative and an esophageal injury still is suspected, an esophagoscopy should be done (40). When the contrast esophagogram must be omitted because of the urgency of the need to repair other injuries, an esophagoscopy can be performed intraoperatively (19, 40).

TREATMENT

The treatment of esophageal injuries should be guided by (*a*) the anatomic location of the injury, i.e., whether it involves the cervical or thoracic esophagus; (*b*) whether the injury or disruption is free or contained and, if contained, whether the cavity drains freely back into the esophagus; (*c*) the severity of the systemic reaction to the injury, which will, to a large extent, be determined by the category of item *b* to which the patient belongs; (*d*) the time interval between the injury and the inception of diagnosis and treatment; and (*e*) whether there is an associated obstructing lesion distal to the injury.

Injuries of the Cervical Esophagus

These injuries constitute a special category. Surgical drainage, with or without definitive repair, is so simple to perform and generally provides such satisfactory results that there is very little place for conservative, nonoperative management (33). Exploration and drainage should be carried out through an obliquely vertical skin incision along the anterior border of the sternocleidomastoid muscle or, alternatively, through a modified collar incision (Fig. 11.2). The dissection proceeds inward, passing anteromedial to the sternocleidomastoid muscle and the internal jugular vein and carotid artery, lateral to the thyroid gland and the trachea, and on down to the esophagus. Only the middle thyroid vein and, at times, the inferior thyroid artery and omohyoid muscle need to be divided. If the perforation can be readily visualized and if the surrounding wall of the esophagus is not too inflamed or friable, the perforation should be sutured. Otherwise, suturing can be omitted. But the essential step is the establishment of adequate drainage, usually with a suction-type drainage system (33). Broad-spectrum antimicrobials should be administered. Oral intake is withheld and provision is made for nutritional support, either through intravenous hyperalimentiaton or a feeding jejunostomy.

When the perforation has been diagnosed late and a retroesophageal or retropharyngoesophageal abscess has formed, the identical surgical approach and method of drainage should be used, but, of course, suture of the perforation should not be attempted. Most of these perforations eventually heal if no distal obstruction is present.

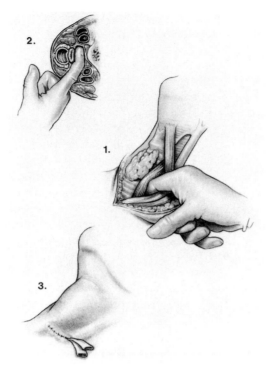

Figure 11.2.   Technique for exploration and drainage of a cervical esophageal perforation. The incision may be either an obliquely vertical approach along the anterior border of the sternocleidomastoid muscle or a transverse, "collar" approach. *1,* the dissection proceeds inward, anteromedial to the sternocleidomastoid muscle, the internal jugular vein, and the carotid artery and lateral to the thyroid gland and the trachea. *2,* cross-sectional view shows operator's finger entering and exploring the space between the esophagus and the prevertebral fascia. *3,* a drain has been placed in the retroesophageal space and brought out through the lateral end of the incision. (Modified from Grillo HC. Esophageal perforation. Surg Rounds 1983;6:50–71).

Injuries of the Thoracic Esophagus

The treatment of injuries of the thoracic esophagus must be individualized according to the category, mentioned earlier, to which the patient belongs.

CONSERVATIVE SUPPORTIVE AND NONOPERATIVE MANAGEMENT

Certain carefully selected patients can be successfully treated by *conservative supportive management* without resorting to thoracotomy and operative repair. Lyons et al. (41) retrospectively compared two groups of patients. The first group (thoracotomy) consisted of 18 patients with esophageal perforations from a variety of causes, mostly spontaneous and instrumental, who were treated by major thoracotomy and suture of the defect. The second group (conservative) consisted of 11 patients with perforations from a variety of causes (but also mostly spontaneous and instrumental) who were treated with various combinations of "minor procedures," such as gastrostomy and chest tube insertion, but without a major thoracotomy. Mortality was 7 of 18 (39%) in the first group but only 1 of 11 (9%) in the second group. Most of the patients in each group apparently had free, rather than contained, perforations. Chest tube drainage was used in 4 of the 11 patients in group two, and cervical mediastinotomy and pericardial drainage in 1 other patient. Since the publication of this report by Lyons et al., we have found very few, if any, reports in which there has been duplication of such a high success rate with the use of conservative-supportive management in patients with free perforation of the thoracic esophagus.

A somewhat better-defined group of candidates for *nonoperative management* has been pointed out by Cameron et al. (42): patients with so-called contained perforations. These authors had several criteria for the selection of patients for their nonoperative management protocol: (*a*) the perforation or disruption must be contained within the mediastinum or between the mediastinum and the visceral pleura; (*b*) the cavity should drain freely back into the esophagus; (*c*) there must be minimal symptoms; and (*d*) there must be minimal signs of clinical sepsis. The authors treated eight patients who met these criteria using an approach that consisted simply of the following: no oral intake; broad-spectrum, combination antibiotic therapy; and intravenous hyperalimentation. The causes of the perforations were leakage from suture lines after esophageal operations (five patients), forceful emesis (two patients), and dilatation for achalasia (one patient). All eight patients survived and were discharged after an average postdisruption stay of 28 days.

An important proviso should be observed when treating a patient nonoperatively: if the patient's condition deteriorates while he/she is undergoing such treatment or if an empyema or a mediastinal abscess develops, a thoracotomy should be performed (11, 17).

Santos and Frater (43) described a type of conservative management intended especially for a patient whose perforation is diagnosed late and who already has an established mediastinitis when first seen. This management consists of copious "transesophageal irrigation" of the mediastinum with swallowed fluid in a patient in whom adequate, wide mediastinal drainage has been effected by the placement of chest tubes. Adequate antimicrobial therapy is, of course, administered concomitantly. If the patient cannot swallow, irrigation of the mediastinum is carried out through a nasogastric tube which is positioned in the esophagus above the perforation and through which saline solution is continually infused. These authors used this method to treat eight patients with tardily diagnosed esophageal perforations from a variety of causes. All three patients whose perforations were in the cervical esophagus and four of five others with thoracic perforations survived. (The fifth patient had resolution of the mediastinitis but died of hepatorenal failure.)

Although these results are impressive, this series is small. We think these authors' experience with "transesophageal irrigation" needs to be corroborated in more patients and by other surgeons before it can be generally recommended for patients with late perforations and established mediastinitis.

Another relatively conservative method for treating patients whose perforations have been diagnosed late or who are poor risks for a major thoracotomy is *intubation*. Berger and Donato (44) accomplished this treatment with a Celestin endoesophageal tube inserted by means of a combination of esophagoscopy and laparotomy with gastrotomy. Barringer and Meredith (45) recommended intubation of the esophagus with the combination of a dual-balloon, Sengstaken-Blakemore tube and a nasogastric tube tied to the balloon tube and positioned so that the tip of the second tube lay in the distal esophagus just proximal to the esophageal balloon, for aspiration purposes. These authors used such a combination of tubes to treat successfully two patients with distal esophageal perforations who were diagnosed late. When the balloons were inflated, the segment of the esophagus containing the perforation was successfully "excluded" until healing could occur.

We have had no experience with the use of the Sengstaken-Blakemore tube for esophageal perforations. We have had, for the most part, unsatisfactory experience with the Celestin and other types of endoesophageal tubes in treating esophageal perforations and esophagorespiratory fistulae; we think there is seldom any indication for their use.

SURGICAL MANAGEMENT OF FREE PERFORATIONS
Thoracotomy and Closure

Although conservative or nonoperative methods have a place in the management of certain selected types of thoracic perforations, particularly contained perforations, most thoracic surgeons agree that the treatment of choice for *free* perforations, i.e., those that are accompanied by pneumothorax, pneumomediastinum, hydrothorax, and systemic sepsis with or without shock, is thoracotomy and closure of the perforation. This procedure carries a high possibility of success if performed within 24 hr (in some instances, within up to 48 hr) of the perforation.

The thoracotomy is performed on the side of the thorax into which the leakage has occurred. A thorough exploration of the mediastinum is carried out and the site of the leak identified. A debridement of any nonviable mucosa and muscularis is performed. Particularly in spontaneous perforations, the mucosal tear tends to be larger than the disruption in the muscularis. The muscular defect should be adequately exposed and, if necessary, extended at each end to allow adequate visualization and closure of the mucosal tear. A two-layer repair is carried out, closing the muscosa with interrupted sutures of fine, absorbable material (chromic catgut or polyglactin) and the muscularis with fine, nonabsorbable suture material. The pleural cavity is thoroughly irrigated with a large volume of sterile saline to remove food particles, debris, and loose fibrin. The lung, if restricted by a fibrin "peel," should be decorticated to ensure obliteration of all pleural dead space. The mediastinum and pleural cavity are carefully drained, using large-bore, carefully placed chest tubes.

With the passage of time after the perforation, the esophageal wall, particularly the muscular layer, becomes markedly inflamed, friable, and necrotic, to the point where sutures placed in it will not hold or will later cut through, with resultant recurrent leakage. This severe tissue damage occurs at variable times after perforation. In some patients, it is evident less than 24 hr—occasionally even as early as 12 hr—after perforation. Most patients will show such tissue change 24 hr or more after perforation, and the vast majority will give evidence of these changes beyond 48 hr postperforation. Even beyond 48 hr, successful primary suture repair of the perforation, after debridement, is still possible in certain selected patients, as shown by Finley et al. (46).

Various ancillary surgical maneuvers have been advocated to deal with the problem of tissue friability with resultant dehiscence and recurrent leakage that is encountered in late repairs of esophageal perforations. The least complex of these maneuvers involves the transfer of flaps of local tissues to reinforce or buttress the suture line in the esophagus. The tissues from which these vascularized flaps (in most cases, pedicled) have been constructed include pleura (33, 47, 48), pericardium (pedicled flaps) (49), pericardium (free graft) (50), pericardial fat pad (pedicled) (51), diaphragm (52, 53), intercostal muscle (54, 55), extracostal chest wall muscle (56, 57), lung (58), omentum (59), a pedicled segment of jejunum (60), and the serosal surface of the fundus of the stomach (61, 62). Gastric fundus has been used both as an onlay "patch" (61) or simply as a buttress to reinforce a sutured closure (62). Other authors (46, 63) in using the gastric fundus patch have added a partial or complete fundoplication or gastric "wraparound" to try to obviate gastroesophageal reflux.

Our own preference is for flaps of pleura or intercostal or other chest wall muscle, rather than for flaps of pericardium, diaphragm, omentum, or abdominal viscera. We are concerned about the serious potential for contamination of the pericardium or the peritoneal cavity when these latter types of flaps are used (46). Gastric flaps have an additional potential drawback, namely, the possibility of gastroesophageal reflux. Finley et al. (46) found that neither a partial nor a complete gastric wrap around the distal thoracic esophagus completely prevented reflux. On the other hand, our experience in a small series of cases with pleural flaps, using a technique similar to that popularized by Grillo (33) and Grillo and Wilkins (47), has been generally satisfactory (Fig. 11.3).

Recently, a number of surgeons (17, 31, 33, 48, 57, 64) have made the recommendation that the suture repairs of *all* esophageal perforations, not just those seen late, should be buttressed with autogenous tissue flaps. We would tend to agree with this position. Although parietal pleura is normally the most readily available and adaptable tissue, the pleura may be too thin in patients treated early after the perforation to be readily mobilized or to form a secure buttress (33, 48). In such instances, a buttressing flap of intercostal muscle or other chest wall muscle must be used.

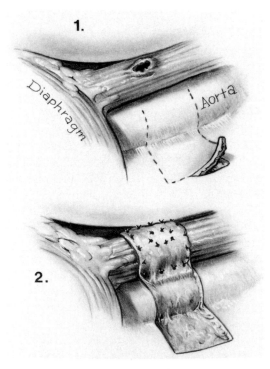

Figure 11.3.   Method of raising and transferring a flap of pleura to buttress the repair of a perforation of the thoracic esophagus. *1,* the flap is dissected with a wide base. *2,* the flap is sutured to the esophagus around the perforation and also at its edges. Not shown is the debridement and suturing of the perforation, which should be performed before the flap is transferred. If the perforation is too large or its edges too friable to permit suture-closure, the flap itself may be used to close the defect. (Modified from Grillo HC. Esophageal perforation. Surg Rounds 1983;6:50–71.)

Exclusion/Diversion and Drainage

Although there has been a recent trend toward extending the indications for debridement and primary repair with local tissue flap buttressing to perforations seen very late, even as late as 8 days (48), there remain some patients with such extensive mediastinitis or with such large perforations that primary repair, even with buttressing, may not be successful. One therapeutic option recommended for such patients is to exclude the esophagus from the alimentary tract, with diversion of saliva and of refluxed gastric contents. In 1956, Johnson et al. (65) used this technique to successfully treat two patients with persistent esophageal fistulas following the failed repair of spontaneous rupture of the esophagus. They first divided the esophagogastric junction and oversewed both ends. Nutrition was maintained by a feeding gastrostomy. Later, after the patient failed to improve sufficiently, they diverted saliva from the fistula by dividing the cervical esophagus, oversewing the distal end, and exteriorizing the proximal end. Ultimately, gastrointestinal continuity was restored using a Roux-Y jejunal loop. In 1970, Abbott et al. (28) reported using a T-tube placed in the esophagus, with the long limb brought out through the perforation and through the chest wall, as a means of producing a controlled fistula or, in other words, a type of diversion. These authors reported a successful outcome in six of nine patients with spontaneous rupture treated by this method. However, a 1989 review of the literature by Gouge et al. (48) disclosed only 12 additional patients so treated, with a 36% mortality rate.

In 1974, Urschel and associates (66) advocated exclusion and diversion *in continuity* to preserve the esophagus for later restoration to the alimentary tract after the perforation had healed. To do so, they created only a side opening in the cervical esophagus, without dividing it, and occluded the distal esophagus with umbilical tape tied over a band of Teflon felt, again without division. After the perforation healed, they restored alimentary tract continuity by closing the cervical esophagostomy and removing the esophageal ligature through a left thoracotomy. Schwartz and McQuarrie (67) utilized the basic technique of Urschel et al. (66) but with certain minor modifications: they created a muscle bridge under the loop cervical esophagostomy to make it more effectively diverting and, for the occluding band, they used Silastic tubing rather than Teflon felt because the former material produced less dense adhesions. Further, they placed the band more distally—around the abdominal esophagus, essentially at the esophagogastric junction—to avoid the contaminated area nearer the perforation.

The exclusion-diversion approach has two serious drawbacks. The first is the prolonged morbidity associated with the procedure; even with the in-continuity modification proposed by Urschel et al. (66), restoring alimentary flow through the esophagus requires a second operation. Urschel (68) recently described an additional technical modification that may obviate the need for reoperation: he occluded the distal esophagus by looping around it heavy Prolene sutures, the ends of which are brought out through a plastic tourniquet tube that exits the abdomen alongside the gastrostomy tube. After the perforation has healed, the occluding Prolene sutures can be removed without a laparotomy. The second disadvantage of exclusion-diversion is that it has a questionable physiologic basis: to prevent gastroesophageal reflux, it produces a distal esophageal obstruction which, in turn, could lead to increased drainage of bacteria-laden mucus through the perforation (57).

Richardson et al. (57) had such poor results with exclusion-diversion in their series of patients that they ultimately abandoned the procedure. On the other hand, Nesbitt and Sawyers (11) achieved a successful outcome in eight of nine patients in whom they used exclusion-diversion. Gouge et al. (48) reviewed 10 reports, detailing experience with exclusion-diversion in 58 patients, published since the 1974 report of Urschel et al. (66). The mortality rate among these 58 patients was 35%.

We believe exclusion-diversion has only a very limited place in the management of esophageal perforation or rupture. We would use the procedure only for patients with extensive mediastinitis or for those with perforations or defects too large to be repaired primarily even with the aid of an autogenous tissue flap. We treated one young woman with mediastinal Hodgkin's disease who sustained a perforation of the midthoracic esophagus during mediastinoscopy with biopsy. Since she presented with advanced mediastinitis and with bilateral empyemas, we elected to employ exclusion and diversion in continuity after the method of Urschel et al. (66) (Fig. 11.4). The perforation healed during the period of defunctionalization without any direct surgical repair. After the second laparotomy to effect deligation of the distal esophagus, the patient recovered fully.

Esophagectomy

Rather than exclusion-diversion of the esophagus, emergency or immediate esophagectomy is an alternative that has been advocated for patients with perforations deemed unsuitable for primary repair and drainage. Esophagectomy is especially indicated in patients with perforations (particularly instrumental perforations) that are associated

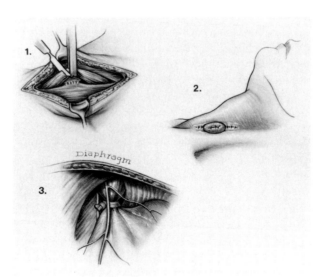

Figure 11.4.   Technique for (reversible) esophageal exclusion and diversion. *1,* the cervical esophagus is approached through the conventional obliquely vertical incision and the vascular plane between the deeper cervical structures. It is partially elevated out of its bed and a short muscle bridge created beneath it by suturing the sternocleidomastoid muscle to the strap muscles. A transverse or oblique incision about 1.5 cm long is made in the anterior wall of the esophagus. *2,* the skin and subcutaneous tissues are sutured down to the mucosal and muscular layers of the esophagus. *3,* the distal esophagus is occluded either by an encircling Silastic band (shown here) or an umbilical tape tied over a band of Teflon felt. Not shown is the gastrostomy which is brought out through the left upper abdominal quadrant. (Modified from Schwartz ML, McQuarrie DG. Surgical management of esophageal perforation. Surg Gynecol Obstet 1980;151:668–670.)

with distal esophageal obstruction. Johnson et al. (69) reported five patients with iatrogenic (instrumental) perforations and associated distal obstructing lesions (three malignant and two benign) who were treated with early esophagogastrectomy and esophagogastrostomy: four of the five survived. Hendren and Henderson (70) performed immediate esophagectomy, with immediate restoration of gastrointestinal continuity by a variety of methods, in five patients—four with benign lesions and one with malignancy—who had sustained instrumental perforation. Despite the fact that three of the patients underwent surgery more than 24 hr after the perforation, all survived. Kerr (71) reviewed the literature up to 1968 and found 19 cases of emergency esophagectomy for instrumental perforation with associated distal obstruction, to which he added three of his own. The patients all were treated by esophageal resection, including the perforation and the obstructing lesion, with immediate restoration of continuity—in most instances by esophagogastrostomy. Even though 14 of the 22 patients had malignant obstructing lesions, 20 of the 22 patients survived.

In 1989, Gouge et al. (48) reviewed six reports in the literature, most published during the preceding 8 yr, that presented experience with a total of 23 patients who underwent urgent esophagectomy. The overall mortality rate was 26%. The mortality rates in recently reported series have varied considerably. Michel et al. (3) had seven survivors among eight patients treated by early esophagectomy. By contrast, Richardson et al. (57) performed esophageal resection in six patients with esophageal leaks or perforations, and five of the six ultimately died. The consensus among many recent authors (17, 24, 32, 69, 72) seems to be that, for esophagectomy to be carried out with a low mortality, it must be performed early, before advanced mediastinal sepsis has developed. Gouge et al. (48) recommend staging the resection and performing the anastomosis at a later stage. Doing so would obviate anastomosis in the presence of sepsis with the attendant increased risk of anastomotic disruption. On the other hand, Yeo et al. (73) performed transhiatal esophagectomy in four patients with esophageal malignancies who had sustained instrumental perforations. The advantage of this procedure is that it allows the anastomosis to be performed in the neck, out of the septic mediastinum. The resection and anastomosis were accomplished in one stage in three of the patients but, in the fourth, who was treated 36 hr after perforation, continuity was restored at a later stage. All four patients survived.

We have used esophagectomy principally to treat patients with perforations associated with carcinomas (three patients) and with caustic ingestion injuries (three patients, all by staged resection and reconstruction). We have also treated three patients with perforations associated with dilation of peptic strictures by resection. However, most of our patients in this category have had dilatable strictures and we have preferred to treat them by primary repair of the perforation and dilation of the stricture.

Concomitant Correction of Underlying Obstruction or Other Disease

Bladergroen et al. (32) found that 63 (50%) of their 127 patients with esophageal perforation or rupture had underlying or associated esophageal diseases. These diseases or lesions included benign strictures due to reflux, paraesophageal hernias, esophageal webs, esophageal rings, carcinomas, achalasia, and lye- or caustic-material-related injuries.

In recent years, several groups of authors (17, 24, 33, 63, 72, 74) have advocated that, if possible, the underlying disease or lesion be corrected concomitantly with the repair (or excision) of the perforation. If the underlying disease is producing distal obstruction, it is imperative that this be relieved at the time of repair of the perforation;

otherwise, releakage will inevitably occur. Thus, if the obstructing lesion is a carcinoma or a severe, long, nondilatable stricture, esophagectomy is the procedure of choice (see above). Esophagectomy also is the indicated procedure for severe caustic injuries with necrosis and perforation of the esophageal wall. When the underlying disease is achalasia and rupture has occurred during attempted balloon or Mosher bag dilation, the perforation should be closed primarily and then a definitive myotomy performed in a location some distance removed from the perforation. Skinner et al. (24) at this point add an antireflux repair to buttress both the perforation repair and the myotomy, but McKinnon and Ochsner (74) apparently do not consider this step to be routinely necessary, nor do we.

If the underlying disorder is a nondilatable stricture in the distal esophagus, there is an alternative to esophagectomy: incise the stricture and the adjacent perforation vertically, orient the incision transversely by placing traction on each lateral edge, and then close the resulting defect using a Thal gastric patch. A Nissen fundoplication is next performed to complete the repair and obviate reflux (63). Although Bush (63) reported good results with such a procedure in three patients, Finley et al. (46) noted that neither a partial nor a complete gastric wrap or fundoplication, when used to supplement a fundic patch, completely prevented reflux.

When the underlying lesion is a dilatable stricture secondary to gastroesophageal reflux, the perforation should be closed and the stricture dilated and, if the diagnosis has been made early and mediastinal sepsis is absent or minimal, an antireflux repair should be performed concomitantly.

THE SHOCK TRAUMA AND UNIVERSITY OF MARYLAND HOSPITAL EXPERIENCE

We reviewed the records of 64 patients with esophageal perforation treated since 1958 (75). The segment of the esophagus involved was cervical in 19 patients, thoracic in 44, and abdominal in 1. In regard to the causative mechanism or agent, 31 (48%) of the patients had perforations that were attributable to intraluminal causes. These causes consisted of endoscopy and/or dilatation of strictures in 22 patients, attempted tracheal intubation in 2, foreign body ingestion in 2, balloon dilatation for achalasia in 2, and ingestion of caustic material in 3. Twenty patients (31%) had perforations that resulted from extraluminal causes: penetrating wounds in 11 patients, blunt trauma in 3, and paraesophageal surgical procedures in 6. Eleven patients (17%) had spontaneous perforations, and 2 (3%) had malignancies of the esophagus that perforated.

Ten of 11 patients (91%) with perforations of the cervical esophagus who were treated within 24 hr survived, while 6 of 8 patients (75%) with such perforations who were treated more than 24 hr after injury survived. Thus, the overall survival for those with cervical esophageal injuries was 16 of 19 (84%). Among the 44 patients with thoracic esophageal perforations, 16 (84%) of 19 who were treated within 24 hr survived, but only 12 (48%) of 25 patients who were treated after 24 hr were survivors. Thus, the overall survivorship among those with thoracic esophageal perforations was 28 of 44 (64%). The single patient with perforation of the abdominal esophagus survived.

In 30 patients, the perforation was treated by primary suture closure, with 25 (83%) surviving. This group included three patients in whom a pleural flap was used to buttress the repair; all three survived. Seventeen patients underwent only drainage of the neck, mediastinum, and pleura, with 10 (59%) surviving. Among nine patients who were treated by total esophagectomy, seven (78%) survived. Of the five patients who were treated by exclusion-diversion, only one (20%) survived. Of the 63 patients with cervical or thoracic perforations, only two carefully selected patients were treated nonoperatively; both survived.

Certain potential risk factors were analyzed to determine if they affected survival. These were: (*a*) *Age.* The median age of the survivors (36 years) was significantly less than that of the nonsurvivors (56 years) ($P = 0.0127$). (*b*) *Location.* The overall survivorship for those with cervical esophageal perforations—16 of 19 (84%)—was better than for those with thoracic esophageal perforations—28 of 44 (64%). However, this difference was not statistically significant, possibly due to the small sample size. (*c*) *Etiology.* When the survival rate among the 31 patients with perforations due to intraluminal causes—which was 84%—was compared with that of the 20 patients with perforations caused by extraluminal agents (75%), the difference was not significant. However, when the survival percentages of the intraluminal and extraluminal groups were compared separately with that of the group of 11 patients with spontaneous perforations, which was only 3 of 11 (27%), the differences were significant, with P values of 0.001 and 0.014, respectively. (*d*) *Time interval between perforation and treatment.* Among 31 patients treated within 24 hr, 27 (87%) survived, whereas among 33 patients treated beyond 24 hr, there were 18 (55%) survivors. Thus, the survival was significantly better for those treated within 24 hr ($P = 0.004$). (e) *Method of surgical treatment.* The small numbers of patients in some of the treatment categories limited the ability to detect significant differences in survival between them. In comparing the two extremes, the survivorship among those treated by primary suture repair of the perforation (25 of 30 (83%)) was better than that of the group treated only by drainage of the neck, mediastinum, and pleura (10 of 17 (59%)). However, this difference was not significant, although it neared significance ($P = 0.064$). (f) *Presence of underlying esophageal disease.* Contrary to what one might expect, the survival among the 30 patients who had an underlying esophageal disease in addition to the perforation (24 of 30 (80%)) was not significantly different from that of the 34 patients who had no underlying disease (21 of 34 (62%)).

Thus, among the key lessons derived from this clinical experience were the importance of diagnosing and treating the perforation within 24 hr; the suggested, but not statistically proved, superiority of primary suture closure as a method of treatment, particularly when it is supplemented by a pleural flap; the good results afforded by urgent esophagectomy when it is used for the proper indications; and the continued poor survival among patients with spontaneous perforation, probably due chiefly to delayed diagnosis.

SUMMARY

Esophageal injury, i.e., perforation or rupture, constitutes a serious, life-threatening clinical entity. Until very recently, this entity was associated with a high mortality rate. The high mortality has been related chiefly to late diagnosis and to failure to institute definitive, effective treatment promptly.

Earlier diagnosis can be achieved if physicians maintain a high index of suspicion of perforation or rupture in patients who are at risk: those who have undergone endoscopy or dilation; those who have suffered penetrating or blunt chest trauma; and those who complain of chest, abdominal, or back pain after sudden emesis. When there is the slightest suspicion that a perforation or rupture has occurred, a contrast esophagogram should be obtained without delay. Although a chest roentgenogram may be helpful if positive, all physicians should be aware that a normal chest roentgenogram does *not* rule out esophageal perforation or rupture.

With regard to therapy, certain patients are suitable candidates for nonoperative treatment. Only those patients who meet all the criteria outlined in this chapter should be so treated. All others should undergo operative treatment. Drainage alone is adequate treatment for most perforations of the cervical esophagus, although the perforation should be sutured as well if it can be identified and the edges are not too friable. For injuries of the thoracic esophagus, drainage of the mediastinum and pleura, although an essential part of the management, does not *alone* constitute adequate treatment. The perforation must be closed primarily (usually, if not invariably, with autogenous tissue buttressing or reinforcement), excluded, or resected. The use of autogenous tissue flaps to buttress the suture line has extended the time interval, during which it is possible to accomplish successful primary repair, beyond the customarily accepted 24–48-hr limit. The recent literature appears to show a trend, also reflected in our own clinical experience, away from exclusion-diversion and toward primary, buttressed repair, as well as a trend toward concomitant rather than delayed correction of any underlying esophageal disease. Thus far, it appears that the use of these approaches, which would have been considered overly aggressive or radical a few years ago, is being attended by reduced, rather than increased, mortality and morbidity. Undoubtedly, recent advances in preoperative and postoperative care, in nutritional support through jejunostomy feedings or total parenteral nutrition, and in antimicrobial therapy also have played an important part in these improved results.

REFERENCES

1. Seiler HH, Brooks JW. Trauma to the esophagus. In: Daughtry DC, ed. Thoracic trauma. Boston: Little, Brown, 1980:151–160.
2. Silvis SE, Nebel O, Rogers G, et al. Endoscopic complications: results of the 1974 American Society for Gastrointestinal Endoscopy survey. JAMA 1976;235:928–930.
3. Katz D. Morbidity and mortality in standard and flexible gastrointestinal endoscopy. Gastrointest Endosc 1969;15:134–141.
4. Michel L, Grillo HC, Malt RA. Operative and nonoperative management of esophageal perforations. Ann Surg 1981;194:57–63.
5. Okike N, Payne WS, Neufeld DM, et al. Esophagomyotomy versus forceful dilation for achalasia of the esophagus: results in 899 patients. Ann Thorac Surg 1979;28:119–125.
6. Hankins JR, Cole FN, Attar S, Satterfield JR, McLaughlin JS. Palliation of esophageal carcinoma with intraluminal tubes: experience with 30 patients. Ann Thorac Surg 1979;28:224–229.
7. Tiller HJ, Rhea WG. Iatrogenic perforation of the esophagus by a nasogastric tube. Am J Surg 1984;147:423–425.
8. Hankins JR, McLaughlin JS. Pericarditis with effusion complicating esophageal perforation. J Thorac Cardiovasc Surg 1977;73:225–230.
9. Dubost C, Kaswin D, Duranteau A, Jehanno C, Kaswin R. Esophageal perforation during attempted endotracheal intubation. J Thorac Cardiovasc Surg 1979;78:44–51.
10. Carlson WJ, Hunter SW, Bonnabeau RC Jr. Esophageal perforation with obturator airway. JAMA 1979;241:1154–1155.
11. Nesbitt JC, Sawyers JL. Surgical management of esophageal perforation. Am Surg 1987;53:183–191.
12. Soderlund C, Wiechel KL. Oesophageal perforation after sclerotherapy for variceal hemorrage. Acta Chir Scand 1983;149:491–495.
13. Huizinga WKJ, Keenan J, Marszalek A. Sclerotherapy for bleeding oesophageal varices—a fatal complication. S Afr Med J 1984;65:436–438.
14. Postlethwait RW. Surgery of the esophagus. 2nd ed. East Norwalk: Appleton-Century-Crofts, 1986:525–540.
15. Gelfand ET, Fisk RL, Callahan JC. Accidental pneumatic rupture of the esophagus. J Thorac Cardiovasc Surg 1977;74:142–144.

16. Randolph H, Melick DW, Grant AR. Perforation of the esophagus from external trauma or blast injuries. Dis Chest 1967;51:121–124.
17. Michel L, Grillo HC, Malt RA. Esophageal perforation (collective review). Ann Thorac Surg 1982;33:203–210.
18. Defore WW Jr, Mattox KL, Hansen HA, et al. Surgical management of penetrating injuries of the esophagus. Am J Surg 1977;134:734–738.
19. Symbas PN, Hatcher CR, Vlasis SE. Esophageal gunshot injuries. Ann Surg 1980;191:703–707.
20. Glatterer MS Jr, Toon RS, Ellestad C, et al. Management of blunt and penetrating external esophageal trauma. J Trauma 1985;25:784–792.
21. Lundberg GD, Mattei IR, Davis CJ, et al. Hemorrhage from gastroesophageal lacerations following closed-chest cardiac massage. JAMA 1967;202:123–126.
22. Hagan WE. Pharyngoesophageal perforations after blunt trauma to the neck. Otolaryngol Head Neck Surg 1983;91:620–626.
23. Wirthlin LS, Malt RA. Accidents of vagotomy. Surg Gynecol Obstet 1972;125:913–916.
24. Skinner DB, Little AG, DeMeester TR. management of esophageal perforation. Am J Surg 1980;139:760–764.
25. Postlethwait RW. Surgery of the esophagus. 2nd ed. East Norwalk: Appleton-Century-Crofts, 1986:178–179.
26. Barrett NR. Spontaneous perforation of the oesophagus: review of the literature and report of three new cases. Thorax 1946;1:48–70.
27. Boerhaave H. Atrocis, nec descripti prius, morbi historia, Secundum Medicae Artis Leges Conscripta. Lugduni Batavorum; Boutesteniana, 1724. English trans., Bull Med Libr Assoc 1955;43:217–240.
28. Abbott OA, Mansour KA, Logan WD, et al. Atraumatic so-called "spontaneous" rupture of the esophagus: a review of 47 personal cases with comments on a new method of surgical therapy. J Thorac Cardiovasc Surg 1970;59:67–83.
29. Cushing H. Peptic ulcers and the interbrain. Surg Gynecol Obstet 1932;55:1–34.
30. Walker WS, Cameron EWJ, Walbaum PR. Diagnosis and management of spontaneous transmural rupture of the oesophagus (Boerhaave's syndrome). Br J Surg 1985;72:204–207.
31. Goldstein LA, Thompson WR. Esophageal perforations: a 15 year experience. Am J Surg 1982;143:495–503.
32. Bladergroen MR, Lowe E, Postlethwait RW. Diagnosis and recommended management of esophageal perforation and rupture. Ann Thorac Surg 1986;42:235–239.
33. Grillo HC. Esophageal perforation. Surg Rounds 1983;6:50–71.
34. DeMeester TR. Perforation of the esophagus [Editorial]. Ann Thorac Surg 1986;42:231–232.
35. James AE Jr, Montali RJ, Chaffee V, Strecker EP, Vessal K. Barium or Gastrografin: which contrast media for diagnosis of esophageal tears? Gastroenterology 1975;68:1103–1113.
36. Dodds WJ, Stewart ET, Vlymen WJ. Appropriate contrast media for evaluation of esophageal disruption. Radiology 1982;144:439–441.
37. McCowan TC, Hillis NL, Diner WC. Esophageal perforation: roentgenographic diagnosis. J Arkansas Med Soc 1985;82:230–234.
38. Faling LJ, Pugatch RD, Robbins AH. The diagnosis of unsuspected esophageal perforation by computed tomography. Am J Med Sci 1981;281:31–33.
39. Heiken JP, Balfe DM, Roper CL. CT evaluation after esophagogastrectomy. AJR 1984;143:555–560.
40. Cheadle W, Richardson JD. Options in the management of trauma to the esophagus. Surg Gynecol Obstet 1982;155:380–384.
41. Lyons WS, Seremetis MC, deGuzman VC, Peabody JW Jr. Ruptures and perforations of the esophagus: the case for conservative supportive management. Ann Thorac Surg 1978;25:346–350.
42. Cameron JL, Kieffer RF, Hendrix TR, Mehigan DG, Baker RR. Selective nonoperative management of contained intrathoracic esophageal disruptions. Ann Thorac Surg 1979;27:404–408.
43. Santos GH, Frater RWM. Transesophageal irrigation for the treatment of mediastinitis produced by esophageal rupture. J Thorac Cardiovasc Surg 1986;91:57–62.
44. Berger RL, Donato AT. Treatment of esophageal disruption by intubation: a new method of management. Ann Thorac Surg 1972;13:27–35.
45. Barringer M, Meredith J. Distal esophageal perforation: esophageal exclusion using a modified Sengstaken-Blakemore tube. Am Surg 1982;48:518–519.
46. Finley RJ, Pearson FG, Weisel RD, Todd TRJ, Ilves R, Cooper J. The management of nonmalignant intrathoracic esophageal perforations. Ann Thorac Surg 1980;30:575–583.
47. Grillo HC, Wilkins EW Jr. Esophageal repair following late diagnosis of intrathoracic perforation. Ann Thorac Surg 1975;20:387–399.
48. Gouge TH, Depan HJ, Spencer FC. Experience with the Grillo pleural wrap procedure in 18 patients with perforation of the thoracic esophagus. Ann Surg 1989;209:612–619.

49. Millard AH. "Spontaneous" perforation of the oesophagus treated by utilization of a pericardial flap. Br J Surg 1971;58:70–72.
50. Hopper CL, Berk PD, Howes EL. Strength of esophageal anastomoses repaired with autogenous pericardial grafts. Surg Gynecol Obstet 1963;117:83–86.
51. Brewer LA III, Carter R, Mulder GA, Stiles QR. Options in the management of perforations of the esophagus. Am J Surg 1986;152:62–69.
52. Rao KVS, Mir M, Cogbill CL. Management of perforations of the thoracic esophagus. Am J Surg 1974;127:609–612.
53. Jara FM. Diaphragmatic pedicle flap for treatment of Boerhaave's syndrome. J Thorac Cardiovasc Surg 1979;78:931–933.
54. Bryant LR. Experimental evaluation of intercostal pedicle grafts in esophageal repair. J Thorac Cardiovasc Surg 1965;50:626–633.
55. Dooling JA, Zick HR. Closure of an esophagopleural fistula using onlay intercostal pedicle graft. Ann Thorac Surg 1967;3:553–557.
56. Lucas AE, Snow N, Tobin GR, Flint LM Jr. Use of rhomboid major muscle flap for esophageal repair. Ann Thorac Surg 1982;33:619-623.
57. Richardson JD, Martin LF, Borzottta AP, Polk HC Jr. Unifying concepts in treatment of esophageal leaks. Am J Surg 1985;149:157–162.
58. Moore TC, Goldstein J, Teramoto S. Use of intact lung for closure of full thickness esophageal defects. J Thorac Cardiovasc Surg 1961;41:336–341.
59. Mathisen DJ, Grillo HC, Vlahakes GJ, Daggett WM. The omentum in the management of complicated cardiothoracic problems. J Thorac Cardiovasc Surg 1988;95:677–684.
60. Mutton T, Goco I, Pennell T. Management of esophageal perforation with a pedicled jejunal patch. Current Surg 1981;38:318–321.
61. Thal AP, Hatafuku T. Improved operation for esophageal rupture. JAMA 1964;41:336–341.
62. Rosoff L, White EJ. Perforation of the esophagus. Am J Surg 1974;128:207–218.
63. Bush RG. Treatment of perforations of the esophagus associated with stricture. Surg Gynecol Obstet 1984;158:498–499.
64. Ajalat GM, Mulder DG. Esophageal perforations: the need for an individualized approach. Arch Surg 1984;119:1318–1320.
65. Johnson J, Schwegman CW, Kirby CK. Esophageal exclusion for persistent fistula following spontaneous rupture of the esophagus. J Thorac Surg 1956;32:827–832.
66. Urschel HC Jr, Razzuk MA, Wood RE, Galbraith N, Pockey M, Paulson DL. Improved management of esophageal perforation: exclusion and diversion in continuity. Ann Surg 1974;179:587–591.
67. Schwartz ML, McQuarrie DG. Surgical management of esophageal perforation. Surg Gynecol Obstet 1980;151:668–670.
68. Urschel HC Jr. Discussion of Gouge TH, Depan HJ, Spencer FC: Experience with the Grillo pleural wrap procedure in 18 patients with perforation of the thoracic esophagus. Ann Surg 1989;209:612–619.
69. Johnson J, Schwegman CW, MacVaugh H. Early esophagogastrostomy in the treatment of iatrogenic perforation of the distal esophagus. J Thorac Cardiovasc Surg 1968;55:24–29.
70. Hendren WH, Henderson BM. Immediate esophagectomy for instrumental perforation of the thoracic esophagus. Ann Surg 1968;168:997–1003.
71. Kerr WF. Emergency oesophagectomy. Thorax 1968;23:204–209.
72. Sarr MG, Pemberton JH, Payne WS. Managment of instrumental perforations of the esophagus. J Thorac Cardiovasc Surg 1982;84:211–218.
73. Yeo CJ, Lillemoe KD, Klein AS, Zinner MJ. Treatment of instrumental perforation of esophageal malignancy by transhiatal esophagectomy. Arch Surg 1988;123:1016–1018.
74. McKinnon WMP, Oschsner JL. Immediate closure and Heller procedure after Mosher bag rupture of the esophagus. Am J Surg 1974;127:115–118.
75. Attar S, Hankins JR, Suter CM, Coughlin TR, Sequeira A, McLaughlin JS. Esophageal perforation: a therapeutic challenge. Presented before the Southern Thoracic Surgical Association, Scottsdale, AZ, 1989, accepted by Ann Thorac Surg).

12 Injuries of the Diaphragm

Aurelio Rodriguez, MD

ANATOMY

The diaphragm is the musculotendinous septum that separates the thoracic from the abdominal cavity. It consists of a central tendon that receives radially oriented muscle fibers originating from the xiphisternum anteriorly, the inferior border of the common cartilage of the 6th to the 10th ribs, and portions of the tips of the 11th and 12th ribs as well. Posteriorly and laterally, the fibers originate from the lumbar fascia adjacent to the quadratus lumborum and the first and second lumbar vertebrae.

The position of the dome of the diaphragm varies with the respiratory cycle. During forced expiration, it reaches the fifth intercostal space anteriorly; during profound inspiration, it extends to the inferior border of the rib cage (Fig. 12.1). The diaphragm has three major openings: the aortic, esophageal, and caval hiatus. The lowest and most posterior is the aortic hiatus. It is intimately related to L1 and the crura, which originate inferiorly, and crosses the aorta to form the esophageal hiatus located more anteriorly. The caval hiatus is located in the right portion of the central tendon.

ETIOLOGY AND INCIDENCE

Blunt and penetrating trauma are the most common causes of diaphragmatic disruption. In the majority of published series (1–4), the frequency of this injury is related to the types of injury treated and the geographic location of the medical facility. In institutions where penetrating injuries are prevalent (1, 2), diaphragmatic disruption is seen more frequently. In contrast, at facilities primarily treating blunt-injured patients (such as the Shock Trauma Center of the Maryland Institute for Emergency Medical Services Systems where 80% of the patient population has experienced blunt trauma), blunt injury of the diaphragm is encountered more often (4–6). It is impossible to determine the exact incidence of diaphragmatic disruption because it is often unrecognized or misdiagnosed, particularly in blunt trauma patients (7, 8).

LOCATION

Diaphragmatic injuries constitute 6% of injuries found during laparotomy for penetrating trauma (5); 80–90% are located in the left hemidiaphragm and 10–20% in the right. This higher incidence of left-sided injuries is probably related to the preponderance of right-handed assailants and the fact that the liver protects the viscera on the right side from herniation.

In blunt trauma, the incidence of this injury during laparotomy is between 1 and 3% (9, 10); 70% are on the left side and 30% on the right (4, 6, 11).

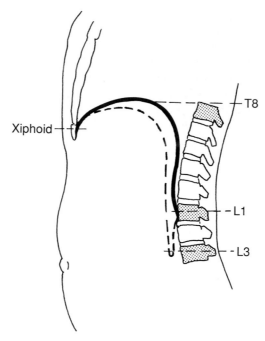

Figure 12.1.   Lateral view showing insertion of diaphragm.

PATHOPHYSIOLOGY IN BLUNT TRAUMATIC DISRUPTION

The precise mechanism is still unknown. The increased intraabdominal pressure produced during a sudden impact creates a probable critical gradient point that subjects the embryologically weak points of this musculotendinous structure to maximum stress (9, 10).

The tears are usually radially located, and the pericardium and esophageal hiatus are rarely compromised (3). Recently, there have been increasing reports of right hemidiaphragm tears (4, 11). The herniation of viscus is more common in blunt trauma, probably due to the extent of the tears. The organs more frequently involved, in order of frequency, are the stomach, colon, spleen, and small bowel.

DIAGNOSIS

The acute phase of diaphragmatic disruptions can be overlooked frequently because of the high incidence of associated injuries that can overshadow it. A high index of suspicion should be maintained when treating a patient with any penetrating wound of the lower chest, particularly from the level of the sixth rib down. In the same fashion, any thoracoabdominal blunt trauma of a sufficient magnitude to produce hemopneu-mothoraces or intraabdominal bleeding should alert the surgeon to the possibility of diaphragmatic rupture.

Penetrating Trauma

As discussed above, the location and trajectory of the penetration should alert the clinician to the possibility of diaphragmatic disruption (2–5). The majority of diagnoses

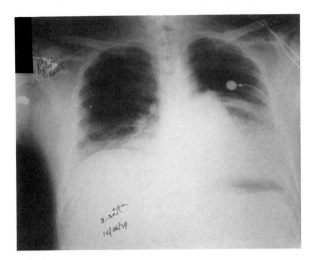

Figure 12.2.   Rupture of the left hemidiaphragm: hemothorax obscuring the rupture.

are made during an emergency laparotomy or thoracotomy. During this procedure, the diaphragm should be examined carefully.

In many cases, the initial clinical manifestations are absent or minimal (e.g., pleuritic pain, shoulder pain, dyspnea, tachypnea, or borborygmus heard in the chest). On the other hand, persistent bleeding from the chest or drainage of gastrointestinal contents from the chest tube during diagnostic peritoneal lavage should be indicative of diaphragmatic rupture. The diagnostic value of roentgenology has been studied by some authors (13, 14); sometimes the combination of several of these procedures increases diagnostic accuracy (13). Chest roentgenology, in particular, is one of the most simple and informative tests (Figs. 12.2–12.4): elevation of the hemidiaphragms, the presence of pleural effusion, mediastinal shift, or abnormal gas bubbles observed above the diaphragm must be correlated carefully with the clinical picture. Chest fluoroscopy has been used in stable patients, and recently, computerized tomography

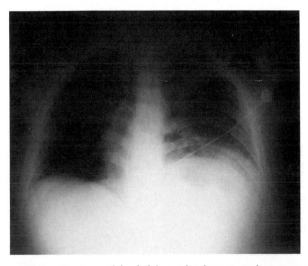

Figure 12.3.   Rupture of the left hemidiaphragm: indistinct contour.

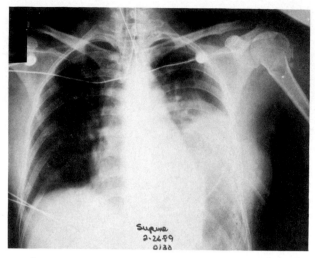

Figure 12.4.   Rupture of the left hemidiaphragm with gastric herniation.

(Fig. 12.5) and magnetic resonance imaging have been used successfully as well (14, 15) (Fig. 12.6).

Blunt Trauma

The frequent association with other intraabdominal and thoracic injuries makes the diagnosis of diaphragmatic disruption more difficult. As in the penetrating injury group, 80% of these injuries are found during exploratory laparotomy, usually following a positive diagnostic peritoneal lavage (4, 5). However, we should not forget that diagnostic peritoneal lavage can have an 11% false-negative rate (16). The use of roentgenographic techniques, as described above, can have the same implications. Some authors have used a pneumoperitoneum technique: 500–1000 ml of air are injected into the peritoneal cavity, with the expectation of being able to see signs of diaphragmatic disruption or pneumothorax in the upright chest (13). Others have injected methylene blue into the peritoneal cavity, with questionable results. Barium

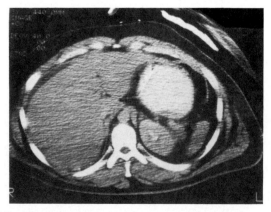

Figure 12.5.   Computed tomography scan: left hemidiaphragm avulsion.

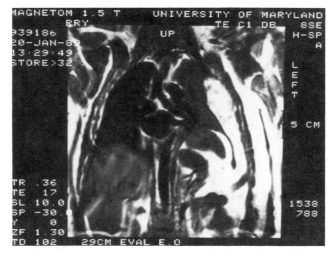

Figure 12.6.   Magnetic resonance imaging: left diaphragmatic avulsion with omentum herniation.

series of the gastrointestinal tract could be helpful in selected cases (Fig. 12.7). In our experience, computerized tomography has been neither very useful nor as precise as magnetic resonance studies (15).

Pelvic Fracture and Ruptured Diaphragm

Some authors have found that 34% of blunt-injured patients with ruptured diaphragms have associated pelvic fractures. Anteroposterior and lateral compression mechanisms have been proposed as the cause (17) (Fig. 12.8).

TREATMENT

Once the diagnosis of diaphragmatic rupture is made, the repair should be done expeditiously—as soon as the patient's hemodynamic condition permits. Prompt

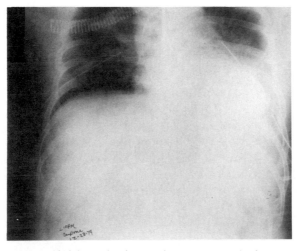

Figure 12.7.   Rupture of left hemidiaphragm: barium series disclosing gastric herniation.

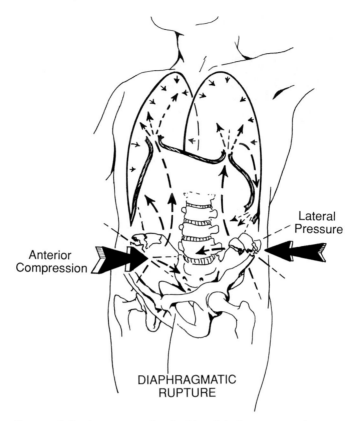

Figure 12.8. Ruptured diaphragm associated with pelvic fracture: mechanisms of production.

treatment will help to avoid the chronic phase and its danger of gastrointestinal incarceration.

The surgical approach preferred in the acute phase is celiotomy since it allows the surgeon to explore the abdomen thoroughly and look for frequent associated injuries. However, in cases in which intraabdominal pathology has been ruled out and the diagnosis is made 1 week later or more, thoracotomy provides an excellent surgical approach.

In any case, the chest and abdomen should be prepared and, if the surgeon has advance knowledge of a herniated viscus, hyperventilation with an Ambu bag during induction of anesthesia should be avoided to prevent overdistention of the viscus. In the majority of cases, the repair is done primarily with interrupted horizontal mattress sutures of a nonabsorbable type (0 Prolene), which are then reinforced with a running suture over the edges to prevent postoperative bleeding from them (Fig. 12.9).

When there is no peripheral edge of the diaphragm to suture, it is necessary to apply pericostal stitches instead. On few occasions, fascia lata, external oblique flaps, or prosthetic grafts such as a mesh of Gore-tex must be used (18, 19).

CHRONIC STAGE OF DIAPHRAGMATIC INJURY

"Chronic" diaphragmatic injuries are those not diagnosed until 30 days or more after penetrating or blunt trauma. A patient can progress to this stage of diaphragmatic rupture with or without herniation of abdominal viscera. Frequently, herniation is

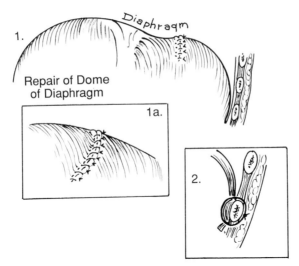

Figure 12.9. Repair techniques for ruptured diaphragm. 1, repair of dome of diaphragm. 2, repair of lateral tear.

intermittent initially; it may become permanent, with consequent impairment of the involved organ's blood supply or strangulation.

Patients with chronic diaphragmatic injury can remain asymptomatic for a long time. However, a protean clinical picture has begun to manifest, consisting of respiratory distress, chronic respiratory infections, empyema, intermittent small bowel obstruction, and finally strangulation of abdominal viscera such as the stomach or small bowel (20, 21).

The chest roentgenogram is very helpful for diagnosis, as in the acute stage, showing the same radiologic findings previously mentioned (Fig. 12.10). The diagnosis can be confirmed with barium studies.

The surgical repair is usually performed through a posterolateral thoracotomy. The adhesions formed between the abdominal and thoracic cavities, as well as visceral herniation, make dissection through a celiotomy very difficult (2).

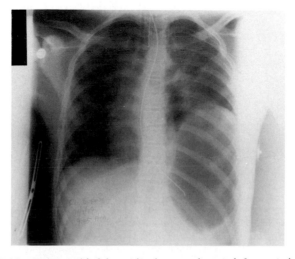

Figure 12.10. Ruptured left hemidiaphragm: chronic left gastric herniation.

Table 12.1.
Complications of Diaphragmatic Disruption

Respiratory	Atelectasis
	Pneumonia
	Emphysema
	Persistent pneumothorax
Intraabdominal	Hemoperitoneum
	Enteric fistulas
	Disruption of the repair (very rare)
Miscellaneous	Pulmonary embolism
	Hepatic failure due to compression of the extrahepatic biliary tree by a high diaphragmatic hematoma

COMPLICATIONS

The complications of diaphragmatic disruption vary in frequency (22, 23). The most commonly encountered are listed in Table 12.1.

The overall mortality is 18% in some series (1, 4, 7). The mortality often is related to the associated injuries.

REFERENCES

1. Wiencek RG Jr, Wilson RF, Steiger Z. Acute injuries of the diaphragm: an analysis of 165 cases. J Thorac Cardiovasc Surg 1986;92:989–993.
2. Symbas PN, Vlasis SE, Hatcher CR Jr. Blunt and penetrating diaphragmatic injuries with or without herniation of organs into the chest. Ann Thorac Surg 1986;42:158–162.
3. Hood RM. Traumatic diaphragmatic hernia (collective review). Ann Thorac Surg 1971;12:311–324.
4. Rodriguez-Morales G, Rodriguez A, Shatney CH. Acute rupture of the diaphragm in blunt trauma: analysis of 60 patients. J Trauma 1986;26:438–444.
5. Miller L, Bennett EV Jr, Root HD, Trinkle JK, Grover FL. Management of penetrating and blunt diaphragmatic injury. J Trauma 1984;24:403–409.
6. Morgan AS, Flancbaum L, Esposito T, Cox EF. Blunt injury to the diaphragm: an analysis of 44 patients. J Trauma 1986;26:565–568.
7. Böttger T, Schröder D, Ungeheuer E. Rupture of the diaphragm: a frequently undetected injury. Aktuel Traumatol 1986;16:180–185.
8. Van Loenhout RM, Carol EJ, Lubbers EJ, Reinders JF, van der Werken C. Misdiagnosed rupture of the diaphragm following blunt tracheoabdominal trauma. Unfallchirurg 1987;13:271–273.
9. Orringer M, Kirsh M. Traumatic rupture of the diaphragm. In: Blunt chest trauma. Boston: Little, Brown, 1977:129–141.
10. Lucido JL, Wall CA. Rupture of the diaphragm due to blunt trauma. Arch Surg 1963;86:989–999.
11. Flancbaum L, Morgan AS, Esposito T, et al. Non-left sided diaphragmatic rupture due to blunt trauma. Surg Gynecol Obstet 1985;161:266–270.
12. Freixinet JL, Segur JM, Mestres CA, et al. Traumatic injuries of the diaphragm: experience in 33 cases. Thorac Cardiovasc Surg 1987;35:215–218.
13. Reinbold WD, Kirchner R, Dinkel E, Kropelin T. Roentgenographic diagnosis in diaphragmatic trauma. Radiologe 1978;27:407–413.
14. Schneider K, Dietz HG, Fendel H. Sonografic diagnosis of diaphragmatic rupture following blunt thoracic abdominal trauma. Z Kinderchir 1987;42:313–316.
15. Mirvis S, Buckman R, Rodriguez A. Magnetic resonance imaging in the diagnosis of diaphragmatic disruption. J Comput Assist Tomogr 1988;12:147–149.
16. DuPriest RW, Rodriguez A, Khaneja SC, et al. Open diagnostic peritoneal lavage in blunt abdominal trauma. Surg Gynecol Obstet 1979;148:890–894.
17. Lewis J, Rodriguez A, Crepps J, Rodriguez G, Young T. Personal communication, 1989.
18. Wyffels PL, Kenny JN. Primary repair of bilateral diaphragmatic rupture with crural involvement. Am J Surg 1984;147:414.

19. Noon GP, Beall AC Jr, De Bakey ME. Surgical management of traumatic rupture of the diaphragm. J Trauma 1966;6:344–352.
20. Dajee A, Schepps D, Hurley EJ. Diaphragmatic injuries. Surg Gynecol Obstet 1981;153:31–32.
21. Payne JH, Yellin AE. Traumatic diaphragmatic hernia. Arch Surg 1982;117:18–24.
22. Negre J, Teerenhovi O, Autio V. Hepatic coma resulting from diaphragmatic rupture and hepatic herniation. Arch Surg 1986;121:950–951.
23. Gastinne H, Venot J, Dupuy JP, Gay R. Unilateral diaphragmatic dysfunction in blunt chest trauma. Chest 1988;93:518–521.

13 Injuries to the Great Thoracic Vessels

Stephen Z. Turney, MD
Aurelio Rodriguez, MD

Due to their immediately highly lethal nature, injuries to the great thoracic vessels are seen relatively infrequently by most thoracic or trauma surgeons. Although the patient population served by the receiving medical facility will determine whether the prevalent injury in this category is blunt or penetrating, the thoracic great vessel injury that has received by far the greatest attention in the medical (and legal) literature is blunt traumatic aortic rupture. We have seen a large number of these latter cases at the Shock Trauma Center of the Maryland Institute for Emergency Medical Services Systems (MIEMSS). In this chapter the emphasis will be on blunt thoracic aortic rupture, plus a review of the management of blunt injury to the other great thoracic vessels, as well as of penetrating wounds of all the great thoracic vessels.

Elsewhere in this book will be found chapters pertinent to great vessel injury, including preoperative evaluation, stabilization, and prioritization of treatment (Chapters 1–3); anesthesia (Chapter 5); and postoperative management (Chapters 6, 7, 17, and 18). In particular, the reader is referred to Chapter 4 (Imaging of Thoracic Trauma) for a review of the radiologic findings and the modalities used in assessment of great vessel trauma, to Chapter 15 (Management of Penetrating Thoracic Trauma) for a general discussion of the operative management of penetrating injuries to the great thoracic vessels, and to Chapter 8 (Heart Assist Devices in Cardiothoracic Trauma) for a discussion of use of cardiopulmonary bypass in management of great vessel injuries. Chapter 19 (Civilian Cardiothoracic Combat Injuries) provides an insightful description of the effects and management of high-velocity missile trauma.

BLUNT TRAUMATIC THORACIC AORTIC RUPTURE

Rupture of the thoracic aorta due to blunt trauma is a leading cause of immediate death in motor vehicular accidents and falls, but it may be survivable if the aortic bloodstream is fortuitously contained long enough by fragile periaortic tissues to permit diagnosis and appropriate management. For victims who die immediately at the scene of the accident from aortic rupture, prevention in the form of safety engineering, traffic and occupational safety education, and law enforcement offers the only hope for the foreseeable future. For those patients who would otherwise die within an hour or so of their accidents, appropriate triage by field medical personnel, attuned to the mechanisms of injury, and immediate transport to trauma centers equipped to handle trauma to the great vessels may improve survivability. It is in the relatively small category of providential early survivors of thoracic aortic rupture who reach the trauma surgeon alive that successful treatment may be possible and where controversy as to optimal management remains. That group is the focus of this section.

Incidence

Ever since Vesalius in the 16th century described a traumatic aortic aneurysm following a fall from a horse (1), autopsy studies have shown the occurrence of aortic rupture to vary considerably with the dominant mode of transportation (2). In modern times, blunt traumatic aortic rupture occurs primarily in motor vehicular, train, and airplane accidents (70–80% of all ruptures), although falls or kicks (8–17%) and blast or crush injuries (2–3%) account for many cases, depending on the autopsy series (3–5). Struck pedestrians account for 6% to as high as 84% of cases, depending on the population sample (1, 4, 5). The incidence of aortic rupture among traffic fatalities was measured in Maryland in 1985, when there were 739 traffic deaths: autopsies were performed in 447, and 105 of these (23.5%) had a ruptured thoracic aorta (6). In other series, rupture of the thoracic or abdominal aorta is reported in 10–16% of all motor vehicular fatalities (4, 7).

Age distribution is that of trauma in general, with children and the elderly included, but most cases are in the young adult age group (3, 7–9). The male-to-female ratio is weighted to the male, being about 1.5:1 in general population autopsy series (7, 10), with the ratio being higher for drivers and lower for passengers and pedestrians (7).

Fifty-five to 68% of the ruptures occur at the aortic isthmus, and 14–21% involve the distal descending thoracic aorta (3, 4, 7, 11). Fewer than 5% of traumatic ruptures involve the abdominal aorta (3). The ascending aorta is the site of rupture in about 19% of cases in autopsy series (3, 4), although very few of these patients reach a trauma facility alive. Multiple ruptures of the thoracic aorta in various combinations are reported in 7–19% of cases (3–5, 7).

Natural History

The natural history of blunt traumatic thoracic aortic rupture was described by Parmley et al. (5), in their classic review of Armed Forces autopsy material in 1957, and by Strassman from the New York City Medical Examiner's Office in 1947 (3), both in the era before thoracic aortic surgery was widely practiced. These are the only relatively modern acute postmortem series nearly untainted by attempts at early surgical intervention, although neither may be representative of the blunt injury population seen in subsequent years when the driver/passenger/pedestrian/falls case mix, highway speeds, and the use of passive restraint devices differ (1, 10, 12, 13). These caveats aside, they found that about 10–20% of ruptured thoracic aorta victims, depending on the site of rupture, survived the initial injury for some period of time, but that 25% (5) or more (3) of these initial survivors died from aortic rupture within 24 hr, and the remainder succumbed at an average rate of about 5% of survivors per day during the first 2 weeks postinjury, leaving only about one-third of the initial survivors, or 6% of the total victims, still alive at that time (5). Thus, untreated chronic traumatic thoracic aortic aneurysms are found only in patients at the tail end of a dismal early survival curve, and these continue to have a fairly steady attrition rate of about 2% of survivors per year from late rupture (14–16a) (Fig. 13.1).

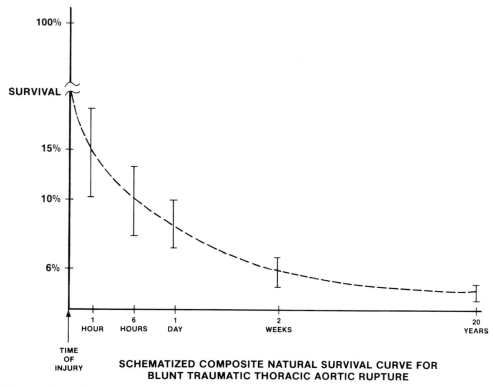

Figure 13.1.   Hypothetical composite survival curve of *untreated* blunt traumatic aortic rupture, with estimated uncertainty limits, based on published autopsy and clinical series and Shock Trauma Center resuscitation outcome experience (3, 5, 8, 14, 16).

Strassman (3) and Parmley et al. (5) found that the death rate from exsanguination for initial survivors was highest in the first several hours postinjury and was estimated to be about 2% (3) to 10% (5) per hour, a rate still being seen in 1985 in the Maryland Shock Trauma Center, where 30% died during attempted initial resuscitation, i.e., within the first several hours following injury (8). These early resuscitative deaths in our facility reflect the natural history of acute traumatic aortic rupture superimposed on a highly developed *system* of emergency medical transport that rapidly delivers the patient, who might otherwise die at the scene or in transport, to the trauma center still alive (17, 18). Statistics such as these are what continue to guide those of us responsible for improving trauma care to manage these patients by aggressive intervention, particularly in the early hours after injury, and challenge us to improve our overall management, from rapid field stabilization, triage, and transport to the resuscitative, diagnostic, and operative phases (19, 19a).

Mechanism of Injury

Although rupture can occur anywhere, the thoracic aorta is particularly vulnerable to rupture from shear and/or burst stresses at principal points, namely the intrapericardial ascending portion adjacent to the aortic annulus and the descending portion just distal to the origin of the left subclavian artery (Fig. 13.2). Of the patients with injuries at this

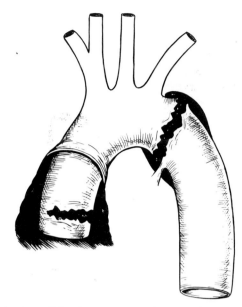

Figure 13.2.   Schematic view of the thoracic aorta showing the common sites of rupture from blunt trauma.

latter site, the aortic isthmus, perhaps 20% survive for some period and constitute more than 90% of those cases coming to surgery (8). The vast majority of ascending aortic rupture victims die immediately from pericardial tamponade, often with associated cardiac rupture (12, 20). Multiple ruptures may be present (21, 22). The question of which stresses lead to which type of rupture is mostly a matter of speculation, since no laboratory model has adequately represented the thoracic aorta of the living human (23). Retrospective review of accident conditions and knowledge of tensile strengths of aortic tissues allow some estimate to be made of the forces necessary to disrupt the aorta (24). However, biomechanical analysis is difficult due to (*a*) normal individual variability of aortic wall elasticity, thickness, and strength, superimposed on preexisting aortic disease, if any; (*b*) compliance of the victim's chest wall and the status of the cardiac cycle at the moment of impact; and (*c*) the forces and conditions of the accident, such as velocity and direction at impact, position of the victim at impact, ejection from the vehicle, use of seat belts and other impact-buffering conditions, and torsional elements (4, 7, 10, 24).

The common location of rupture at the embryologic aortic isthmus and the frequent finding of the ligamentum arteriosum at the rupture margin lend support to the hypothesis that weaker ductus arteriosus remnant tissue in this region predisposes the aorta to rupture here. Also, the ligamentum may serve as a fulcrum for deceleration forces moving the arch away (forward or to either side) from the descending aorta, which is relatively fixed in enveloping prevertebral fascia. The rapid rise of intraluminal aortic pressure from a direct blow to the chest with the appropriate conditions of aortic valve closure and limitation of distal run-off such as partial kinking of the femoral arteries at the flexed hip can produce forces sufficient to burst the aorta from within (24). Some combination of rapid deceleration shear forces and/or intraluminal burst pressure may be active in any given case. The rupture margin may be clean and smooth or uneven and ragged (see below). It is conjectured that intraluminal burst is associated with longitudinal tearing, whereas stretch and torsional shear stress often results in circumferential rupture (7, 23, 25).

In addition to these deceleration/burst mechanisms, direct disruptive forces are associated with rupture in the descending thoracic aorta at the site of a thoracic spine dislocation, usually in the supradiaphragmatic area (4). Numerous iatrogenic misadventures have been reported as causes of thoracic aortic rupture or damage, such as from the balloon of an intraaortic balloon pump (26), by an empyema drainage tube (27), by attempted venipuncture (28), incidental to cardiac catheterization (29), following intraoperative aortic clamping (30, 31), and during closed-chest cardiac massage (32). Corrosive esophagitis can involve the aorta in extreme cases (33, 34). See the section on penetrating wounds of the great thoracic vessels below for more discussion.

Diagnosis

For the acute case, a high index of suspicion engendered by recognition that an appropriate mechanism of injury is present is a prerequisite for prompt diagnosis. Although external signs of chest injury are usually present, there may be no such evidence in a given case (35–37). For this reason, *every* victim of blunt trauma associated with deceleration should have a baseline chest film taken as soon as possible upon admission to a trauma facility (19, 38). The only exception is the patient who requires immediate lifesaving surgery, which preempts any diagnostic workup. For the hemodynamically unstable patient, this means that the diagnosis is often made at emergency left thoracotomy.

Radiographic findings of a widened mediastinum and/or obscured aortic knob are presumptive signs of aortic rupture and *must* be evaluated further (19, 35–37) (Figs. 2.4, 4.2a). Often, these findings, present on an initial film taken in the supine position because the patient cannot be sat up for one reason or another, will disappear on a repeat upright posterior-anterior chest film (Fig. 4.2b). If the findings persist, and if there is *any* question about the diagnosis, then further diagnostic workup is done as soon as possible. This will usually be an aortogram (Figs. 2.5, 4.6b, 4.8), although other imaging modalities may be considered in a given case, depending on available radiographic equipment and manpower and the condition of the patient. The reader is referred to Chapter 4 (Imaging of Thoracic Trauma) for a complete description of the radiographic signs and modalities in blunt aortic rupture.

A coarctation effect may be present, probably due to a flap valve mechanism at the distal segment of the aortic wall of the rupture site (39–42) (Fig. 13.3). Peripheral

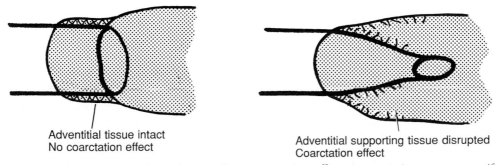

Adventitial tissue intact
No coarctation effect

Adventitial supporting tissue disrupted
Coarctation effect

Figure 13.3. Hypothetical mechanism for a coarctation effect. A coarctation may occur if adventitial tissue is disrupted around the distal stump, allowing the unsupported intima and media to collapse into the lumen, forming a flap valve.

embolism is rarely reported (42a, 42b). Femoral and pedal pulses should be palpated in every patient with suspected aortic rupture, particularly if upper extremity hypertension is present on admission.

Symptoms of chronic traumatic thoracic aortic aneurysms depend on size and location of the aneurysm, and diagnosis frequently is incidental to discovery on routine x-ray film. They usually appear on the chest film as distinct, often calcified, circumscribed lesions (14) but may mimic lung cancer (43) or ascending or descending thoracic aortic dissection (44). They may impinge on the bronchus or trachea (45–46a), the left pulmonary artery (47), the recurrent laryngeal nerve, or the esophagus (48). A history of blunt chest trauma is usually obtainable in retrospect (48a).

Associated Injuries

Associated injuries are very common, due to the powerful forces involved in causing the aortic rupture in the first place (24, 30, 49). Severe brain and maxillofacial injuries; rupture of the diaphragm, trachea, or esophagus; contusions and lacerations of the lung and heart; lacerations of the liver, spleen, bowel, and mesentery; injuries to retroperitoneal organs; and multiple rib and other fractures are commonly reported (5, 7, 18, 30, 33, 50, 51). In his medical examiner's study, Greendyke (7) reported an average of 2.3–3.3 visceral lacerations and 3.9–4.4 fractures/victim, the higher figure in each category being for pedestrians. In our clinical report of 115 cases over 15 yr, the 83 patients in the last 10 yr had a mean Injury Severity Score (ISS) of 18.2 (range, 0–50), excluding the aortic injury in order to eliminate its bias, which would have added either 25 or 36 to the ISS, depending on an arbitrary quirk of the Abbreviated Injury Score (AIS) from which the ISS is computed (8). This corresponds to an average per case of at least one other severe injury and one or more minor or moderate injuries in addition to the aortic rupture.

Treatment Prioritization

In the hemodynamically *stable* patient in whom the diagnosis of aortic rupture has been made by aortogram, immediate surgical repair of the rupture will usually precede other procedures, such as major orthopedic, maxillofacial, or abdominal operations (30, 52, 52a). Concomitant procedures are often possible, such as placement of an intracranial pressure monitoring bolt, reduction of a posterior hip dislocation, or insertion of skeletal traction pins, especially during preparation for thoracotomy. A positive peritoneal lavage for blood does not of itself warrant laparotomy before thoracotomy in the hemodynamically stable patient. On the other hand, the presence of an acute intracranial hemorrhage with signs of increased intracranial pressure may warrant preaortic neurosurgical attention.

In the hemodynamically *unstable* patient in whom the chest film does not indicate major bleeding from the aortic rupture site, and in whom another source of hemorrhage is identified, the latter site may receive operative attention first: for example, an exploratory laparotomy for a positive peritoneal lavage, radiographically controlled selective arterial embolization for major retroperitoneal bleeding, or control of extensive maxillofacial bleeding. Of course, if the chest film suggests major intrathoracic blood loss by virtue of the appearance of a very wide mediastinum and/or large hemothorax (left or right), then immediate thoracotomy is mandatory (8, 52). In that case, even if there is also major hemorrhage below the diaphragm, supradiaphragmatic aortic cross-clamping can be continued after the aorta is repaired while the other bleeding is assessed intraabdominally, by way of a thoracoabdominal extension or a separate laparotomy incision.

Surgical Management

The first successful repairs of chronic blunt traumatic aortic rupture were reported as cases or small series in the 1950s, using tangential excision or excision and grafting, often with homograft (2, 53–55). The first attempts at management in the acute phase were reported in that era (5, 54). Adjuncts used were surface hypothermia, total cardiopulmonary bypass, or left atrial-femoral artery bypass. High mortality associated with the use of bypass techniques utilizing total body anticoagulation on these trauma victims led to trials of other techniques to attempt to mitigate the deleterious effects of thoracic aortic cross-clamping on the distal organs, particularly the spinal cord. During the 1960s many more cases were reported, and the use of passive aortic-aortic shunts became more common (15, 42, 55–69). Aortic clamping and repair without shunt or bypass came into more common use in the early 1970s (30, 70–72). In the intervening years, numerous other case reports and small series attest to the continuing occurrence of major complications, particularly paraplegia, and to trials of various modalities, especially femoral vein–artery bypass (73, 73a), heparinless left atrial-femoral artery bypass (74, 75), and heparinless aortic-aortic shunts (76), to protect the patient during aortic repair (77–100).

PREOPERATIVE PREPARATION

The patient is prepared for emergency surgery. Unless there is significant hemodynamic instability, preparation can be done in a deliberate, orderly fashion. Preoperative assessment of other major injuries is carried out, except that studies that can await the completion of aortic surgery are deferred. Baseline routine blood gas analyses, blood chemistries, hematology, coagulation profile, and urinalysis are obtained. Blood is sent for typing and cross-matching of 10 units or more (packed red blood cells) as soon as aortic rupture is diagnosed.

In most cases, the patient will have no major preexisting disease, although, if possible, the surgeon should be aware of the use of medications; the presence of entities such as diabetes, renal disease, and pulmonary and arteriosclerotic disease; and the performance of previous surgical procedures, which can complicate the operative and postoperative management.

Because of the high amount of litigation concerning traumatic aortic rupture, it is especially important that the patient and his/her family be thoroughly informed of the procedures, risks, and alternatives preoperatively if at all possible. The preoperative neurologic assessment and the extent of the information provided in the informed consent process must be fully documented on the medical record. The highly lethal nature of traumatic aortic injury needs to be emphasized, as well as the major risks of intraoperative and postoperative death, paraplegia, paraparesis, vocal cord paralysis, infection, renal failure, adult respiratory distress syndrome, and other complications. The likely use of a synthetic aortic graft and its potential for infection and pseudoaneurysm formation must be explained. The planned use of shunt/bypass versus simple aortic clamping and the relative advantages and disadvantages of the use of each, along with the experience and preference of the surgeon and institution, must be discussed candidly. These discussions and the signing of the institutional informed operative consent form should always be done in the presence of witnesses. If the patient is to be transferred to another facility for the aortic surgery, the risks of the time delay and of jostling in transit, and the limited monitoring potential must be stressed, and signed consent obtained. In Maryland, such interhospital transfers to the Shock Trauma Center are usually made by helicopter, weather permitting, to reduce transit time.

The patient may have aortic hypertension and may be restless and combative due to head injury or to apprehension, especially secondary to acute alcohol or drug intoxication. In this case, rapid neurologic assessment must be carried out and the patient sedated, medically paralyzed, intubated, and mechanically ventilated to mitigate the increased stress on the rupture site from undue systolic ejection force and aortic hypertension, as well as torso motion. In the Shock Trauma Center, the neurologic assessment is always made by the in-house staff neurosurgeon, who then follows the patient intraoperatively and postoperatively as required.

Antihypertensive drug therapy may be necessary in addition to sedation and anesthesia, in which case a short-acting agent such as intravenous sodium nitroprusside is started and carefully titrated. The mean aortic blood pressure should be kept at about 90 mm Hg. Volatility in aortic blood pressure can easily ensue due to the counter-mechanisms of normal homeostatic hypovolemic compensation and vasoactive drug intervention. It is extremely important to avoid both hypertension due to the fragile aortic rupture site and hypotension and its deleterious effects on vital organ, especially spinal cord, perfusion. For these reasons, powerful antihypertensive agents should be avoided where possible. A mild or moderate degree of aortic hypertension may be tolerable if preparation for surgery is proceeding smoothly and rapidly, whereas the use of intravenous sodium nitroprusside in inexperienced hands or without adequate nursing or medical supervision may be more hazardous than the hypertension.

Preparations for anesthesia are described in detail in Chapter 5 (Anesthesia in Thoracic Trauma). It is imperative that the surgeon and anesthesiologist establish good, amicable communications. Planning for preferred drugs, procedures, and strategies must be discussed thoroughly and agreed upon ahead of time. The surgeon and anesthesiologist should both feel free to interact in areas where responsibilities may overlap. Thus, during surgery, the surgeon should be able to immediately alert the anesthesiologist to loss of lung ventilation or darkening of blood color in the operative field, and the anesthesiologist should notify the surgeon of unexpected changes in the patient's blood pressure, blood gases, or intracranial pressure. If left heart bypass requiring the attendance of a cardiopulmonary perfusionist is to be used, coordination among the surgeon, anesthesiologist, and perfusionist must also be arranged before-hand.

Large-bore intravenous access is guaranteed using catheters placed in two or more large veins such as the subclavian and femoral. Electrocardiographic and core temperature monitoring are always established. A Foley catheter is inserted and urine output monitoring instituted. Continuous proximal aortic pressure monitoring is mandatory and is almost always accomplished through a right radial artery catheter (avoiding the left subclavian artery, which will likely be temporarily clamped during aortic repair). Distal aortic pressure monitoring through the femoral artery (often via a catheter kindly left in place by the aortographer) is done when feasible. Central venous pressure monitoring is highly desirable, usually through a subclavian vein catheter. A pulmonary artery (PA) catheter for monitoring PA and PA wedge pressure, thermal dilution cardiac output, and mixed venous oxygen saturation is desirable, though not mandatory. Cerebrospinal fluid (CSF) monitoring is instituted if CSF pressure is to be managed intraoperatively. Procedures such as placement of an intrathecal or PA catheter should not be attempted by inexperienced personnel in cases such as these, where unnecessary preoperative delays cannot be tolerated.

Prophylactic antibiotic therapy is instituted with a broad-spectrum agent, in anticipation of using a vascular prosthesis. The operating and scrub nursing staff are apprised of the plans for surgery. The nursing staff protocols for thoracotomy and aortic surgery are implemented. Several sizes of sealed, sterile aortic grafts are made available, from which one will be selected intraoperatively. Suture material, shunt/bypass cannulas and tubing, and vascular clamps are selected at this time. The planned procedures are reviewed with the nurses so that they can anticipate the surgeon's needs. If autotransfusion is to be used, the apparatus off and on the operative field must be readied now.

OPERATIVE TECHNIQUES

The patient is anesthetized and positioned for a left posterolateral thoracotomy. A single- or double-lumen endotracheal tube is used, depending on the preference and experience of the anesthesiologist and surgeon. Vital signs are watched carefully during and after induction of anesthesia and positioning, and adjustments made to anesthesia, volume replacement, or vasoactive drug rates as necessary. It is often during this phase of preoperative preparation that a tenuous aortic rupture site bleeds massively or a compensated hypovolemic state decompensates. It may be necessary to abandon routine procedures in such a case and do a "crash" thoracotomy under less than sterile conditions. Otherwise, routine careful skin preparation and draping are done.

The posterolateral thoracotomy is made in the fourth intercostal space in the case of the usual aortic isthmic rupture or in the fifth or sixth interspace for a lower lesion. The thoracotomy incision should be generous in length in order to give optimal exposure. It is not our practice to excise a rib. Hemostasis as meticulous as time permits is obtained in the chest wall incision prior to entering the pleural space. Electrocautery or argon beam cautery is used liberally.

The pleura is entered, and the color and amount of free blood are noted and measured. A small amount of partially clotted bright red blood is commonly present in the pleural space, often associated with rib fractures rather than the aortic rupture, per se. The blood may be dark from a bleeding lung injury. A large amount of bright red blood in the pleural space is often the portent of an intrapleural aortic rupture in progress. It is particularly important for the surgeon to take note of the patient's vital signs at such a moment in order to decide how rapidly to proceed from there. If the vital signs are stable and the rate of volume replacement is not great, then the surgeon should proceed deliberately, taking time for careful exposure, dissection, and hemostasis along the way. However, if the vital signs are highly unstable, it may be necessary to move more rapidly in order to stop hemorrhage at the aortic rupture site.

Exposure of the mediastinum requires careful deflation and retraction of the lung. If a double-lumen endotracheal tube is in place, deflation of the left lung is accomplished readily by the anesthesiologist. For a single-lumen endotracheal tube, the anesthesiologist and surgeon must coordinate the maneuver of decompressing the airway while gently squeezing the lung. In either case, care must be taken to not superimpose operative upon traumatic pulmonary contusion. Care is taken to take down any adhesions that may be present without tearing the lung.

The lung, diaphragm, and chest wall are inspected and palpated carefully through the thoracotomy; contusions, lacerations, and fractures are noted. The pericardium is

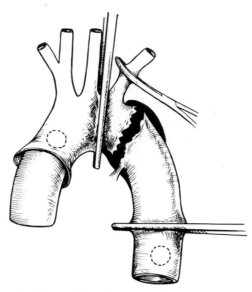

Figure 13.4. Typical sites for applying clamps to achieve hemostasis in a traumatic rupture at the aortic isthmus. The preferred cannulation sites for aortic-aortic bypass are outlined. The pericardial reflection is shown. (From Turney SZ, Attar S, Ayella R, Cowley RA, McLaughlin J. Traumatic rupture of the aorta: a five-year experience. J Thorac Cardiovasc Surg 1976;72:727–732.)

examined quickly to ensure that there is no tamponade or rupture. The lung is retracted inferiorly and the mediastinal hematoma assessed. The hematoma's longitudinal extent and width are estimated. It may be relatively small and confined to the aortic rupture site, sometimes being present only along one side of the aorta. However, the hematoma often extends the entire depth of the mediastinum and onto the aortic arch, obliterating the normal landmarks, such as the vagus and phrenic nerves, the left subclavian artery, and the aorta itself. It may extend well down the descending aorta, even below the diaphragm. Palpation rarely reveals the actual rupture site due to the thickness of the hematoma wall. Bright red oozing may be seen coming from fissures in the pleural surface as it is stretched by the hematoma. At this point, particular attention should once again be paid to the extent of bleeding from the hematoma and the stability of the patient's vital signs in order to determine the urgency of gaining aortic control.

In principle, isolation of the thoracic aortic rupture site entails dissection with cross-clamping above and below plus occlusion of any branches between the two aortic clamps (Fig. 13.4). The proximal aortic clamp is usually placed between the left subclavian and left common carotid arteries unless the rupture site is unusually distal to the left subclavian artery, in which case the proximal clamp can be placed below the latter, allowing an additional measure of flow through the left subclavian collaterals during the aortic cross-clamping period. If the rupture site is more proximal, as into the base of the left subclavian artery, then the proximal clamp site may be between the left common carotid and innominate arteries (see discussion below on gaining additional proximal stump length).

Proximal control can first be approached intrapericardially, particularly if an aortic-aortic shunt or left atrial bypass is planned. If neither shunt nor bypass is to be used, then it is usually not necessary to open the pericardium. If they are, then the left lung is retracted posteriorly and the pericardium is incised longitudinally over its upper half anterior to the left phrenic nerve. The distal ascending aorta is dissected free from the main pulmonary artery and encircled with a cotton tape. In a difficult case, the pericardial incision is extended past the aortic reflection onto the lateral arch, facilitating exposure to the latter.

An adequate periaortic arch tunnel for the proximal clamp can best be made digitally medial to the left subclavian artery and left vagus nerve, staying within the adventitial plane but outside the hematoma wall (Fig. 13.5). Unless this space is made widely, the aortic wall may not conform to the proximal clamp, preventing its full occlusion. This dissection is begun by opening the mediastinal pleura with scissors near the thoracic outlet at the palpable left subclavian artery. With the artery as a guide, the pleura is incised caudad to the aortic arch, staying on the medial side of the artery. Fairly brisk bleeding is encountered commonly as the engorged mediastinal space is opened, but the aortic hematoma cavity usually will not be found at this level. This bleeding will usually taper off quickly as the dissection proceeds. The surgeon should monitor the arterial blood pressure continuously by palpation of the aortic arch, the pulse rate, and rhythm and, as an indicator of the adequacy of ventilation by the anesthesiologist, the brightness of the color of the blood in his field of vision. The dissection should be

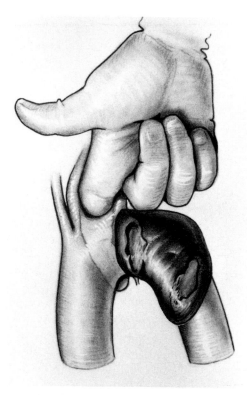

Figure 13.5.   Maneuver to digitally dissect and dilate a periaortic tunnel around the aortic arch between the left common carotid artery and the left subclavian artery in the presence of an acute traumatic rupture at the aortic isthmus. The extent of the still-intact hematoma surrounding the rupture site is illustrated. It is important to avoid entering the hematoma while making a generous tunnel for the proximal aortic cross-clamp.

interrupted to restore adequate ventilation and blood volume when necessary, unless bleeding is excessive, in which case the operator must proceed with deliberate haste.

A cotton tape is placed around the left subclavian artery, where it will be clamped later. The highest intercostal vein, crossing the base of the subclavian artery, is ligated and divided. The left vagus nerve can almost always be identified and is a useful landmark to the space between the bases of the left subclavian and common carotid arteries. Using the spreading tips of the scissors and the tip of the index finger as sharp and blunt dissectors, the lateral surface of the aortic arch is exposed. This dissection is carried first to the convexity, then to the concavity of the arch aided by a large right-angle instrument such as a renal pedicle clamp. The index finger and the gently spreading tips of the clamp are used alternately to develop this plane carefully. The darker color of the proximal border of the hematoma wall commonly is seen as the periadventitial layers facing the operator are dissected under direct vision. Great care must be taken to avoid entering the hematoma. The index finger should freely encircle the arch. A cotton tape is placed for later ease of access to this plane. Opposition of the thumb to the index finger within the tunnel can be used to gain temporary proximal control in the emergency situation where there is otherwise uncontrollable bleeding from the proximal stump.

The aorta distal to the rupture site is then dissected and encircled with a cotton tape. Care must be taken to stay below the rupture site, but not so distal as to include more than one or two sets of intercostal arteries in the isolated aortic segment. Often, the aortogram can be used as a guide to estimate the distal extent of the rupture, although the extent of the hematoma below this can be determined only in situ. Here again, dark staining of the adventitia warns of the proximity of the hematoma. Intercostal arteries that will be above the distal aortic clamp are looped with 2-0 silk for temporary occlusion. Due to obscuration of the intercostal vessels by the hematoma, this may not be possible until after the aortic clamps are applied. Temporary occlusion of these intercostal arteries is important in order to avoid often substantial back bleeding into the operative field and to prevent the spinal artery "steal" phenomenon (see the section on spinal cord injury below).

Once dissection of the major aortic clamp sites is completed, the cannulations for shunt or bypass, if they are to be used, are done. For a passive aortic-aortic shunt, the proximal cannulation site is best done intrapericardially near the pericardial reflection on the lateral surface of the aorta facing the operator. The distal site is 2–3 cm below the distal aortic clamp site. At each site, purse string or felt pledget-reinforced horizontal mattress sutures are placed in the adventitial aortic tissue. A short longitudinal stab wound is made with a no. 11 knife blade and the opening dilated to the cannula size, usually 8.5 mm for a Sarns (Morris) cannula. Dilators for this purpose are available from the shunt manufacturer. Shunt tubing is filled with heparinized saline solution and clamped. The cannulas are then inserted, taking care to direct the tip toward the heart for the proximal and toward the abdomen for the distal cannula (Fig. 13.6). Great care is taken to prevent air from entering the aorta during cannulation, especially at the aortic arch. The cannulas are secured to the cannulation sutures by temporary ties. Cannulation tubings are connected, expressing all air bubbles, and are left clamped until aortic clamps are placed. It is not necessary to instill heparin in the distal aorta. This may be harmful to the multitrauma patient.

In the case of left atrial-aortic bypass, the femoral artery is usually the preferred site for distal perfusion and may be prepared concomitantly with the thoracotomy. Alternatively, distal perfusion may be accomplished by aortic cannulation like that

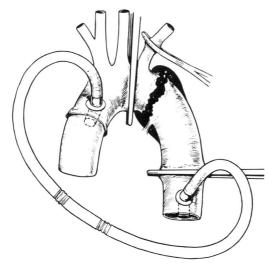

Figure 13.6.   Placement of a passive aortic-aortic shunt to bypass a traumatic rupture of the descending thoracic aorta. The shunt tubing, initially primed with heparinized saline solution and clamped, was unclamped as the aortic clamps were applied. See text. (From Turney SZ, Attar S, Ayella R, Cowley RA, McLaughlin J. Traumatic rupture of the aorta: a five-year experience. J Thorac Cardiovasc Surg 1976;72:727–732.)

described for aortic-aortic bypass. The left atrial appendage is exposed through the pericardiotomy, made as described above. A purse string suture is placed near the base of the appendage, which is clamped and opened, dividing muscle bands that might impede insertion and function of the atrial cannula. The femoral/aortic cannula is placed first, then the atrial cannula, each with attached heparinized saline-filled tubing. Great care must be taken to avoid damage to the left atrium and to prevent entrance of air into the left atrium. Connections are made to the centrifugal pump with the assistance of the cardiopulmonary perfusionist. If femoral vein-femoral artery bypass with an oxygenator is to be used (73) (Fig. 8.7), the arterial and venous cannulations are done in the proximal femoral vessels near the inguinal ligament. Since systemic heparinization is required by this technique, its applicability in the acute multitrauma patient is limited.

It is our practice to ask the anesthesiologist to administer 12.5 g of mannitol intravenously immediately prior to aortic cross-clamping and to repeat the dose after 15 min of cross-clamping. The proximal aortic clamp is applied, a time-lapse clock started running, and shunt/bypass, if used, begun. The clamp is carefully ratcheted tight while palpating the clamp tips beneath the aortic arch with an opposing index finger to ensure complete aortic occlusion. The subclavian artery and distal aortic clamps are then applied. A moderate to severe rise in proximal aortic blood pressure may occur, particularly if shunt/bypass is not used. The hypertension will usually wane with time and operative bleeding, but the anesthesiologist may need to be admonished to not vasodilate the patient excessively, nor to give excessive blood transfusion. The anesthesiologist calls out the accrued aortic cross-clamp time at 5-min intervals.

The mediastinal hematoma is opened rapidly longitudinally with a no. 10 knife blade over the lateral aspect of the presumed rupture site. A gush of blood under pressure is anticipated, so the surgeon should protect himself and his assistants with a shielding hand and suction. The extent of the aortic rupture is appraised quickly. If bleeding persists, intercostal arteries above the distal aortic clamp may need to be occluded with temporary looped sutures, and the aortic clamps may need to be repositioned. Occasionally, with a more proximal rupture, the bleeding is found to originate at the proximal aortic clamp stump, so that the clamp must be "walked" proximally by applying a second clamp proximal to the first, then releasing the first and applying it proximal to the second, etc. until sufficient proximal stump length is obtained (Fig. 13.7).

With the aorta opened and bleeding controlled, the full extent of rupture is determined. Fig. 13.8 illustrates examples of tears of different degrees and locations. Tears may be total and circumferential with the proximal and distal stumps retracted and separated by several centimeters. They may be partial, whether circumferential or longitudinal, whether medial, posterior, or lateral. The free edges of the rupture may be clean and smooth, as if freshly incised, or ragged and torn, with dangling strips of aortic tissue. The surrounding hematoma may be localized sharply to the rupture site or widely extensive into the surrounding mediastinal tissue. The ligamentum arteriosum is frequently found attached to the proximal or distal free edge of the rupture site.

In most cases, the rupture is converted from one of these types into a clean proximal and distal stump suitable for interposition of a tubular synthetic aortic prosthesis of woven Dacron or polytetrafluoroethylene. It is rare in our experience to find a rupture suited to primary repair without undue tension on the suture line, because of retraction of the aortic wall and stiffening of the periaortic tissue by the hematoma (101–105). Occasionally, a small laceration separate from a major disruption can be sutured primarily, although we would usually consider it wiser to trim the intervening tissue and convert it into a single larger lesion. Bridging aortic tissue in

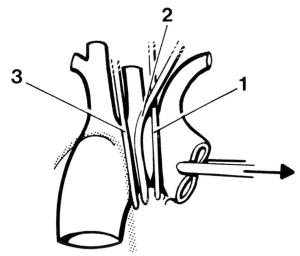

Figure 13.7. Techniques to gain extra proximal stump length. "Walking" the proximal clamp from position 1 to 2 or to position 3 may gain more stump length on the convexity than the concavity of the aortic arch. In position 3, the left common carotid artery is occluded, a potentially dangerous but sometimes necessary maneuver. Also shown is the *gentle* application of traction with vascular forceps on the proximal stump in the direction of the arrow while repositioning the proximal cross-clamps.

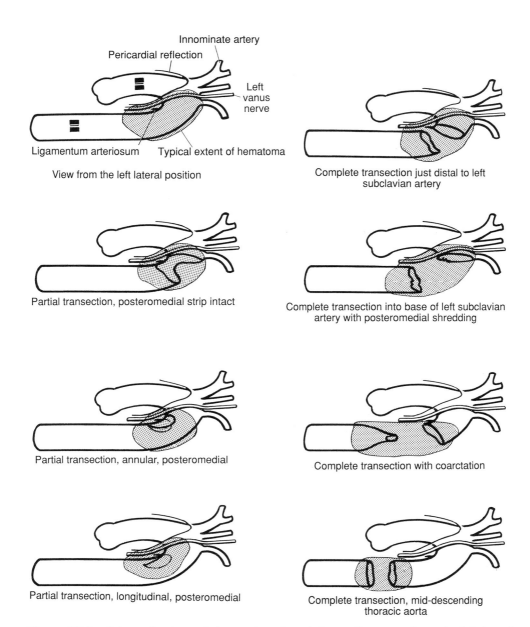

Figure 13.8. Schematic views of the aortic arch and descending aorta from the left lateral perspective, showing common variations of an acute traumatic rupture of the descending aorta. **A,** view from the left lateral position. Possible aortic cannulation sites are illustrated. **B,** complete transection just distal to the left subclavian artery. **C,** partial transection, with a posteromedial strip of aortic wall left intact. **D,** complete transection into the base of the left subclavian artery with posteromedial shredding of the proximal stump. **E,** partial transection, annular, posteromedial. **F,** complete transection with coarctation effect. **G,** partial transection, longitudinal, posteromedial. **H,** complete transection, mid-descending thoracic aorta.

partial disruptions should usually be divided to convert the lesion into a complete one. An exception might be made in the presence of extensive arteriosclerotic disease, where it is not possible to safely suture a tubular graft in place, particularly proximally. A patch repair with woven Dacron or polytetrafluoroethylene might suffice in that situation if the rupture is on the lateral aorta. If the rupture is medial, patch repair might be inordinately difficult, if not impossible.

The aortic graft is selected according to the diameter of the patient's aorta. Usually, a graft in the range of 16–22-mm diameter is selected, commonly a 20-mm graft in a male or 18-mm in a female. The graft is sewn in place quickly, using simple running suture technique, usually without pledget reinforcement (Fig. 13.9). We prefer double-armed 300 monofilament polypropylene suture with a larger taper needle. Sutures are taken widely and deeply, incorporating periaortic fibrous tissue for added support, but taking care to avoid the underlying esophagus, particularly at the proximal suture line.

The proximal suture line is placed first; the tubular graft is stretched to a slight tension and cut to a length that will not result in too much suture line tension nor in bowing or kinking; and then the distal suture line is begun. Prior to completion of the distal suture line, the proximal aortic clamp is released to flush out debris or clot, then reapplied. Similarly, the distal clamp is released briefly, and the suture line is completed.

Great care is taken in the proximal suture line, particularly medially, in the region of the ligamentum arteriosum, where the aortic tissue is frequently weak, thin, and easily torn. If tearing should occur, it may be necessary to begin the suture line again, repositioning the aortic clamp by "walking" it (see above). A few felt pledget-reinforced mattress sutures may be necessary to bolster this area. The proximal suture line may be tested before beginning or completing the distal suture line by clamping the graft with a vascular clamp and briefly releasing the proximal aortic clamp. Significant bleeding points are usually controlled by simple 4-0 sutures. The distal suture line is tested in a similar manner.

Extensive bleeding may occur from multiple suture needle holes, particularly in the face of a bleeding diathesis, and require wrapping the suture lines with felt strips and packing with a thrombogenic material such as Surgicel cotton. Much of this sort of bleeding can be obviated by careful attention to clotting factor replacement during transfusions, correcting platelet deficiencies, and maintaining body temperature through use of fluid administration and anesthesia gas-warming devices.

Once the anastomoses are completed, the distal aortic and subclavian artery clamps are removed and the proximal aortic clamp is released slowly, allowing the patient and anesthesiologist to adjust to the restoration of normal aortic blood flow. Concomitantly, shunt/bypass is discontinued. Temporary intercostal artery loops are released. If it is clear that there is no significant suture line leak, shunt/bypass cannulas are removed and cannulation sites closed by tying down the preplaced sutures (Fig. 13.9). If bleeding is a problem, the cannulas should be left in place until the need for shunt/bypass has passed.

The surgeon should palpate the aorta throughout the early postclamp period to ensure adequate pressure. It may be necessary to partially reapply the proximal aortic clamp to allow time for volume replacement. Presence of a thrill at the graft site is unusual and, in the absence of a significant pressure gradient across the graft, can be disregarded. If a significant gradient is present (> 30 mm Hg), then serious consideration should be given to revising the offending suture line if the patient's

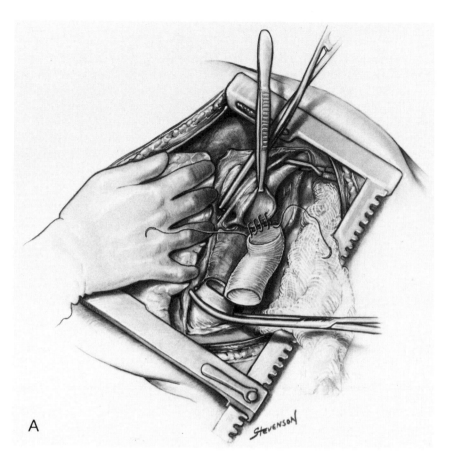

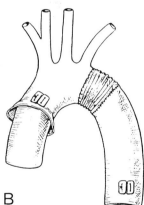

Figure 13.9. **A,** technique of suture placement in the fragile posteromedial proximal aortic stump. The lateral aortic wall facing the surgeon is retracted gently by the first assistant. Clamps are shown on the aortic arch proximal to the left subclavian artery and on the latter artery. The recurrent laryngeal branch of the left vagus nerve is shown passing behind the ligamentum arteriosum, which is still attached to the proximal aortic stump. **B,** appearance of the aorta following reconstruction with a tubular synthetic graft correctly sized to the aortic diameter and to the length of the rupture site defect. Simple running suture technique was used, taking wider and deeper bites than illustrated here. Aortic cannulation sites, if used, are shown having been closed using tied-down felt pledget-reinforced horizontal mattress sutures taken superficially in the aortic wall. (**B** from Turney SZ, Attar S, Ayella R, Cowley RA, McLaughlin J. Traumatic rupture of the aorta: a five-year experience. J Thorac Cardiovasc Surg 1976;72:727–732.)

condition warrants. If the patient is hemodynamically stable and the total aortic cross-clamp time has been less than about 30 min, it may be safe to reclamp the aorta and revise the anastomosis, assuming the revision can be accomplished quickly. If there is any question about the patient tolerating more aortic surgery at this time, revision can await another day.

Prior to closure of the thoracotomy, the aortic graft is covered with mediastinal pleura, if possible, with a few interrupted absorbable sutures. The graft, if properly sized, should follow the normal aortic contour. An anterior and a posterior chest tube are left, taking care that neither impinges on the repair site, and the thoracotomy is closed.

Surgical Alternatives

In the patient who is considered a high risk for aortic repair but whose aortic injury is otherwise stable, medical management in the form of antihypertensive and ß-blocking agents may be considered, at least for an interim period while the patient remains a high operative risk (106, 107). Examples are patients with ongoing sepsis (106), severe associated closed head injury, and traumatic aortic valve insufficiency (107). Lesions that appear radiographically to involve only the intima and to not extend through the media, but that have an associated periaortic hematoma, probably should be explored surgically on the presumption that the radiographic appearance is not revealing the full extent of rupture. However, in such a case, the radiographic evidence would probably weigh on the side of medical management in the high-operative-risk patient.

While it is highly unusual in our experience to use this modality due to the known natural history of traumatic aortic rupture, each case should be individualized so that any patient with questionable survival potential can be considered a possible candidate for nonsurgical management. If the diagnosis has been made late, and the period of early higher rate of exsanguinating rupture has past (i.e., after 6–8 hr postinjury), serial chest films show a stable mediastinal shadow with no evidence of accumulating hemothorax, and the patient has one or more other conditions that would otherwise contraindicate a major thoracotomy, then medical management should be considered. In any case, careful observation and meticulous control of pharmacologic agents are mandatory. Reassessment for definitive surgical repair should be made frequently, with an aggressive surgical posture being appropriate.

Outcome
SURGICAL MORTALITY

Blunt thoracic aortic rupture is a highly lethal injury, as reflected in the 80–90% death rate at time of injury, as well as in the 30% mortality during initial resuscitation of survivors of initial injury in the MIEMSS Shock Trauma Center, where the patient population is biased toward more severely injured patients (see section on natural history above). For survivors of resuscitation, i.e., patients undergoing definitive emergency aortic repair, 12% died intraoperatively and 21% postoperatively in our series (8). Operative mortality is reported in the 15–29% range in other series and reviews (76, 108, 108a).

Operative deaths are usually from uncontrollable hemorrhage, often from shunt cannulation attempts (30), but usually from false aneurysm rupture before control can be obtained or from bleeding from nonaortic sites. Autotransfusion and rapid infusion techniques incorporating integral heat exchangers should be available for these cases (8, 109). Although not specifically recommended for this situation, Crawford et al. (31)

have recently described use of the technique described by Lillehei et al. (110) of profound hypothermia via partial cardiopulmonary bypass (femoral vein–femoral artery) through a posterolateral exposure to manage difficult aortic arch problems, including intraoperative hemorrhage. Even with use of a modern membrane oxygenator, centrifugal pump, and countercurrent heat exchanger for this purpose, total body heparinization would still be required (111), although in a desperate situation, the risk of bleeding elsewhere in the acute multiple-trauma patient might well be taken.

SPINAL CORD INJURY

Paraplegia or paraparesis is the most serious complication following otherwise successful repair of traumatic aortic rupture. The incidence is 2–22%, depending on the series reported (8, 75, 76, 108). Paraplegia usually is noted as soon as the patient awakens from anesthesia. It may improve inexplicably after days or weeks, leaving the patient with only a paraparesis of varying degree (111a).

In order to better understand the genesis of, and controversies surrounding, this complication, a more detailed discussion follows.

Knowledge of the collateral circulation of the thoracic aorta and of the spinal cord is particularly important in understanding the development of spinal cord ischemia in these cases. The arterial blood supply of the spinal cord (Fig. 13.10) is derived from the basilar artery, and segmentally from the intercostal and lumbar arteries, in communication with the anterior (and, to a lesser degree, the posterior) spinal artery. The anterior spinal artery is frequently incomplete, particularly in the lower thoracic segment, so that spinal cord perfusion then depends upon spinal branches of the lower intercostal and lumbar arteries. These connect to the anterior radicular arteries (to the anterior spinal artery) and the posterior radicular arteries (to the posterior spinal arteries) within the spinal canal (Fig 13.11). The spinal branches at any level may be missing, minute, or large; if large, they are referred to as arteria radicularis magna, the so-called artery(ies) of Adamkiewicz. The size and distribution of all these various arteries apparently depend on the volume of spinal cord being perfused in a given segment and the sizes of the possible combinations of collateral connections (112, 113).

In addition to anatomic variations, dynamic variation in perfusion occurs with changing perfusion pressures and vasoactive milieu (113–115). In the surgical setting, a high head of pressure proximal to the aortic cross-clamp may be desirable when perfusing the spinal cord through narrow spinal artery connections in some cases. Cross-clamping the thoracic aorta proximal to the arteria radicularis magna may produce a "steal" phenomenon through the latter into the lower-pressure distal aorta. This shunting of arterial blood away from the spinal arterial network may be aggravated by the use of vasodilating agents during surgery, which are intended to reduce left ventricular afterload and promote increased collateral flow, but which instead increase the systemic venous blood pool and lower distal aortic pressure further (115a).

It is logical to assume that a strategy to maintain aortic pressure distal to the cross-clamp by the use of vasoactive agents, shunt, bypass (with or without hypothermia (116–117b)), or balloon or clamp occlusion at the aortic bifurcation or below should theoretically help maintain good distal cord perfusion through segmental collaterals, as well as prevent the steal phenomenon. Unfortunately, paraplegia still occurs with use of these adjuncts (8, 71, 114, 117c).

Since the spinal cord will tolerate ischemia for about 30 min at normothermia (112, 113), simple aortic cross-clamping without use of adjunct in cases where total cross-clamp time is likely to be within that time frame has many proponents (8, 30, 70,

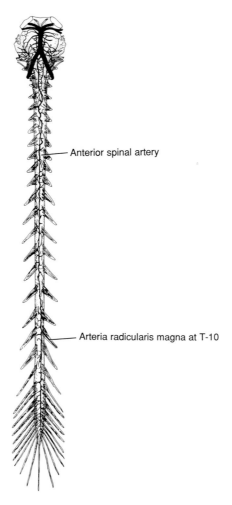

— Anterior spinal artery

— Arteria radicularis magna at T-10

Figure 13.10.   The human spinal cord demonstrating the extreme desegmentation of the vascular pattern. Shown are the anterior spinal artery, the cervical and thoracic segmental radicular branches, and an arteria radicularis magna at the T-10 level. (Adapted from an adaptation of Kadyi from Adams HD, van Geertruyden HH. Neurologic complications of aortic surgery. Ann Surg 1956;144:574–610.)

71, 108, 118–118d). In our series of 83 patients seen at the Shock Trauma Center over the 10-year period from 1976 through 1985, no statistically significant difference was seen in the incidence of paraplegia in 6 of 34 (17.6%) patients in whom aortic-aortic shunts were used versus the 4 of 17 (23.5%) patients who were unshunted (8). Even in this series, the largest in the literature, and one of the few with enough cases to be subjected to statistical analysis, the cases were not randomized, and no firm conclusions can be drawn about the relative merits of shunting. Nonetheless, it remains our conviction that, in competent hands, simple cross-clamping without shunt/bypass is as safe as any other method currently available and has the major advantages of rapidity and simplicity. The issue will remain controversial as long as paraplegia occurs in these cases.

As a result of the persistent occurrence of postoperative paraplegia, modalities

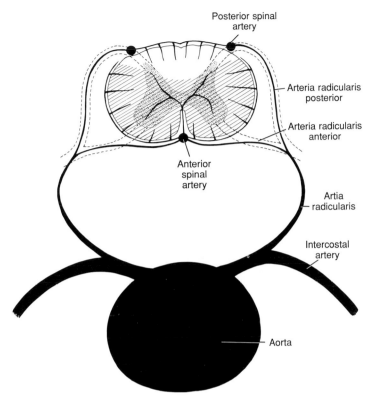

Figure 13.11.   Cross-sectional arterial blood supply to the spinal cord demonstrating the large anterior area (*shaded*) receiving its blood supply via the spinal branch (arteria radicularis) of a pair of intercostal arteries, the anterior radicular arteries, and the anterior spinal artery. The paired posterior spinal arteries are shown supplied by the posterior radicular arteries. (Adapted from Adams HD, van Geertruyden HH. Neurologic complications of aortic surgery. Ann Surg 1956;144:574–610.)

other than shunt/bypass in recent years have been studied or advocated to detect, treat, or prevent spinal cord ischemia and injury during thoracic aortic surgery, including that done for traumatic rupture (115). These include agents to ameliorate reperfusion hyperemia and damage, such as allopurinol and superoxide dismutase, direct spinal artery vasodilation with intrathecal papaverine, control of elevated cerebrospinal fluid pressure (and hence an increase in transcerebrospinal perfusion gradient) using intraoperative CSF pressure monitoring and drainage, intraoperative distal aortic pressure monitoring, and monitoring of somatosensory and/or motor-evoked potentials to detect critical spinal cord ischemia during surgery (113–115, 119, 120–120c). To date, no clear reproducible advantage is ascribable to any of these modalities in clinical practice.

In our series, all 10 cases of paraplegia occurred with aortic cross-clamp times exceeding 30 min, and no cases of paraplegia occurred with cross-clamp times of less than 30 min, although the difference did not achieve true statistical significance in the analysis. Hypotension during aortic cross-clamping occurred in 6 of the 10 paraplegia cases and this did not achieve statistical significance either. However, the avoidance of hypotension during periods of spinal cord ischemia and the limiting of duration of aortic cross-clamping are both potentially within the realm of the surgeon's control and should be in the forefront of the surgeon's thoughts throughout the period of aortic repair.

OTHER COMPLICATIONS

Renal failure (120d, 120e), severe sepsis, and adult respiratory distress syndrome are other major, relatively common life-threatening complications seen postoperatively. In our experience, one or more major complications (including paraplegia/paraparesis) occurred in 21 of 51 (41.2%) of operating room survivors (8). (See the discussion of risk factors below.) The treatment of these complications is beyond the scope of this text.

Vocal cord paralysis (30), persistent hypertension (121), reexploration of the chest for bleeding, suture line pseudoaneurysm, jaundice, phrenic nerve palsy, pericarditis, pulmonary thromboembolism, chylothorax, cholecystitis, surgical wound infection, and aortoesophageal fistula (122) are less serious or reported infrequently (8). Taking care to avoid injury of the left vagus and recurrent laryngeal nerves should prevent most cases of vocal cord palsy, although difficulties in exposure from periaortic hematoma and bleeding may make damage to these nerves unavoidable. Most cases of postoperative hypertension resolve in a few days, but persistent hypertension can usually be treated satisfactorily medically (121). A suture line stricture should be ruled out by aortography in all cases of persistent hypertension. Suture line pseudoaneurysm was detected on routine chest film 2 weeks to 5 months following aortic repair in 3 of our 51 operative survivors (6%), all of whom required reoperation. Follow-up visits with chest roentgenograms should be done on all cases.

RISK FACTORS FOR DEATH OR MAJOR COMPLICATION

Table 13.1 summarizes an analysis of risk factors made in our series of 81 cases from the 10-year period of 1976 through 1985 (8). Contrary to the findings of Sturm et al. (123) in their report of risk factors in 37 patients reported in 1984, age of the injured patient did not influence outcome in our series.

A higher ISS was associated with higher intraoperative and postoperative mortality and the appearance of renal failure in our series. Higher postoperative mortality was also associated with use of shunt adjunct during aortic repair and direct transfer from the scene of injury as opposed to transfer from another hospital. The strongest statistical predictors for death during admission resuscitation attempts were a low (< 90 mm Hg) admission systolic blood pressure, a large (> 500 ml) presenting hemothorax, lesser (nonthoracic surgery-boarded) surgeon's qualifications, and the necessity to perform other major surgery prior to attempted aortic repair.

Adult respiratory distress syndrome occurred more frequently in patients treated by less qualified surgeons and with use of shunt adjunct during aortic repair. Aortic cross-clamp time of longer than 30 min was only very weakly associated with development of postoperative paraplegia, as discussed above. Renal failure was associated with higher ISS, as noted above, and with transfer directly from the scene of injury. There were no statistically significant predictors of sepsis in our analysis.

Blunt Injuries to the Brachiocephalic Vessels

Blunt injuries to the intrathoracic brachiocephalic vessels are uncommon. The innominate artery was found ruptured at aortogram in about 4% of 510 aortic and brachiocephalic artery cases in a radiologic review by Fisher et al. in 1981 (124). A similar incidence of subclavian, common carotid, and combinations of brachiocephalic artery and aortic injuries was found, for a combined incidence of brachiocephalic artery

Table 13.1.
Summary of Risk Factors for Death or Major Complication in 83 Patients with Rupture of the Thoracic Aorta Due to Blunt Trauma Treated at the Shock Trauma Center from 1976 through 1985[a]

Risk Factor	Complication	Death
Age	N/C	N/C
Female sex	N/C	DA*
Higher ISS	R*	DS*, DP*
Admission systolic blood pressure <90 mm Hg	N/C	DA***
Presenting hemothorax >500 ml	C†	DA***
Nonthoracic surgeon	A*, C*	DA***, DP†
Other surgery first	N/C	DA**
Aortic cross-clamp time >30 min	P?†	N/C
Use of shunt/bypass	A*	DP*
Transfer from scene of injury	R†	DP*

[a]N/C, no correlation. R, severe renal failure; A, adult respiratory distress syndrome; P, paraplegia/paresis; C, any combination of R, A, P, and severe sepsis. DA, death during resuscitation; DS, death during aortic surgery; DP, death within 30 postoperative days. χ^2 P value: †<0.1 (= 0.18 in paraplegia associated with aortic cross-clamp time), *<0.05, **<0.01, ***≤0.001. ISS, Injury Severity Score.

injury of about 8%. Castagna and Nelson (125) found 36 case reports in a major surgical literature review in 1975 (125), 22 involving the innominate artery. Symbas (73) reported only four cases of rupture of the brachiocephalic arteries in his extensive experience in 1989.

The mechanism of injury is conjectured to be some combination of deceleration, chest compression, and extension or rotation of the neck (73, 126). Decreased distal pulse is present in less than 50% of the cases, due to continued vessel patency or extensive collateral circulation (125). A widened upper mediastinum on chest x-ray film is the principal radiologic sign. Aortography is the definitive test and must be done in all suspected cases. The aortographic findings may be overt or subtle; they include false aneurysm, filling defect, and complete obstruction (124). Avulsion or tear at or near the origin of a brachiocephalic vessel is a common finding (86, 125, 127–130).

Prompt surgical repair is required for the same reasons given above for blunt traumatic aortic injury, namely to prevent the inevitable fatal intrapleural or intraperi-cardial rupture or the consequences of an expanding chronic aneurysm. Too little is known of the natural history of brachiocephalic vessel injury to be dogmatic about the timing of surgery, although an avulsion at or near the aortic arch, or adjacent to the pleural space, probably should be treated with the same sense of urgency as an aortic rupture. Operative mortality cannot be judged reliably from the case report material available for review (125).

The surgical approach depends on the location of the injury (130a). Median sternotomy with extension into the neck gives good access to the innominate and proximal left common carotid arteries, whereas right or left thoracotomy offers the best exposure to the intrathoracic right and left subclavian arteries, respectively. Lesions distal to the aortic origin can be isolated by simply clamping the involved vessel and its branches above and below the lesion. The innominate or left common carotid artery may be clamped in most cases, although establishing distal perfusion by a temporary aortic-carotid shunt in the patient with intact neurologic function is recommended, if feasible, especially for the common carotid artery (126, 129, 131). A distal carotid artery stump pressure of less than about 50 mm Hg (at normal aortic pressure) may indicate the need for a shunt (132).

Similarly, reconstruction should be done if at all possible. For more distal lesions, primary repair or repair with interposed synthetic graft may be possible without bypass techniques. For lesions at or near the vessel's aortic take-off, an aortic side clamp may suffice for proximal control. In this case, the length and condition of the proximal stump will determine if it can be used in the vessel reconstruction or be simply oversewn, often with felt pledget buttressing. If it is oversewn, reconstruction is carried out by a jump graft, usually from the aorta to the distal stump.

For lesions at the aortic take-off that cannot be managed by aortic cross-clamp or side-clamp due to their size or location, some form of cardiopulmonary bypass is required. Profound hypothermia and circulatory arrest may be ideal in this circumstance, providing maximal exposure for a lesion that probably can be repaired relatively quickly (130–133a). In each such case, the danger to the acute multitrauma patient of systemic anticoagulation required for cardiopulmonary bypass must be weighed against the risk of the lesion rupturing intrapericardially or intrapleurally or causing distal ischemia or embolism.

Penetrating Wounds of the Great Thoracic Vessels

Nearly 90% of victims of penetrating cardiac and aortic wounds die within 1 hr of injury (134, 134a). Despite this, penetrating injuries to the great thoracic vessels are reported in relatively large series from urban trauma centers (73, 135–136b) and combat zones (137) (see Chapter 19, Civilian Cardiothoracic Combat Injuries). These lesions are, by their nature, diagnosed and treated on an individual basis. Due to the uncertainties of trajectory, there is no characteristic finding that simplifies diagnosis. See Chapter 15 (Management of Penetrating Thoracic Trauma) for a detailed review of the overall assessment of the patient with penetrating thoracic injury.

The principle of rapid operation in the hemodynamically unstable patient in whom the missile or blade path can be surmised overrides all other diagnostic studies (136, 138–140). In the more stable patient, angiography should be done in all cases in which vascular injury is suspected by virtue of missile trajectory and in the presence of hematoma formation and active bleeding. It is important to precisely define the extent of injury, if at all possible, in order to permit logical preoperative planning and to avoid missing unsuspected injuries.

Of course, the patient with intrapericardial hemorrhage and tamponade from an ascending aortic or pulmonary artery laceration will probably require immediate median sternotomy or anterolateral thoracotomy if he or she is to survive. Similarly, a patient with a laceration of the descending thoracic aorta with massive left hemothorax and shock should undergo immediate thoracotomy. On the other hand, a patient with a smaller (< 1000 ml) left hemothorax without hemodynamic instability, and continuing left chest tube drainage of less than 100–200 ml/hr, can probably undergo definitive workup. Such a patient must be watched very carefully, however, since a precariously clotted wound may bleed unexpectedly (140a), requiring urgent exploration before the workup can be completed. All patients with suspected major vascular injuries such as these must be typed and cross-matched immediately for large amounts of blood, and the operating room staff must be notified of the possibility of pending emergency surgery.

Choice of incision depends on the site of the injuries (73, 141). For anterior wounds and wounds known to involve the ascending aorta, the proximal brachiocephalic vessels, and the main pulmonary artery, a median sternotomy, with division of the left innominate vein if necessary, will usually offer the best exposure (Fig. 15.4). Extension of the sternotomy into the neck may be required to gain exposure to the common carotid vessels or into the supraclavicular area for the subclavian vessels. For more lateral wounds and those involving the subclavian vessels and the descending thoracic aorta, a posterolateral thoracotomy may be more appropriate (Fig. 15.5). Through-and-through wounds involving both pleural cavities may be approached best through bilateral anterolateral thoracotomies with sternal division or by median sternotomy with anterolateral thoracotomy extension into one or both sides after initial bilateral intrapleural exploration through the sternotomy incision. Thoracoabdominal wounds may be approached by a thoracoabdominal incision with division of the diaphragm (142).

Immediate control of hemorrhage from a disrupted major vessel is of paramount importance. As discussed in the section on blunt brachiocephalic injuries above, gaining enough control to permit repair may be as simple as using a vascular side-clamp or as complex as preparing the patient for total cardiopulmonary bypass while temporarily applying local pressure. The wound may have temporarily tamponaded or sealed with clot, which may allow time for careful dissection to gain control of the vessel. If there is active bleeding, digital compression will usually be possible while vascular control is attempted quickly. Active bleeding from through-and-through wounds or multiple wounds may require attempts at rapid application of vascular clamps proximal as well as distal to the cluster of holes, where possible.

In general, the technique of repair is determined by the nature of the injury (143), with simple suture sufficing in small clean lacerations (144). Debridement and patch or tubular graft interpositions may be required in more severe injuries. High-velocity gunshot wounds usually have a wider zone of damage requiring more extensive debridement. Aortic tissue friability often requires that sutures be buttressed with felt pledget material. A controlled drop in the arterial blood pressure by appropriate use of a vasodilating agent such as sodium nitroprusside may be helpful in safely securing a side clamp to the aorta, particularly to the ascending aorta.

Wounds to the venae cavae should be repaired if at all possible, using prosthetic material, if necessary. For wounds involving both arteries and veins, or vessels and the trachea or esophagus, interposition of a muscle, pleural, or pericardial flap may help prevent late fistula formation.

Cardiopulmonary bypass, with or without profound hypothermia and circulatory arrest, may be required to repair injuries to the ascending aorta, the aortic arch and its proximal brachiocephalic branches, the main pulmonary artery, and the venae cavae (136). Use of cardiopulmonary bypass in the desperate emergency situation is likely to succeed only if the pump team is already in the operating room on a standby basis (145). Temporary compressive occlusion of the bleeding site may be required until the cannulas are inserted and bypass commenced. Total body heparinization in this setting is somewhat different from that of the blunt trauma victim, in whom hidden bleeding may occur and for whom other modalities of shunt or bypass are available. Of course, the victim of multiple gunshot wounds may have undiagnosed injuries from which bleeding is increased by heparinization, but the lifesaving potential of repair of an intrapericardial or aortic arch injury under cardiopulmonary bypass usually supersedes this concern.

A major sequela of penetrating wounds of the great vessels is the appearance of an arterial-venous (146, 147), aortic-right ventricular or aortic-atrial (148), or aortic-pulmonary fistula (149–151), which may be delayed days or weeks after injury. Presence of a thrill and murmur and development of signs of congestive heart failure usually lead to angiographic investigation and repair (73). All patients with penetrating wounds of the chest should have follow-up examination a month or so following injury, even if asymptomatic, for assessment of possible fistula formation. The repair technique depends on the location of the fistula and usually requires cardiopulmonary bypass for cardiac chamber fistulae.

Chronic traumatic false aneurysm from a penetrating wound may occur in any injured vessel (73, 152). In general, surgical repair will be required once the diagnosis is made since progressive enlargement will almost surely continue. Arterial embolism of missiles is another rarely reported sequela of thoracic vascular missile injury. Embolism has been reported primarily to the iliac and femoral artery distribution, but also to the carotid and brachial arteries (149, 153–155). Local extrication of the embolus is usually indicated.

REFERENCES

1. Moar JJ. Traumatic rupture of the thoracic aorta: an autopsy and histopathological study. S Afr Med J 1985;67:383–385.
2. Gerbode F, Braimbridge M, Osborn JJ, Hood M, French S. Traumatic thoracic aneurysms: treatment by resection and grafting with the use of an extracorporeal bypass. Surgery 1957;42:975–985.
3. Strassman G. Traumatic rupture of the aorta. Am Heart J 1947;33:508–515.
4. Sevitt S. Traumatic ruptures of the aorta: a clinico-pathological study. Injury 1977;8:159–173.
5. Parmley LF, Mattingly TW, Manion WC, Jahnke EJ. Nonpenetrating traumatic injury of the aorta. Circulation 1957;17:1086–1101.
6. Dischinger PC, Cowley RA, Shankar BS, Smialek JE. The incidence of ruptured aorta among vehicular fatalities. Proc Am Assoc Automot Med 1988;32:15–22.
7. Greendyke RM. Traumatic rupture of the aorta: special reference to automobile accidents. JAMA 1966;195:527–530.
8. Cowley RA, Turney SZ, Hankins JR, Rodriguez A, Attar S, Shankar BS. Rupture of thoracic aorta due to blunt trauma: a 15-year experience. J Thorac Cardiovasc Surg, in press, 1990.
9. Nashef SA, Talwalkar NG, Jamieson MP. Aortic arch rupture in a child following minor blunt trauma. Thorac Cardiovasc Surg 1987;35:240–241.
10. Newman RJ, Rastogi S. Rupture of the thoracic aorta and its relationship to road traffic accident characteristics. Injury 1984;15:296–299.
11. Pickard LR, Mattox KL, Espada R, Beall AC, DeBakey ME. Transection of the descending thoracic aorta secondary to blunt trauma. J Trauma 1977; 17:749–753.
12. Sturm JT, McGee MB, Luxenberg MG. An analysis of risk factors for death at the scene following traumatic aortic rupture. J Trauma 1988;28:1578–1580.
13. Arajarvi E, Santavirta S, Tolonen J. Aortic ruptures in seat belt wearers. J Thorac Cardiovasc Surg 1989;98:355–361.
14. Finkelmeier BA, Mentzer RM, Kaiser DL, Tegtmeyer CJ, Nolan SP. Chronic traumatic aortic thoracic aneurysm. J Thorac Cardiovasc Surg 1982;84:257–266.
15. Rittenhouse EA, Dillard DH, Winterscheid LC, Merendino KA. Traumatic rupture of the thoracic aorta: a review of the literature and a report of five cases with attention to special problems in early surgical management. Ann Surg 1969;170:87–100.
16. Bennett DE, Cherry JK. The natural history of traumatic aneurysms of the aorta. Surgery 1967;61:516–523.
16a. Fleming AW, Green DC. Traumatic aneurysms of the thoracic aorta: report of 43 patients. Ann Thorac Surg 1974;18:91–101.
17. Cowley RA, Turney SZ. Blunt thoracic injuries: the ruptured aorta. In: Cowley RA, Conn A, Dunham CM, eds. Trauma care: surgical management. Philadelphia: Lippincott, 1987:172–181.
18. Bodily K, Perry JF Jr, Strate RG, Fischer RP. The salvageability of patients with post-traumatic rupture of the descending thoracic aorta in a primary trauma center. J Trauma 1977;17:754–760.
19. Ayella RJ, Hankins JR, Turney SZ, Cowley RA. Ruptured thoracic aorta due to blunt trauma. J Trauma 1977;17:199–205.
19a. Hartford JM, Fayer RL, Shaver TE, et al. Transection of the thoracic aorta: assessment of a trauma system. Am J Surg 1986;151:224–229.
20. Lynch RP. Cardiovascular disease following trauma. Cardiovasc Clin 1972;4:263–280.

21. Asfaw I, Ramadan H, Talbert JG, Arbulu A. Double traumatic rupture of the thoracic aorta. J Trauma 1985;25:1102–1104.
22. Cimochowski GE, Barcia PJ, DeMeester TR, Griffin LH, Fishback ME. Multiple transections of the thoracic aorta secondary to blunt trauma. Ann Thorac Surg 1973;15:536–540.
23. Jackson FR, Berkas EM, Roberts VL. Traumatic aortic rupture after blunt trauma. Dis Chest 1968;53:577–583.
24. Sevitt S. The mechanisms of traumatic rupture of the thoracic aorta. Br J Surg 1977;64:166–173.
25. Lasky II. Human aortic laceration secondary to impact. Leg Med 1974;0:3–29.
26. O'Rourke MF, Shepherd KM. Protection of the aortic arch and subclavian artery during intra-aortic balloon pumping. J Thorac Cardiovasc Surg 1973;65:543–546.
27. Koutras P, Kwon Y, Holland RH, Webb WR. An unusual cause of perforation of the aorta. Ann Thorac Surg 1969;8:575–579.
28. Iserson KV, Copeland J. Pulmonary and aortic punctures—complications of an attempt at internal jugular venipuncture. J Emerg Med 1984;1:227–231.
29. Primm RK, Karp RB, Schrank JP. Multiple cardiovascular injuries and motor vehicle accidents. JAMA 1979;241:2540–2541.
30. Turney SZ, Attar S, Ayella R, Cowley RA, McLaughlin J. Traumatic rupture of the aorta: a five-year experience. J Thorac Cardiovasc Surg 1976;72:727–732.
31. Crawford ES, Coselli JS, Safi HJ. Partial cardiopulmonary bypass, hypothermic circulatory arrest, and posterolateral exposure for thoracic aortic aneurysm operation. J Thorac Cardiovasc Surg 1987;94:824–827.
32. Bodily K, Fischer RP. Aortic rupture and right ventricular rupture induced by closed chest cardiac massage. Minn Med 1979;62:225–227.
33. Lacombe M, Coquillard JP, Andreassian B, Baumann J. Acute traumatic rupture of the thoracic aorta with secondary necrosis of the esophagus. Ann Thorac Surg 1971;11:171–175.
34. McCabe RE Jr, Scott JR, Knox WG. Fistulization between the esophagus, aorta, and trachea as a complication of acute corrosive esophagitis: report of a case. Am Surg 1969;35:450–454.
35. Attar S, Ayella RJ, McLaughlin JS. The widened mediastinum in trauma. Ann Thorac Surg 1972;13:356–363.
36. Gundry SR, Burney RE, Mackenzie JR, et al. Assessment of mediastinal widening associated with traumatic rupture of the aorta. J Trauma 1983;23:293–299.
37. Gundry SR, Burney RE, Mackenzie JR, Jafri SZ, Shirazi K, Cho KJ. Traumatic pseudoaneurysm of the thoracic aorta. Arch Surg 1984;119:1055–1060.
38. Kram HB, Appel PL, Wohlmuth DA, Shoemaker WC. Diagnosis of traumatic thoracic aortic rupture: a 10-year retrospective analysis. Ann Thorac Surg 1989;47:282–286.
39. Griffin JS, Ochsner JL, Bower PJ. Posttraumatic coarctation of the aorta: diagnostic clues. Am J Cardiol 1973;31:391–392.
40. Verdant A. Major mediastinal vessel injury: an underestimated lesion. Can J Surg 1987;30:402–404.
41. Young MW, Lau SH, Stein E, Damato AN. Pseudocoarctation of the aorta. Am Heart J 1969;77:259–262.
42. Mason CB, Hobson GC. Deceleration injury of the thoracic aorta: brachial hypertension in an accident victim may indicate an injury to the aorta. Hawaii Med J 1967;26:312–316.
42a. Vander Salm TJ, Cutler BS. Traumatic aortic rupture: presentation as a femoral embolus. J Cardiovasc Surg (Torino) 1980;21:501–502.
42b. Roon AJ, Sauvage LR. Blue toe syndrome—a warning sign of unsuspected vascular injury. Surgery 1983;93:722–724.
43. Stulz P, Perruchoud A, Hasse J, Grädel E. Traumatic aneurysms of the thoracic aorta simulating bronchogenic neoplasms. Arch Int Med 1983;143:174–175.
44. Coates GR, Stapleton D. Unusual presentation of traumatic transection of aorta: case report. J Tenn Med Assoc 1987;80:421–422.
45. Bolvig L, Anresen J. Haemoptysis associated with traumatic rupture of the thoracic aorta. Scand J Thorac Cardiovasc Surg 1981;15:221–222.
46. Dosios TJ. Bronchoscopic findings in traumatic rupture of the thoracic aorta [Letter]. J Thorac Cardiovasc Surg 1988;96:342–343.
46a. Verdant A. Chronic traumatic aneurysm of the descending thoracic aorta with compression of the tracheobronchial tree. Can J Surg 1984;27:278–279.
47. Hamby RI, Gulotta SJ, Gruber F. Taumatic aortic aneurysm complicated by obstruction of the left pulmonary artery. Vasc Surg 1967;1:179–183.
48. Di Summa M, Ottino GM, Trucano G, et al. Traumatic rupture of the thoracic aorta: report of two unusual cases. J Cardiovasc Surg (Torino) 1981;22:181–186.
48a. McCollum CH, Graham JM, Noon GP, DeBakey ME. Chronic traumatic aneurysms of the thoracic aorta: an analysis of 50 patients. J Trauma 1979;19:248–252.

49. Hankins JR, Attar S, Turney SZ, Cowley RA, McLaughlin JS. Differential diagnosis of pulmonary parenchymal changes in thoracic trauma. Am Surg 1973;39:309–318.
50. Pupello DF, Mark JB, Iben AB. Surgical treatment of traumatic rupture of the thoracic aorta and diaphragm. Calif Med 1970;112:27–29.
51. Georgiade G, Riefkohl R, Serafin D, Georgiade N. A silent but lethal injury associated with facial trauma. Plast Reconstruct Surg 1981;67:665–667.
52. Mattox KL. Descending thoracic aortic transection. In: Pickard LR, ed. Decision making in surgery of the chest. Philadelphia: Saunders, 1989:150–151.
52a. Borman KR, Aurbakken CM, Weigelt JA. Treatment priorities in combined abdominal and aortic trauma. Am J Surg 1982;144:728–732.
53. Harden CA. Resection and Orlon graft of multiple aortic aneurysms due to trauma. J Thorac Surg 1956;32:251–253.
54. Spencer FC, Guerin PF, Blake HA, Bahnson HT. A report of fifteen patients with traumatic rupture of the thoracic aorta. J Thorac Cardiovasc Surg 1961;41:1–22.
55. Garamella JJ, Schmidt WR, Jensen NK, Lynch MF. Traumatic aneurysms of the thoracic aorta. N Engl J Med 1962;266:1341–1348.
56. Kirsh MM, Kahn DR, Crane JD, et al. Repair of acute traumatic rupture of the aorta without extracorporeal circulation. Ann Thorac Surg 1970;10:227–236.
57. Clarke CP, Brandt PW, Cole DS, Barratt-Boyes BG. Traumatic rupture of the thoracic aorta: diagnosis and treatment. Br J Surg 1967;54:353–358.
58. Conn JH, Hardy JD, Chavez CM, Fain WR. Challenging arterial injuries. J Trauma 1971;11:167–177.
59. Deiraniya AK, Taylor DG. Traumatic rupture of the thoracic aorta. Injury 1970;2:93–98.
60. DeMeules JE, Cramer G, Perry JF Jr. Rupture of aorta and great vessels due to blunt thoracic trauma. J Thorac Cardiovasc Surg 1971;62:438–442.
61. Kiser JC, Peterson TA, Fulks RW, Johnson FE. Repair of traumatic rupture of the aortic arch [Letter]. JAMA 1968;204:404.
62. Moffat RC, Krome RL, Berkas EM. Transection of the thoracic aorta: recognition and immediate repair. Vasc Surg 1969;3:154–160.
63. Richardson RL Jr, Pate JW, Butterick OD, Wells V. Traumatic rupture of the thoracic aorta: a follow-up report. Am Surg 1969;35:624–626.
64. Wilder RJ, Fishbein RH. Complete transection of the aorta. JAMA 1964;188:176–178.
65. Kahn AM, Joseph WL, Hughes RK. Traumatic aneurysms of the thoracic aorta: excision and repair without graft. Ann Thorac Surg 1967;4:175–181.
66. Keen G, Bradbrook RA, McGinn F. Traumatic rupture of the thoracic aorta. Thorax 1969;24:25–31.
67. Keen G. Closed injuries of the thoracic aorta. Ann R Coll Surg Engl 1972;51:137–156.
68. Mulder DG, Grollman JH Jr. Traumatic disruption of the thoracic aorta: diagnostic and surgical considerations. Am J Surg 1969;118:311–316.
69. Pate JW, Butterick OD, Richardson RL. Traumatic rupture of the thoracic aorta. JAMA 1968;203:1022–1024.
70. Appelbaum A, Karp RB, Kirklin JW. Surgical treatment for closed thoracic aortic injuries. J Thorac Cardiovasc Surg 1976;71:458–460.
71. Crawford ES, Rubio PA. Reappraisal of adjuncts to avoid ischemia in the treatment of aneurysms of descending thoracic aorta. J Thorac Cardiovasc Surg 1973;66:693–704.
72. Najafi H, Javid H, Hunter J, Serry C, Monson D. Descending aortic aneurysmectomy without adjuncts to avoid ischemia. Ann Thorac Surg 1980;30:326–335.
73. Symbas PN. Cardiothoracic trauma. Philadelphia: Saunders, 1989:160–230.
73a. Mitchell RL, Enright LP. The surgical management of acute and chronic injuries of the thoracic aorta. Surg Gynecol Obstet 1983;157:1–4.
74. Olivier HF, Maher TD, Liebler GA, Park SB, Burkholder JA, Magovern GJ. Use of the BioMedicus centrifugal pump in traumatic tears of the thoracic aorta. Ann Thorac Surg 1984;38:586–591.
75. Hess PJ, Howe HR, Robiscek F, et al. Traumatic tears of the thoracic aorta: improved results using the BioMedicus pump. Ann Thorac Surg 1989;48:6–9.
76. Verdant A, Page A, Cossette R, Dontigny L, Page P, Baillot R. Surgery of the descending thoracic aorta: spinal cord protection with the Gott shunt. Ann Thorac Surg 1988;46:147–154.
77. Heberer G. Ruptures and aneurysms of the thoracic aorta after blunt chest trauma. J Cardiovasc Surg (Torino) 1971;12:115–120.
78. Inberg MV, Laaksonen V, Scheinin TM, Slätis P, Vänttinen E. Early repair of traumatic rupture of the thoracic aorta: report of two cases. Scand J Thorac Cardiovasc Surg 1972;6:287–292.
79. Kirsh MM, Behrendt DM, Orringer MB, et al. The treatment of acute traumatic rupture of the aorta: a 10-year experience. Ann Surg 1976;184:308–316.

80. Kirsh MM, Sloan H. Blunt chest trauma: general principles of management. Boston: Little, Brown, 1977:179–211.

81. Shek JL. Nonpenetrating traumatic rupture of thoracic aorta. Vasc Surg 1971;5:211–214.

82. Gazzaniga AB, Khuri EI, Mir-Sepasi HM, Bartlett RH. Rupture of the thoracic aorta following blunt trauma. Arch Surg 1975;110:1119–1123.

83. Hallén A, Hansson HE, Nordlund S. Thoracic injuries: a survey of 765 patients treated at the University Hospital, Uppsala, during the years 1956–1969. Scand J Thorac Cardiovasc Surg 1974;8:34–45.

84. Iyengar SR, Charrette EJ, Lynn RB, McArthur R. Traumatic rupture of the thoracic aorta. Can J Surg 1972;15:350–359.

85. Kosak M. Traumatic rupture of the aorta caused by deceleration. J Cardiovasc Surg (Torino) 1971;12:131–139.

86. Langlois J, Binet JP, Jegou D. Traumatic rupture of the thoracic aorta and its branches. J Cardiovasc Surg (Torino) 1971;12:83–92.

87. Michaud P, Chassignolle J, Termet H, et al. Traumatic aneurysms of the aorta: analysis of 11 observations. J Cardiovasc Surg (Torino) 1971;12:121–130.

88. O'Sullivan MJ Jr, Folkerth TL, Morgan JR, Fosburg RG. Posttraumatic thoracic aorta aneurysm: recognition and treatment. Arch Surg 1972;105:14–18.

89. Roe BB. Cardiac trauma including injury of great vessels. Surg Clin North Am 1972;52:573–583.

90. Wilson RF, Arbulu A, Bassett JS, Walt AJ. Acute mediastinal widening following blunt chest trauma: critical decisions. Arch Surg 1972;104:551–558.

91. Toledo A. Transected thoracic aorta: experience at one hospital. Rev Surg 1976;33:68–70.

92. Svensson LG, Antunes MD, Kinsley RH. Traumatic rupture of the thoracic aorta: a report of 14 cases and review of the literature. S Afr Med J 1985;67:853–857.

93. Symbas PN, Tyras DH, Ware RE, Diorio DA. Traumatic rupture of the aorta. Ann Surg 1973;178:6–12.

94. Sutorius DJ, Schreiber JT, Helmsworth JA. Traumatic disruption of the thoracic aorta. J Trauma 1973;13:583–590.

95. Stafford G, O'Brien MF. Traumatic rupture of the thoracic aorta. Aust NZ J Surg 1977;47:175–179.

96. Soyer R, Brunet A, Piwnica A, et al. Traumatic rupture of the thoracic aorta with reference to 34 operated cases. J Cardiovasc Surg (Torino) 1981;22:103–108.

97. Skotnicki SH, Vincent J, Buskens FG, van der Meer JJ. Traumatic rupture of the thoracic aorta. Acta Chir Belg 1982;82:485–491.

98. Tegner Y, Bergdahl L, Ekeström S. Traumatic disruption of the thoracic aorta. Acta Chir Scand 1984;150:635–638.

99. Feliciano DV, Mattox KL. Traumatic aneurysms. In: Rutherford RB, ed. Vascular surgery. 2nd ed. Philadelphia: Saunders, 1984:848–855.

100. Ruberti U, Odero A, Arpesani A, et al. Acute ruptures of the thoracic aorta: personal experience. J Cardiovasc Surg (Torino) 1987;28:81–84.

101. McBride LR, Tidik S, Stothert JC, et al. Primary repair of traumatic aortic disruption. Ann Thorac Surg 1987;43:65–67.

102. McGough EC, Hughes RK. Acute traumatic rupture of the aorta: a reemphasis of repair without a vascular prosthesis. Ann Thorac Surg 1973;16:7–10.

103. Orringer MB, Kirsh MM. Primary repair of acute aortic disruption. Ann Thorac Surg 1983;35:672–675.

104. Schmidt CA, Jacobson JG. Thoracic aortic injury: a 10-year experience. Arch Surg 1984;119:1244–1246.

105. Stothert JC Jr, McBride L, Tidik S, Lewis L, Codd JE. Multiple aortic tears treated by primary suture repair. J Trauma 1987;27:955–956.

106. Akins CW, Buckley MJ, Daggett W, McIlduff JB, Austen WG. Acute traumatic disruption of the thoracic aorta: a 10-year experience. Ann Thorac Surg 1981;31:305–309.

107. Pezzella AT, Todd EP, Dillon ML, Utley JR, Griffen WO. Early diagnosis and individualized treatment of blunt thoracic aortic trauma. Am Surg 1978;44:699–703.

108. Mattox KL, Holzman M, Pickard LR, Beall AC, DeBakey ME. Clamp/repair: a safe technique for treatment of blunt injury to the descending thoracic aorta. Ann Thorac Surg 1985;40:456–463.

108a. Smith RS, Chang FC. Traumatic rupture of the aorta: still a lethal injury. Am J Surg 1986;152:660–663.

109. Sassano JJ. The rapid infusion system. In: Winter PM, Yang YG, eds. Hepatic transplantation: anesthetic and peri-operative management. New York: Praeger, 1986:120–134.

110. Lillehei CW, Todd DB, Levy MJ, Ellis RJ. Partial cardiopulmonary bypass, hypothermia, and total circulatory arrest. J Thorac Cardiovasc Surg 1969;58:530–544.

111. Kantor KR, Pennington G, Weber TR, Zambie MA, Braun P, Martychenko V. Extracorporeal membrane oxygenation for postoperative cardiac support in children. J Thorac Cardiovasc Surg 1987;93:27–35.

111a. Lynch C, Weingarden SI. Paraplegia following aortic surgery. Paraplegia 1982;20:196–200.

112. Adams HD, van Geertruyden HH. Neurologic complications of aortic surgery. Ann Surg 1956;144:574–610.

113. Svensson LG, Rickards E, Coull A, Rogers G, Fimmel CJ, Hinder RA. Relationship of spinal cord flow to vascular anatomy during thoracic aortic cross-clamping and shunting. J Thorac Cardiovasc Surg 1986;91:71–78.

114. Svensson LG, Von Ritter CM, Groeneveld HT, et al. Cross-clamping of the thoracic aorta. Ann Surg 1986;204:38–47.

115. Laschinger JC, Izumoto H, Kouchoukos NT. Evolving concepts in prevention of spinal cord injury during operations on the descending thoracic aorta and thoracoabdominal aorta. Ann Thorac Surg 1987;44:667–674.

115a. Gelman S, Reves JG, Fowler K, Samuelson PN, Lell WA, Smith LR. Regional blood flow during cross-clamping of the thoracic aorta and infusion of sodium nitroprusside. J Thorac Cardiovasc Surg 1983;85:287–291.

116. Symbas PN, Pfaender LM, Drucker MH, Lester JL, Gravanis MB, Zacharopoulos L. Cross-clamping of the descending aorta: hemodynamic and neurohumeral effects. J Thorac Cardiovasc Surg 1983;85:300–305.

117. Coles JG, Wilson GJ, Sima AF, et al. Intraoperative management of thoracic aortic aneurysm: experimental evaluation of perfusion cooling of the spinal cord. J Thorac Cardiovasc Surg 1983;85:292–299.

117a. Molina JE, Cogordan J, Einzig S, et al. Adequacy of ascending aorta–descending aorta shunt during cross-clamping of the thoracic aorta for prevention of spinal cord injury. J Thorac Cardiovasc Surg 1985;90:126–136.

117b. Frantz PT, Murray GF, Shallal JA, Lucas CL. Clinical and experimental evaluation of left ventriculoiliac shunt bypass during repair of lesions of the descending thoracic aorta. Ann Thorac Surg 1981;31:551–557.

117c. Wadouh F, Arndt C-F, Metzger H, Hartmann M, Wadouh R, Borst HG. Direct measurement of oxygen tension on the spinal cord surface of pigs after occlusion of the descending aorta. J Thorac Cardiovasc Surg 1985;89:787–794.

118. Katz NM, Blackstone EH, Kirklin JW, Karp RB. Incremental risk factors for spinal cord injury following operation for acute traumatic aortic transection. J Thorac Cardiovasc Surg 1981;81:669–674.

118a. van Niekerk JL, Heijstraten FM, Goris RJ, Buskens FG, Eijgelaar A, Lacquet LK. Spinal cord injury following surgery for acute traumatic rupture of the thoracic aorta. Thorac Cardiovasc Surg 1986;34:30–34.

118b. Crawford ES, Walker HSJ, Saleh SA, Normann NA. Graft replacement of aneurysm in descending thoracic aorta: results without bypass or shunting. Surgery 1981;89:73–85.

118c. Crawford ES, Fenstermacher JM, Richardson W, Sandiford F. Reappraisal of adjuncts to avoid ischemia in the treatment of thoracic aortic aneurysms. Surgery 1970;67:182–196.

118d. Antunes MJ. Acute traumatic rupture of the aorta: repair by simple aortic cross-clamping. Ann Thorac Surg 1987;44:257–259.

119. Knight RQ, Devanny JR. Spinal cord ischemia and paraplegia in the multiple-trauma patient with aortic arch injury: case report. Spine 1987;12:624–627.

120. Kouchoukos NT, Lell WA, Karp RB, Samuelson PN. Hemodynamic effects of aortic clamping and decompression with a temporary shunt for resection of the descending thoracic aorta. Surgery 1979;85:25–30.

120a. Nguyen H, Maggio R, Savino J, Agarawal N, Cerabena T, Berman E. Prevention of complications by monitoring distal aortic perfusion pressure in traumatic aortic rupture. Crit Care Med 1989;17:S41.

120b. Kirshner DL, Kirshner RL, Hegeness LM, DeWeese JA. Spinal cord ischemia: an evaluation of pharmacologic agents in minimizing paraplegia after aortic occlusion. J Vasc Surg 1989;9:305–308.

120c. Maeda S, Miyamoto T, Murata H, Yamashita K. Prevention of spinal cord ischemia by monitoring spinal cord perfusion pressure and somatosensory evoked potentials. J Cardiovasc Surg 1989;30:565–571.

120d. Joob AW, Harman PK, Kaiser DL, Kron IL. The effect of renin-angiotensin system blockade on visceral blood flow during and after thoracic aorta cross-clamping. J Thorac Cardiovasc Surg 1986;91:411–418.

120e. Sturm JT, Billiar TR, Luxenberg MG, Perry JF. Risk factors for the development of renal failure following surgical treatment of traumatic aortic rupture. Ann Thorac Surg 1987;43:425–427.

121. Fox S, Pierce WS, Waldhausen JA. Acute hypertension: its significance in traumatic aortic rupture. J Thorac Cardiovasc Surg 1979;77:622–625.

122. Gomez-Alonzo A, Lozano F, Cuadrado F, Almazan A. Traumatic aorto-esophageal fistula [Letter]. J Thorac Cardiovasc Surg 1984;87:148–149.

123. Sturm JT, Billiar TR, Dorsey JS, Luxenberg MG, Perry JF. Risk factors for survival following surgical treatment of traumatic aortic rupture. Ann Thorac Surg 1985;39:418–421.

124. Fisher RG, Hadlock F, Ben-Menachem Y. Laceration of the thoracic aorta and brachiocephalic arteries by blunt trauma. Radiol Clin North Am 1981;19:91–110.

125. Castagna J, Nelson RJ. Blunt injuries to branches of the aortic arch. J Thorac Cardiovasc Surg 1975;69:521–532.
126. Kirsh MM, Orringer MB, Behrendt DM, Mills LJ, Tashian J, Sloan H. Management of unusual traumatic ruptures of the aorta. Surg Gynecol Obstet 1978;146:365–370.
127. Danielson GK, Wood R, Holloway JB Jr. Traumatic avulsion of the innominate artery from the aorta: successful immediate repair utilizing cardiopulmonary bypass. Ann Thorac Surg 1968;5:451–458.
128. Dula DJ, Hughes HG, Majernick T. Traumatic disruption of the brachiocephalic artery. Ann Emerg Med 1983;12:639–641.
129. O'Neill MJ Jr, Myers JL, Brown GR, Harrison JL, DeMuth WE Jr. Avulsion of the innominate artery from the aortic arch associated with a posterior tracheal tear. J Trauma 1982;22:56–59.
130. Franz JL, Simpson CR, Penny RM, Grover FL, Trinkle JK. Avulsion of the innominate artery after blunt chest trauma: an application of an old technique. J Thorac Cardiovasc Surg 1974;67:478–480.
130a. Faro RS, Monson DO, Weinberg M, Javid H. Disruption of aortic arch branches due to nonpenetrating chest trauma. Arch Surg 1983;118:1333–1336.
131. Chandler WF. Carotid artery injuries. Mount Kisco, NY: Futura Publishing, 1982:96–98.
132. Baker WH. Shunting and nonshunting during carotid artery endarterectomy. In: Ernst CB, Stanley JC, eds. Current therapy in vascular surgery. Toronto: BC Becker, 1987:27–29.
133. Dumanian AV, Hoeksema TD, Santschi DR, Greenwald JH, Frahm CJ. Profound hypothermia and circulatory arrest in the surgical treatment of traumatic aneurysm of the thoracic aorta. J Thorac Cardiovasc Surg 1970;59:541–545.
133a. Lowery RC Jr, Ergin MA, Galla J, Lansman S, Griepp RB. Successful treatment of multiple simultaneous great vessel disruptions. Ann Thorac Surg 1986;41:672–674.
134. Parmley LF, Mattingly TW, Manion WC. Penetrating wounds of the heart and aorta. Circulation 1958;17:953–973.
134a. Jones TK, Barnhart GL, Greenfield LJ. Cardiopulmonary arrest following penetrating trauma: guidelines for emergency hospital management of presumed exsanguination. J Trauma 1987;27:24–31.
135. Reul GJ Jr, Beall AC Jr, Jordan GL Jr, Mattox KL. The early operative management of injuries to great vessels. Surgery 1973;74:862–873.
136. Reul GJ Jr, Rubio PA, Beall AC Jr. The surgical management of acute injury to the thoracic aorta. J Thorac Cardiovasc Surg 1974;67:272–281.
136a. Borlase BC, Metcalf RK, Moore EE, Manart FD. Penetrating wounds to the anterior chest: analysis of thoracotomy and laparotomy. Am J Surg 1986;152:649–653.
136b. Weaver FA, Suda RN, Stiles QM, Yellin AE. Injuries to the ascending aorta, aortic arch and great vessels. Surg Gynecol Obstet 1989;169:27–31.
137. Billy LJ, Amato JJ, Rich NM. Aortic injuries in Vietnam. Surgery 1971;70:385–391.
138. Richardson JD, Flint LM, Snow NJ, Gray LA Jr, Trinkle JK. Management of transmediastinal gunshot wounds. Surgery 1981;90:671–676.
139. Siemens R, Polk HC Jr, Gray LA Jr, Fulton RL. Indications for thoracotomy following penetrating thoracic injury. J Trauma 1977;17:493–500.
140. McQuaide JR. Penetrating wounds of the aorta. S Afr Med J 1967;41:234–238.
140a. Manwaring JH. Delayed hemorrhage after stab wounds of aorta. J Thorac Cardiovasc Surg 1974;67:788–791.
141. Hewitt RL, Smith AD, Becker ML, Lindsey ES, Dowling JB, Drapanas T. Penetrating thoracic injuries of the thoracic outlet. Surgery 1974;76:715–722.
142. Dart CH Jr, Braitman HE, Larlarb S. Gunshot penetrating injuries of the descending thoracic aorta. West J Med 1981;134:442–446.
143. Hardy JD, Raju S, Neely WA, Berry DW. Aortic and other arterial injuries. Ann Surg 1975;181:640–653.
144. Ramanathan T, Somasundaram K, Yong NK. Successful repair of a penetrating wound of the thoracic aorta. Thorax 1975;30:348–351.
145. Lodi R, Bondioli A, Domenichini G, et al. Simultaneous penetrating wounds of the myocardium and aorta caused by firearms: surgical treatment. Thorax 1979;34:819–821.
146. Martinez E, Meller J, Godoy M, Herrmann JL, Buffolo E. Arteriovenous fistula of the thoracic aorta: report of a case presenting with superior vena caval obstruction. Thorax 1981;36:315–318.
147. Symbas PN, Sehdeva JS. Penetrating wounds of the thoracic aorta. Ann Surg 1970;171:441–450.
148. McNalley MC, Sugg WL. Traumatic communication between aorta, right atrium and left atrium: a case report. J Thorac Cardiovasc Surg 1967;54:150–152.
149. Lam CR, McIntyre R. Air-pistol injury of pulmonary artery and aorta: report of a case with peripheral embolization of pellet and residual aorticopulmonary fistula. J Thorac Cardiovasc Surg 1970;59:729–732.
150. Snow N, Johnson P. Traumatic fistula between the descending thoracic aorta and the left main pulmonary vein. J Trauma 1985;25:263–265.

151. Dively WL, Daniel RA Jr, Scott HW Jr. Injuries to ascending aorta and aortic arch. J Thorac Cardiovasc Surg 1961;41:23–33.
152. Astolfi D, di Carlo D, di Eusanio G, Marcelletti C. Repair of traumatic aortic arch to innominate vein fistula under deep hypothermia and circulatory arrest. Thorax 1976;31:753–756.
153. Trimble C. Arterial bullet embolism following thoracic gunshot wounds. Ann Surg 1968;168:911–916.
154. Stanford W, Crosby VG, Pike JD, Lawrence MS. Gunshot wounds of the thoracic aorta with peripheral embolization of the missile: a case report. Ann Surg 1967;165:139–141.
155. Burkitt DS, Dhasmana JP, Mortensen NJ, Wisheart JD. "Bullet embolism" to the popliteal artery following air rifle injury to the thoracic aorta: case report. Br J Surg 1984;71:61.

14 Blunt Injuries of the Heart and Pericardium

Aurelio Rodriguez, MD
Stephen Z. Turney, MD

MYOCARDIAL CONTUSION

The era of high-speed motor vehicles has brought about a tremendous increase in blunt cardiac trauma. Although it is estimated that this type of injury accounts for only 5% of the 50,000 deaths due to automobile crashes every year in the United States, the detection and treatment of myocardial contusion tax the clinical skills of the physicians in charge of the initial evaluation (1). Despite being the most common lesion found clinically in patients with nonpenetrating trauma (2), myocardial contusion is frequently overlooked. Its exact frequency has not been determined: some series report 15% in autopsy findings (3) and others cite 10–38% based on clinical diagnosis (4, 5). However, in the studies that detected higher frequencies, the diagnostic modalities differed so much that it is difficult to compare them.

Pathophysiology

The lesions associated with myocardial contusion can have different degrees of intensity depending on the mechanism of injury, e.g., vehicular crashes, industrial accidents, blows to the chest, balls traveling at high speeds, animal kicks, and sports injuries. The damage can range from small areas of epicardial or subendocardial ecchymosis to transmural lesions, including heart rupture (1). The severity of the injury does not seem to depend upon whether impact occurred during systole or diastole. Furthermore, the thickness of pathology specimens does not seem to correlate with the functional disturbance (6), probably because the patients who die immediately after the impact do not have the chance to develop massive interstitial edema and hematoma.

The pathologic findings in acute myocardial contusion are very similar to those found in myocardial infarction. However, there are some distinguishing features: the amount of hemorrhage is more prominent in acute myocardial contusion (6, 7), and the disintegration of muscle fibers that occurs in the first 24 hr after a myocardial contusion is not seen in ischemic myocardial necrosis. In addition, contusion presents an abrupt change between normal and abnormal myocardium whereas the changes are more gradual with infarction; in later stages, it is virtually impossible to differentiate the two scars.

261

Physiologically, the causes of arrhythmias are unclear. All types have been reported (8). In animal studies, arrhythmias are frequently the cause of death following myocardial contusion. In other experimental studies, arrhythmias occurred in 50% of cases.

Reduction in cardiac output by 30–40% after experimentally induced myocardial contusion has been reported. Clinically, using impedance cardiography, a 50% reduction of cardiac output has been observed by others (9–11). Although some studies have shown that the administration of alcohol causes significant depression of the ventricular performance of the heart and makes it prone to arrhythmias, others have not shown this correlation (12).

Diagnosis

Currently, there are no generally accepted criteria for making the diagnosis of myocardial contusion.

SYMPTOMS AND PHYSICAL EXAMINATION

Patients can be asymptomatic or can present with chest pain, usually radiating to the shoulder or interscapular space; however, in many circumstances this pain is of chest wall origin. Bruises on the anterior chest are present only in 30% of the patients. An electrocardiogram could show a variety of cardiac dysrhythmias: nonspecific ST or T wave abnormalities, atrial flutter, ventricular tachycardia, or ventricular fibrillation. Conduction defects, e.g., sinoatrial or atrioventricular blocks, may also be present. Unfortunately, these alterations of the cardiac rhythm could be nonspecific; they may be related to hypovolemia, hypoxia, and/or electrolyte imbalance occurring during the first moments of initial resuscitation (13–15). In a few cases, a cross-sectional echocardiogram can detect unsuspected myocardial and pericardial changes (15, 16).

CARDIAC ENZYMES

Elevation of CPK-MB (creatinine phosphokinase-MB) isoenzymes is an unreliable indicator of blunt cardiac injury in the opinion of some authors (17–19). They note that it is not unusual to observe high levels of CPK-MB when myocardial contusion is absent and vice versa. Keller and Shatney (17) found that 2 of 7 patients with an abnormal multigated angiogram (MUGA) scan and 4 of 11 patients with normal studies had elevated MB fractions. Two of three patients with severe power cardiac failure secondary to myocardial contusion had CPK-MB/CPK ratios of less than 2%. The same authors express concern regarding the isoenzyme levels that are considered diagnostic. Several investigators have expressed different levels, e.g., > 6 IU. Tenzer (20) believes that a CPK-MB fraction above 5% is indicative of this diagnosis. On the other hand, Kron and Cox (21) and Kettunen (13) suggest values equal to or above 6% of total CPK. Contrary to these negative opinions, others (22–25) have found that measurement of cardiac enzyme (CPK-MB) concentration not only is the most commonly applied test to determine myocardial contusion but also is sensitive and specific for myocardial lesions. They believe levels above 5% of the total CPK are associated with 70% of electrocardiographic abnormalities.

Frazee et al. have employed CPK-MB assessments to screen patients in conjunction with two-dimensional echocardiography to differentiate concussion from contusion (24). Concussion is suggested when the enzymes are abnormally elevated with a normal echocardiogram, and contusion should be suspected when both tests are abnormal.

Cardiac enzyme concentrations should be measured at admission and every 6 hr during the subsequent 24–48 hr.

NUCLEAR MEDICINE SCANS

A great deal of attention was given to the value of scans employing technetium-99 pyrophosphate in the diagnosis of myocardial contusion; however, this test proved to be neither specific nor reliable (26). Recently, several authors (27–29) have advanced radionuclide angiograms (MUGA) as a sensitive and specific technique. This procedure allows evaluation of the ejection fraction from the right ventricle (normal, 55) and of the motility of the ventricular walls (Figs. 14.1–6).

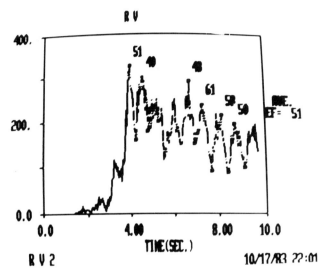

Figure 14.1.   Normal ejection fraction from right ventricle.

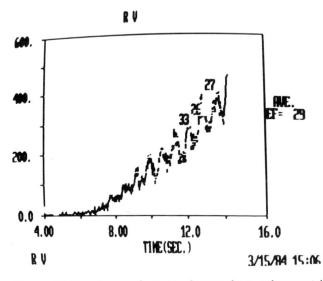

Figure 14.2.   Abnormal ejection fraction from right ventricle.

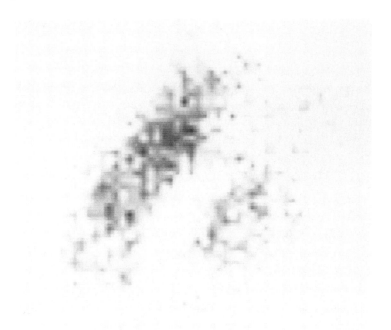

Figure 14.3. MUGA scan: end diastolic normal contraction.

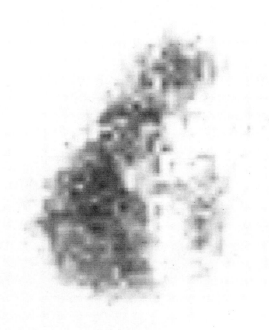

Figure 14.4. MUGA scan: end diastolic abnormal contraction.

Figure 14.5.   MUGA scan: end systolic normal contraction.

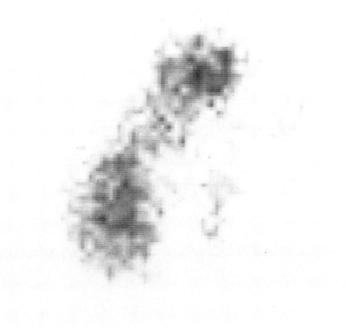

Figure 14.6.   MUGA scan: end systolic abnormal contraction.

ECHOCARDIOGRAM

Two-dimensional echocardiography is considered one of the diagnostic "gold standards" by some clinicians (16, 23, 24, 30). This test not only allows the evaluation of ejection fraction and ventricular cardiac contractility but also gives information about the state of the valves and amount of fluid in the pericardium (Figs. 14.7, 14.8).

CARDIAC HEMODYNAMICS

Cardiac hemodynamics can be assessed through cardiac output measured with a Swan-Ganz catheter or impedance plethysmography; unfortunately, this information makes no major contribution to the elusive diagnosis.

In summary, the diagnosis of myocardial contusion is difficult because of the lack of universally accepted criteria. Therefore, we believe that, when myocardial contusion is

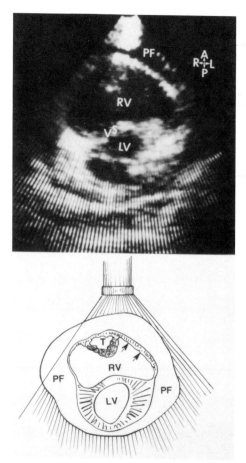

Figure 14.7. Echocardiogram showing right ventricular contusion (parasternal short-axis view). The right ventricle is dilated and the free wall is thinned *(arrows)*. In real time, the free wall was hypokinetic. Note the mural thrombus (*T*) underlying the right ventricular wall. Moderate size pericardial fluid (*PF*) is also present. *RV,* right ventricle; *LV,* left ventricle; *VS,* ventricular septum; *A,* anterior; *P,* posterior; *R,* right; *L,* left. (Courtesy of Dr. Peter Mucha.) (From Miller FA, Seward JB, Gersh BJ, Tajik AJ, Mucha P Jr. Two-dimensional echocardiographic findings in cardiac trauma. Am J Cardiol 1982;50:1022–1027.)

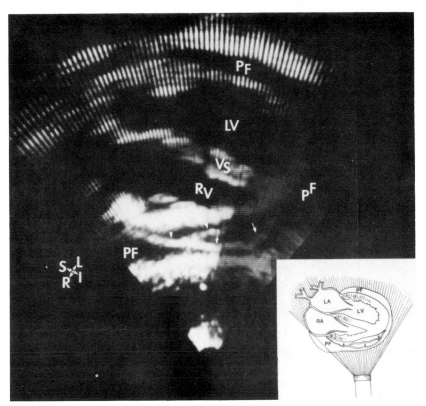

Figure 14.8. Echocardiogram showing pericardial effusion with strands. Subcostal four-chamber view shows that the right ventricle (*RV*) and left ventricle (*LV*) are surrounded by a large collection of pericardial fluid (*PF*). *RA,* right atrium; *LA,* left atrium; *VS,* ventricular septum; *S,* superior; *I,* inferior; *R,* right; *L,* left. (Courtesy of Dr. Peter Mucha.) (From Miller FA, Seward JB, Gersh BJ, Tajik AJ, Mucha P Jr. Two-dimensional echocardiographic findings in cardiac trauma. Am J Cardiol 1982;50:1022–1027.)

suspected, (*a*) a screening test should be done for nonspecific manifestations of the lesion, i.e., an electrocardiogram (ECG) followed by measurement of CPK-MB enzymes, and (*b*) patients with positive screening test results should undergo other more physiologic, dynamic, and specific evaluations, i.e., MUGA or two-dimensional echocardiogram.

Treatment and Outcome

The primary danger associated with myocardial contusion is the potential for arrhythmias. The efficacy of many of the extreme precautionary measures previously used (bedrest and prolonged continuous cardiac monitoring) is being questioned (9). A single screening test or combination of tests that can prognosticate the development of serious arrhythmias or hemodynamic intraoperative deterioration has not been found (31).

Flancbaum et al. (32) have shown that patients with myocardial contusion can tolerate major surgical procedures provided they are monitored adequately during the operation. Different questions arise in the emergency department when patients present with a history of severe anterior chest blow, e.g., from hitting a steering wheel, and chest pain. We believe that if the ECG is normal, or becomes normal after the correction of hypovolemia or hypoxia, these patients do not need to be treated as having myocardial contusion and consequently do not require cardiac monitoring. Otherwise, if the ECG is abnormal, serial cardiac enzyme determinations should be ordered and the patient should be kept in a cardiac monitoring bed (not ICU) for 48 hr or until the results of the cardiac enzyme assessments are known. At that point, the decision must be made whether to perform a more specific test (MUGA or two-dimensional echocardiogram) if the CPK-MB fraction is elevated or to obtain a cardiology consultation for assessment of other causes of the arrhythmias if the ECG abnormalities persist in conjunction with normal enzyme levels. A patient who is "confirmed" to have a myocardial contusion by MUGA or two-dimensional echocardiogram should be kept in the hospital on cardiac monitoring for at least 2 weeks, after which the test should be repeated. In the majority of cases, the MUGA or two-dimensional echocardiogram becomes normal in 3–4 weeks. Various sequelae of myocardial contusion have been described (ventricular aneurysms, coronary artery fistulas (33)), but we have not identified any in 15 yr in more than 2,500 patients with blunt thoracic trauma.

PERICARDIAL INJURIES

Traumatic pericardial tears are not common in patients with blunt thoracic trauma. Our previous review of the literature (34) from 1939 to 1983 identified only 142 patients with this diagnosis. Recently (35), we reviewed the experience in our institution over the past 10 yr (1978–1989) and identified 22 patients with pericardial tears due to blunt trauma.

Pathophysiology

The frequent association of these injuries with myocardial contusion or heart rupture probably indicates a similar mechanism of production: severe precordial impaction or a hydraulic mechanism such as sudden increase of intraabdominal pressure. The usual locations of the tears, in order of frequency, are as follows: left pleuropericardial rupture parallel to the phrenic nerve, 64%; diaphragmatic pericardial tears, 18%, right pleuropericardial tears, 9%; and superior mediastinal tears, 9% (35). These figures correlate fairly well with those presented in the literature. The extent of the tear can range from millimeters to almost the whole length of the pericardium; in our experience, the smallest was 2 cm long. Herniation of the heart through the defect is not uncommon. We found 6 of 22 patients with herniation of the heart, mostly on the left pleuropericardial side.

Diagnosis

The preoperative diagnosis of pericardial tears may be difficult, particularly if the tear is small. The patient can be asymptomatic; however, a pericardial rub can be heard in the precordium. In 1866, a characteristic murmur was reported by Morel-Lavalee (36). The murmur was described as sounding like a splashing wheel ("bruit de moulin"). We were unable to identify clinical records of this sound in our review.

If the tear is large enough to allow herniation of the heart through the defect, severe compromise of cardiac function ensues.

Chest roentgenography may be one of the important screening tests in making the diagnosis of pericardial tears (35) (Figs. 14.9–14.10). Radiographic findings such as

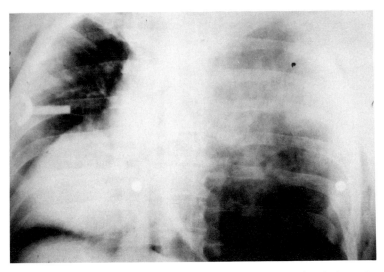

Figure 14.9.   Ruptured pericardium: heart herniation toward right hemithorax.

pneumopericardium, heart displacement, or bowel gas in the pericardial sac are very suggestive. Electrocardiography, fluoroscopy, and computerized tomography (CT) have also been used in an attempt to diagnose pericardial tears, however, in general, they have not been very reliable. In a stable patient in whom pericardial tear is suspected, a subxiphoid pericardial window allows identification of blood in the pericardium. This suggests pericardial or myocardial injury and should be followed by a thoracotomy. If the return pericardial fluid is pink or serosanguineous, we recommend irrigation of the pericardium with a Robinson catheter: 100–150 ml of warm saline is instilled into the pericardial sac. If the return continues to be pink or bloody, we proceed with a diagnostic midsternotomy (Figs. 14.11–14.12).

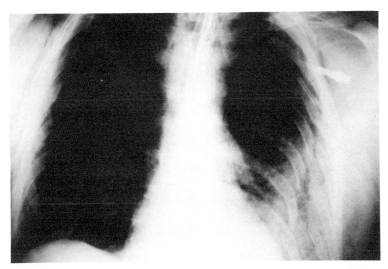

Figure 14.10.   Pericardial rupture: heart returning to normal position after placing the patient in an upright position.

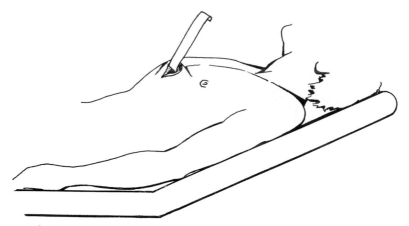

Figure 14.11.   Semi-Fowler's position for the pericardial window and irrigation.

Treatment

The treatment of pericardial tears is dependent on their location and the presence or absence of herniation. If the tear is located in the diaphragmatic part of the pericardium, it should be closed. If it is in a pleuropericardial location, repair should be attempted if the tear is small or there is a history of heart dislocation. However, if swelling of the heart makes the repair technically difficult or if a medium-size tear is found, the defect can be opened the entire length of the pericardium to avoid heart strangulation (Fig. 14.13).

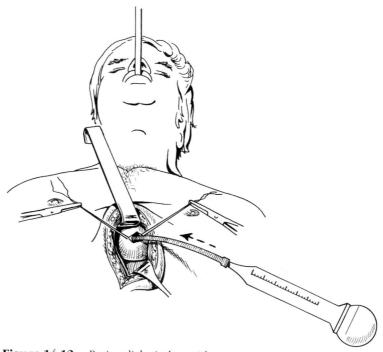

Figure 14.12.   Pericardial window with irrigation of the pericardial sac.

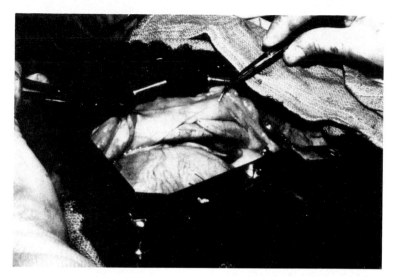

Figure 14.13. Right pleural pericardial rupture found at surgery in the patient depicted in Figure 14.12.

Posttraumatic Pericardial Syndrome

A substantial number of patients develop this syndrome, characterized by chest pain, fever, and elevation of the white cell count. These manifestations are indistinguishable from those that follow elective pericardiotomy or myocardial infarction. The pathogenesis of the postpericardiotomy syndrome remains unknown. Hypotheses regarding an immunologically based inflammatory reaction to blood, bacteria, viruses, or damaged tissue have been postulated (1).

The diagnosis is made by exclusion of other causes of chest pain and fever. Echocardiography should corroborate the diagnosis by disclosing pericardial thickness and effusion. We recommend that an echocardiogram be obtained immediately after surgery to be used as a baseline for comparison with subsequent findings.

The treatment of postpericardiotomy syndrome is symptomatic. This entity is self-limiting and lasts 2–4 weeks. Antiinflammatory medications such as acetylsalicylic acid are usually sufficient in the majority of cases. Steroids and drainage of pericardial fluid are rarely necessary.

Suppurative Pericarditis

This condition is found more commonly in patients with penetrating wounds of the heart and pericardium. However, in patients who underwent emergency thoracostomies with pericardiotomies performed under nonsterile conditions, the diagnosis should be entertained in the presence of a septic course and symptoms of cardiac tamponade. Echocardiography is valuable for localizing the site and extent of fluid accumulation. The definite diagnosis can be made after examination of the fluid obtained by pericardiocentesis.

The treatment is surgical drainage of the pericardial sac through a posterolateral thoracotomy. Anterior pericardiectomy from right phrenic to left phrenic nerves and drainage of the surgical field toward the left hemithorax are recommended.

Constrictive Pericarditis

Occurring rarely after blunt thoracic trauma, constrictive pericarditis has an unknown etiology. Some authors have suggested that the presence of blood, lipids, bacteria, or viruses (1) could be responsible for this dense fibrous thickness of the pericardium. The clinical manifestations may appear weeks or years after the original injury (34, 36–40).

The diagnosis should be suspected in a patient who presents with a low cardiac output syndrome, including low blood pressure and low urine output. A roentgenogram may disclose a small heart with or without calcifications. An echocardiogram or CT scan will show the thickening of the pericardium. Cardiac catheterization will confirm the diagnosis.

Treatment of constrictive pericarditis is surgical: pericardiectomy of the anterior pericardium, including the relief of the part covering the pulmonary veins and superior and inferior vena cava, is indicated. Early digitalization is recommended to minimize postoperative congestive heart failure (40).

BLUNT TRAUMATIC CARDIAC RUPTURE

Until about the beginning of this century, blunt traumatic rupture of the heart was reported almost exclusively in autopsy series (35). Since then, several reviews of small series have demonstrated that this injury is not necessarily fatal (41, 42).

Remarkable improvements in emergency medical systems, with stabilization in the prehospital care period and rapid transport to a medical facility, are probably responsible for the improved survivability. The incidence of cardiac rupture in patients sustaining blunt trauma is very low, ranging from 0.5–0.7% (5). During the past 10 yr, among 16,000 blunt trauma patients admitted to the Shock Trauma Center of the Maryland Institute for Emergency Medical Services Systems, 0.3% had cardiac and/or pericardial rupture (35).

Pathophysiology

Several mechanisms of blunt cardiac rupture have been postulated (42, 43), and some of them correlate with the cardiac chambers that are injured (Figs. 14.14–14.19). The oldest mechanism described is direct precordial impaction with a massive transmission of energy to the heart. A second mechanism—implying a hydraulic effect—is explained as a sudden increase in the venous pressure transmitted to the heart, the atrium in particular. This is secondary to a massive force transmitted from the abdomen and lower extremities. These patients usually do not present with evidence of external chest trauma. A compressive mechanism is responsible for the entrapment of the heart between the sternum and vertebral column. An acceleration/deceleration mechanism could be responsible for atriocaval and pulmonary vein tears.

In this era of terrorism and drug-related bombings, injuries resulting from blast mechanisms are seen more frequently. A tremendous blast effect can be transmitted to the thorax and thus to the heart chambers. Fractures of the bony structures (sternum and ribs) caused by blasts or compression also have the potential to injure the cardiac chambers (penetrating mechanism).

Some authors (1) have implied that factors determining ventricular versus atrial ruptures are related to the point in the cardiac cycle that injury is incurred. Ventricular rupture is more common during late diastole or early systole, and atrial rupture is more common in late systole, when all valves are closed and no exit is available for the increased intrachamber pressure.

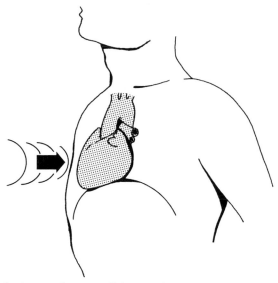

Figure 14.14.   Mechanism of blunt cardiac rupture: direct precordial impact.

Diagnosis

Preoperative diagnosis of cardiac rupture is very rare and demands a very high index of suspicion, particularly with patients who have mechanisms of injury such as chest compression and deceleration and a clinical picture of upper torso cyanosis or symptoms and signs of acute cardiac tamponade or massive hemothorax. Patients who are hemodynamically stable should be examined via a pericardial window (subxiphoid pericardiotomy) (see Chapter 2 for technique).

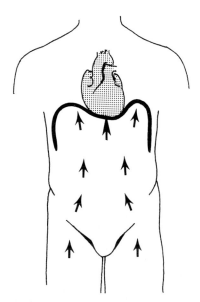

Figure 14.15.   Mechanism of blunt cardiac rupture: hydraulic effect.

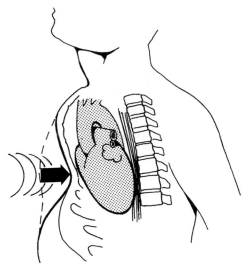

Figure 14.16.   Mechanism of blunt cardiac rupture: compressive mechanism.

Borja and Lansing (44) demonstrated a 25% incidence of false-negative pericardiocentesis results in patients with hemopericardium. The failure to obtain blood during a pericardiocentesis does not rule out cardiac rupture; likewise, the return of blood during pericardiocentesis is not proof that the blood is coming from the cardiac chambers or pericardium. Due to all these difficulties in the interpretation of pericardiocentesis fluid return, we prefer to create a pericardial window.

In the majority of the published series and in ours (35, 45, 46), the diagnosis of pericardial or cardiac chamber rupture was made by emergency thoracotomy. In the MIEMSS series (35), in 43 (73%) of 59 patients, the diagnosis was made by left anterolateral emergency thoracotomy. Interestingly, 30 of 59 patients arrived in our admitting area in cardiac arrest.

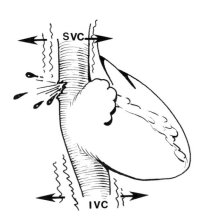

Figure 14.17.   Mechanism of blunt cardiac rupture: deceleration mechanism. *SVC,* superior vena cava; *IVC,* inferior vena cava.

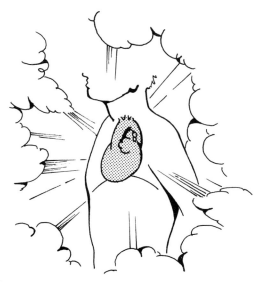

Figure 14.18.   Mechanism of blunt cardiac rupture: blast mechanism.

Treatment

If the patient presents with evidence of cardiac tamponade or shock, and an emergency thoracotomy is deemed necessary, the most versatile and quickest incision should be chosen: anterolateral thoracotomy with extension to the other hemithorax if necessary. This procedure is described in Chapter 15.

ATRIAL INJURIES

The atrium is a low-pressure chamber. Consequently, bleeding from it can be controlled temporarily with finger pressure or balloon catheter (Fig. 14.20). Definite

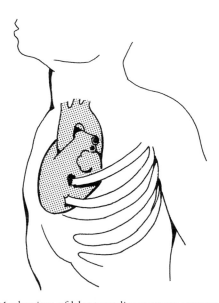

Figure 14.19.   Mechanism of blunt cardiac rupture: penetrating mechanism.

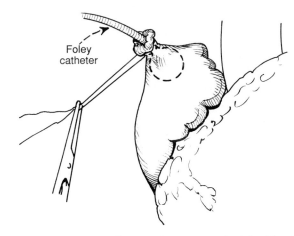

Figure 14.20. Blunt atrial rupture: balloon catheter control of the bleeding and purse string suture placement.

treatment consists of the application of a vascular clamp, which is released as soon as the injury is repaired with 4–0 vascular nonabsorbable interrupted sutures (47, 48). We prefer to reinforce the suture with the application of pledgets (Figs. 14.21–14.23).

VENTRICULAR INJURIES

The right ventricle is the most commonly injured chamber. Lacerations less than 0.5 cm long can be repaired with a simple nonabsorbable 3–0 suture. Longer lacerations may require the use of Teflon pledgets for reinforcement. If the lacerations are close to a coronary artery, it is advisable to close the laceration with mattress sutures underneath the coronary vessels (Figs. 14.24, 14.25).

Outcome

Most of the series in the literature agree that patients who arrive at the emergency department in cardiac arrest secondary to heart rupture die. However, patients who

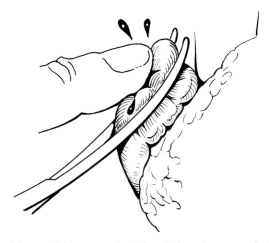

Figure 14.21. Blunt atrial rupture: digital and clamping control of the bleeding.

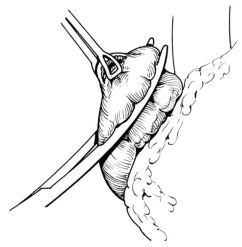

Figure 14.22.   Blunt atrial rupture: repositioning of the clamp in preparation for repair sometimes is necessary.

sustain cardiac arrest in the emergency department have a 50% chance of survival, as found in our series (35). We found that one-third of patients with a ruptured heart or pericardium will survive long enough for us to do a diagnostic evaluation.

TRAUMATIC VENTRICULAR SEPTAL DEFECT

The development of a ventricular septal defect due to blunt trauma is a rare occurrence. At Grady Memorial Hospital (1), in a period of 10 yr, only one patient with this injury was seen. At our institution, in the same period of time, we have not had any case secondary to blunt trauma.

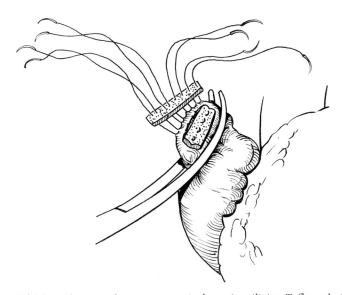

Figure 14.23.   Blunt atrial rupture: surgical repair utilizing Teflon pledgets.

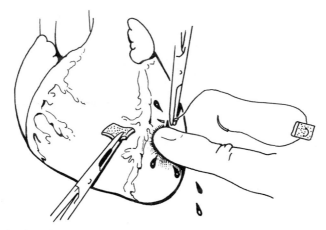

Figure 14.24. Blunt ventricular rupture: surgical repair utilizing Teflon pledgets.

Pathophysiology

Inkley and Barry (49) proved by catheterization that the tear of the septum occurs during the most vulnerable period of the cardiac cycle: late diastole or early systole. At this point, the valves are closed and there is a maximal increase in the intrachamber pressures without an exit. Mechanisms such as compression of the heart between the sternum and the spine or deceleration are responsible for a sudden increase of intracardiac pressures; subsequent ventricular septal tears are more likely located in the muscular septum near the apex (50, 51). Delayed ruptures can also occur secondary to disruption of an infarcted segment within a previously damaged vessel. Multiple perforations have also been described (50). This injury is usually accompanied by a left-to-right shunt, causing an increase in the pulmonary blood flow and consequent congestive heart failure.

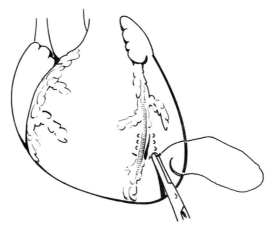

Figure 14.25. Blunt ventricular rupture: surgical repair using horizontal mattress sutures placed under the coronary vessel.

Diagnosis

Due to the associated myocardial contusion, patients with ventricular septal defect secondary to blunt trauma present with severe heart failure. This clinical picture is very similar to that in patients with ventricular septal defect secondary to myocardial infarction (1): chest pain, dyspnea, orthopnea, cyanosis, and a systolic thrill along the left sternal border are not uncommon. A holosystolic murmur loud enough to be heard throughout the precordium is characteristic. The symptomatology can be delayed for days, hours, or even weeks or months. Explanation of this phenomenon is controversial, but it is probably related to the initial postcontusion low cardiac output. The differential diagnosis should be made with traumatic mitral or tricuspid regurgitation secondary to laceration of the papillary muscles or chorda tendineae. Modalities other than the clinical picture have been used to confirm the diagnosis; some of them, such as the chest roentgenogram, electrocardiogram, and two-dimensional echocardiography, have not proven to be very reliable or sensitive (52). The conclusive diagnosis of ventricular septal defect secondary to blunt chest trauma can be accomplished only by cardiac catheterization and angiocardiography (53). These procedures can be done on an elective or emergency basis, according to the clinical condition of the patient.

Treatment

In addition to stabilizing cardiopulmonary function in patients with ventricular septal defect secondary to blunt trauma, one of the most important decisions to make is the determination of the urgency of surgery. Do the indications warrant immediate surgery, delayed surgery, or no surgical intervention at all?

A patient with severe congestive heart failure despite aggressive medical therapy and a left-to-right shunt greater than 2:1 (pulmonary-to-systemic blood flow ratio) should have surgical intervention expeditiously. If the patient has severe symptomatology related to a myocardial contusion, 1–2 weeks of intraaortic balloon support is advisable before elective surgical intervention. The assumption is that, at this point, hemodynamic derangements due to the myocardial contusion have subsided. Patients with small shunts (less than 1.5:1 pulmonary-to-systemic flow ratio) and mild and controlled clinical symptomatology should be monitored closely with the speculation that the defect could close spontaneously (1) or worsen and require a semiemergency surgical repair. Teflon pledgets are recommended for a more safe and stable repair (Fig. 14.26).

INFERIOR VENA CAVA AVULSIONS

These injuries are very rare and have an enormous mortality. Clinically, the patients present in severe shock or cardiac arrest; however, some patients are moderately hypotensive and relatively hemodynamically stable for 30–60 min. This incongruency is due to the low venous pressure system, which allows an artificial temporary seal of the tear at the junction of the inferior vena cava and right atrium.

Treatment

Application of two balloon catheters to facilitate the approximation and repair has been described. However, in reality, the injuries are uniformly fatal even when they are recognized very early in the resuscitation period, which is usually the case. In our

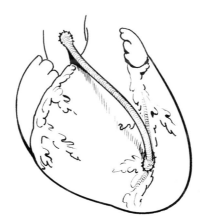

Figure 14.27. Blunt coronary artery injury: surgical repair using a reverse saphenous bypass graft from the aorta to the distal coronary artery.

REFERENCES

1. Symbas PN. Cardiothoracic trauma. Philadelphia: Saunders, 1989:55–58.
2. Liedtke AJ, DeMuth WE Jr (citing Spelman J). Nonpenetrating cardiac injuries: a collective reivew. Am Heart J 1973;86:687–697.
3. Kissane RW. Traumatic heart disease: nonpenetrating injuries. Circulation 1952;6:421–425.
4. Jones JW, Hewit RL, Drapanas T. Cardiac contusion: a capricious syndrome. Ann Surg 1975;181:567–574.
5. Shorr RM, Crittenden M, Indeck M, Hartunian SL, Rodriguez A. Blunt thoracic trauma: analysis of 515 cases. Ann Surg 1987;206:200–205.
6. Moritz AR, Atkins JP. Cardiac contusion: an experimental and pathological study. Arch Pathol 1938;25:445–462.
7. Kissane RW. Traumatic heart diseases, especially myocardial contusion. Postgrad Med 1954;15:114–119.
8. Stein PD, Sabbah HN, Viano DC, Vostal JJ. Response of the heart to nonpenetrating cardiac trauma. J Trauma 1982;22:364–373.
9. Beresky R, Klingler R, Peaske L, et al. Myocardial contusion: when does it have clinical significance? J Trauma 1988;28:64–68.
10. Mashiko K. Clinical and pathophysiological study of myocardial contusion. Nippon Geka Gakkai Zasshi 1983;84:1138–1148.
11. Sutherland CR, Cheng HW, Hollyday PL, et al. Hemodynamic adaptation to acute myocardial contusion complicating blunt chest trauma injury. Am J Cardiol 1986;157:291–293.
12. Stein PD, Sabbah HN, Przyblski J, et al. Effect of alcohol upon arrhythmias following nonpenetrating cardiac impact. J Trauma 1988;28:465–471.
13. Kettunen P. Cardiac damage after blunt chest trauma: injury diagnosed by CPK MB plus EKG. Int J Cardiol 1986;6:355–374.
14. Mayfield W, Hurley EJ. Blunt cardiac trauma. Am J Surg 1984;148:162–167.
15. Markiewicz W, Best LA, Burstein S, Peleg H. Echocardiographic evaluation after blunt trauma of the chest. Int J Cardiol 1985;8:269–276.
16. Berk WA. EKG findings in nonpenetrating chest trauma: a review. J Emerg Med 1987;5:209–211.
17. Keller KD, Shatney CH. Creatinine phosphokinase MB assays in patients with suspected myocardial contusion: diagnosis test or test of diagnosis? J Trauma 1988;28:58–63.
18. Soliman MH, Waxman K. Value of a conventional approach to the diagnosis of traumatic cardiac contusion after chest injury. Crit Care Med 1987; 15:218–220.
19. Beggs CN, Helhoy TS, Evans LL, et al. Early evaluation of cardiac injury by 2D echo in patients with blunt chest trauma. Ann Emerg Med 1987;16:542–545.
20. Tenzer ML. The spectrum of myocardial contusion: a review. J Trauma 1985;25:620–627.
21. Kron IL, Cox PM Jr. Cardiac injury after chest trauma. Crit Care Med 1983;11:524–526.
22. Kumar SA, Puri VN, Mettal VK, Cortez J. Myocardial contusion following nonfatal chest trauma. J Trauma 1983;23:327–331.

23. King RM, Mucha P Jr, Seward JB, Gersh BJ, Farnell MB. Cardiac contusion: a new diagnositic approach utilizing two-dimensional echocardiography. J Trauma 1983;23:610–614.
24. Frazee RC, Mucha P Jr, Farnell MB, Miller FA. Objective evaluation of blunt cardiac trauma. J Trauma 1986;26:510–520.
25. Fabian TC, Mangiante EC, Pattern CR, et al. Myocardial contusion in blunt trauma: clinical characteristics, means of diagnosis and implications in patient management. J Trauma 1988;28:50–57.
26. Rodriguez A, Shatney C. The value of technetium^{99m} pyrophosphate scanning in the diagnosis of myocardial contusion. Am Surg 1982;48:472–474.
27. Rosenbaum RC, Johnston CC. Posttraumatic cardiac dysfunction: assessment with radionuclide ventriculography. Radiology 1986;160:91–94.
28. Schamp DJ, Plotnik GD, Croteau D, Rosenbaum RC, Johnston GS, Rodriguez A. Clinical significance of radionuclide angiographically-determined abnormalities following acute blunt chest trauma. Am Heart J 1988;116:500–504.
29. Soutter DI, Rodriguez A. Cardiac contusion: diagnosis and management. Trauma Q 1988;4:16–23.
30. Miller FA, Seward JB, Gersh BJ, Tajik AJ, Mucha P Jr. Two-dimensional echocardiographic findings in cardiac trauma. Am J Cardiol 1982;50:1022–1027.
31. Waxman K, Soliman MH, Braunstein P, et al. Diagnosis of traumatic cardiac contusion. Arch Surg 1986;121:689–692.
32. Flancbaum L, Wright J, Siegel JH. Emergency surgery in patients with posttraumatic myocardial contusion. J Trauma 1986;26:795–803.
33. Haas GE, Parr GV, Trout RG, et al. Traumatic coronary artery fistula, 2 years after cardiac injury. J Trauma 1986;26:854–857.
34. Clark DE, Wiles CE III, Lim MK, Dunham CM, Rodriguez A. Traumatic rupture of the pericardium. Surgery 1983;93:495–503.
35. Fulda G, Brathwaite CEM, Rodriguez A, Turney SZ, Dunham CM, Cowley RA. Blunt traumatic rupture of the heart and pericardium: a ten-year experience (1979–1989). Presented at the American Association for the Surgery of Trauma Congress, Chicago, 1989.
36. Morel-Lavallee. Rupture de pericarde; bruit de roue hydraulique; bruit de moulin. Gaz Med Paris 1866;19:695–696, 729–730, 771–772, 803–808.
37. McKusick VA. Chronic constrictive pericarditis: some clinical and laboratory observations. Bull Johns Hopkins Hosp 1952;90:3–26.
38. de Vernejoul R, Bouisson P, Courbier R, Tricot R. Les péricardites constrictives posttraumatiques. Presse Med 1957;65:241–243.
39. McKusick VA, Kay JH, Isaacs JP. Constrictive pericarditis following traumatic hemopericardium. Ann Surg 1955;142:97–103.
40. Phillips TF, Rodriguez A, Cowley RA. Right ventricular outflow obstruction secondary to right-sided tamponade following myocardial trauma. Ann Thorac Surg 1983;36:353–358.
41. DesForges O, Ridder WP, Lenoli RJ. Successful suture of ruptured myocardium after nonpenetrating injury. N Engl J Med 1955;252:567–569.
42. Bright EF, Beck CF. Nonpenetrating wounds of the heart: a clinical and experimental study. Am Heart J 1935;10:293–321.
43. Parmley LF, Marrion WC, Mattingly TW. Nonpenetrating rupture of the heart. Circulation 1958;18:371–396.
44. Borja AK, Lansing AM. Traumatic rupture of the heart: a case successfully treated. Ann Surg 1970;171:438–440.
45. Calhoun JH, Hoffman TH, Trinkle JK, Harman PK, Crowers FL. Management of blunt rupture of the heart. J Trauma 1986;26:495–502.
46. Leavitt BJ, Meyer JA, Morton JR, et al. Survival following nonpenetrating rupture of the cardiac chamber. Ann Thorac Surg 1987;44:532–535.
47. Getz BS, Davies E, Steinberg SM, et al. Blunt cardiac trauma results in right atrial rupture. JAMA 1986;255:761–763.
48. Griffort GL, Zeok JV, Mallory W, et al. Right atrial rupture due to blunt chest trauma. South Med J 1984;77:715–716.
49. Inkley SR, Barry FM. Traumatic rupture of the intraventricular septum proved by cardiac catheterization. Circulation 1958;18:916–917.
50. Campbell GS, Vernier R, Varco RL, Lillehei CW. Traumatic ventricular septal defect: report of two cases. J Thorac Surg 1959;37:496–501.
51. DesForges G, Abelmann WH. Interventricular septal defect due to blunt trauma: report of a case repaired surgically under total cardiopulmonary bypass. N Engl J Med 1963;268:128–131.

52. Sklar J, Clarke D, Campbell D, Pearce B, Appareti K, Johnson M. Traumatic ventricular septal defect and lacerated mitral leaflet: two-dimensional echocardiographic demonstration. Chest 1982;81:247–249.
53. Guilfoil PH, Doyle JT. Traumatic cardiac septal defect: report of a case in which diagnosis is established by cardiac catheterization. J Thorac Surg 1953;25:510–515.
54. Protais E, Simon JC, Herreman F, Fouchard J. Valvular cardiopathy due to nonpenetrating injury apropos of a surgical case of aortic insufficiency. Rev Med Interne 1986;7:259–264.
55. Kokubo M, Hirose M, Tanabe H, et al. A case of tricuspid regurgitation. Kyobu Geka 1986;39:731–734.
56. Takahasi K, Maruyama A, Ainai S, Momokawa T, Fujita T, Takeyama M. An operated case of traumatic tricuspid regurgitation. Kyobu Geka 1986;39:809–812.
57. Brady PW, Deal CW. An unusual case of mitral incompetence, posttraumatic paraprosthetic. J Trauma 1988;28;259–266.
58. Perroth MG, Hazan E, Lecompte Y, et al. Chronic tricuspid regurgitation and bifistular block due to blunt chest trauma. Am J Med Sci 1986;291:2119–2125.
59. Pellegrim RV, Copeland CE, DiMarco RF, et al. Blunt rupture of both atrioventricular valves. Ann Thorac Surg 1986;42:471–472.
60. Goulah RD, Rose MR, Stroba M, et al. Coronary dissection following catheterization with systemic embolization. Chest 1988;93:887–888.
61. Haas GE, Parr GU, Trout RG, et al. Traumatic coronary fistula—atrial. J Trauma 1986;26:854–857.

15 Management of Penetrating Thoracic Trauma

Vincent K. H. Tam, MD
Alfred S. Casale, MD
Timothy G. Buchman, PhD, MD

This chapter describes the resuscitation, stabilization, and definitive care of the patient with penetrating thoracic trauma within the familiar framework of the Advanced Trauma Life Support management protocols (1). Although most life-threatening injuries associated with penetrating thoracic trauma can be identified and treated during the primary survey, others may not become apparent until later in the stabilization phase. The diagnostic and therapeutic paradigms are based solely on readily available clinical data routinely collected during a trauma resuscitation. The presentation is limited to methods employed in our clinical practice, often without mention of valid alternatives. Emphasis is placed on strategy and decisions, providing technical detail for common lifesaving interventions.

EMERGENCY DEPARTMENT PHASE
Airway

Hospital treatment begins with the primary survey and resuscitation of the patient. Protection or provision of an airway has highest priority. An apneic patient or a patient who has an altered mental status (and thus an unprotected airway) should be immediately tracheally intubated. Both oxygenation and ventilation are thus supported. Other patients with an obvious need for urgent surgical intervention should also be considered for prompt tracheal intubation. Although nasotracheal intubation can be accomplished expeditiously by some practitioners, we prefer the orotracheal route because of its familiarity and reliability in experienced hands. Orotracheal intubation is relatively safe, provided the cervical spine is either proven uninjured or appropriately protected and stabilized with in-line traction. The struggling patient is often managed with a fast-acting depolarizing muscle relaxant (such as succinylcholine), used alone or in combination with the anesthetic ketamine. Cricoid pressure (Sellick's maneuver) (2) is always used to prevent regurgitation and aspiration. In every instance, the surgeon must be prepared to provide a surgical airway in the event of intubation failure.

The internal diameter of the endotracheal tube should be at least 8 mm to allow for the subsequent performance of fiberoptic bronchoscopy, if necessary, and for optimal clearance of secretions. There is never an indication for the use of a double-lumen endobronchial tube at this early point during the resuscitation.

Breathing

Examination of the patient's breathing should begin with a rapid yet careful inspection of bilateral chest expansion and a search for penetrating wounds. Breath sounds should be auscultated over the midaxillary lines to avoid confusion with transmitted bronchial breath sounds. The chest wall should be palpated for subcutaneous emphysema or rib fractures and for increased tympany. Shotgun blast injuries may cause large chest wall defects that should be inspected and covered with an occlusive dressing, followed immediately by tube thoracostomy in an uninjured area. Sucking chest wounds should be managed in a similar fashion. Any penetrating chest wound associated with dyspena, ipsilateral subcutaneous emphysema, or hemodynamic instability demands immediate needle and subsequent tube thoracostomy on the side of the injury without waiting for radiologic studies, presuming the presence of a tension pneumothorax. Tracheal deviation suggests either *ipsilateral* pulmonary collapse or *contralateral* tension pneumothorax or hemothorax (Fig. 15.1). Immediate needle thoracostomy followed by tube thoracostomy on the contralateral side (*away* from the tracheal deviation) should be considered and performed if tension pneumothorax cannot be excluded.

Circulation

The circulatory system should be examined using a "look, listen, and feel" approach. Jugular venous filling should be assessed. Central cyanosis, if present, should be noted. Heart sounds are frequently difficult to auscultate. A rapid qualitative assessment of the patient's blood pressure can be made by palpating the carotid, femoral, and radial pulses for both rate and strength. The peripheral circulation is evaluated by blanching the nail bed and observing capillary refill.

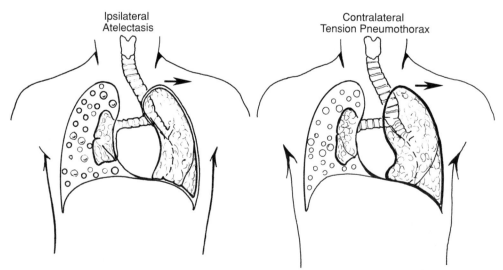

Figure 15.1.   Tracheal deviation: ipsilateral to pulmonary collapse and contralateral to a tension pneumothorax.

Monitoring

Cool, tachycardiac patients with poor capillary refill are in shock until proven otherwise. Electrocardiogram monitoring is essential but, in patients with a palpable pulse, pulse oximetry (3) is more useful and should be initiated first. The pulse oximeter gives data concerning arterial oxygen saturation, heart rate, and regularity of rhythm, providing clues both to the patient's oxygen delivery and to peripheral perfusion. Intubated patients should be mechanically ventilated and continuously monitored with pulse oximetry and end-tidal CO_2 analysis in addition to periodic arterial blood gas determinations.

Venous Access

Venous access both above and below the diaphragm must be secured. If technically feasible, the preferred "first" cannula is a 14-gauge, 2-inch catheter inserted into the antecubital fossa opposite the side of injury. Next a no. 8.5 French "introducer" is placed in either the internal jugular or subclavian vein on the side of injury for rapid infusion access above the diaphragm. (Use the opposite side if a thoracic inlet injury is suspected.) If the patient is in obvious shock, a second no. 8.5 French introducer should be inserted into one femoral vein (4) to provide venous access below the diaphragm. Additional procedures performed in the inguinal area (for instance, arterial cannulation or puncture) should be restricted to the same side as the femoral venous catheter, leaving one groin undisturbed to facilitate the later use of femoral–femoral cardiopulmonary bypass or saphenous vein harvest. If the patient is in shock (irrespective of cause), 2 liters of balanced salt solution should be rapidly infused over 2 min. The central venous pressure (CVP) transduced either directly through the large-bore neck catheter or through a separate central venous catheter will commonly rise to 15–20 cm of water but will rapidly fall to or below the normal range within a few minutes if the patient has unobstructed venous return to the heart.

Shock: Mechanisms and Management

Shock associated with penetrating thoracic trauma occurs by several mechanisms. Hemorrhage, often from relatively small blood vessels such as the internal mammary artery and the intercostal artery, is the leading cause of shock in penetrating thoracic trauma. Each hemithorax may hold up to 2.5 liters of blood.

The second mechanism is mechanical embarrassment of venous return to the heart. The causes are *(a)* pericardial tamponade and *(b)* mediastinal shift due to tension pneumothorax or hemothorax. *Given a thoracic trauma patient in shock, the presence of jugular venous distention or rising CVP strongly suggests obstruction of venous return.* Whether the underlying mechanism is hypovolemia, embarrassment of venous return to the heart, or something less common, the initial therapy is *always* rapid volume infusion. Next, tube thoracostomy should be performed first on the side of the injury and then, if there is no immediate improvement, on the opposite side. Despite the lateral location of an entrance wound, a single missile or knife wound can traverse the mediastinum and cause a tension hemothorax or pneumothorax on the opposite side. The absence of jugular venous distention or muffled heart sounds in the hypotension patient does *not* exclude pericardial tamponade. When shock persists despite initial volume infusion and tube thoracostomy, another round of rapid volume infusion (2 liters over 2 min) is indicated. The patient will be either persistently hypovolemic or in pericardial tamponade. In this instance, quick CVP determination may help discriminate between these possibilities.

If pericardial tamponade is suspected, there are two management options. With profound shock (either no detectable pulse or rapidly falling blood pressure), an immediate left anterior thoracotomy should be performed in the emergency room to evacuate blood from the pericardium, to digitally control the wound, and to temporarily clamp the descending thoracic aorta. With diminished or adequate blood pressure, a subxiphoid exploration should be performed in the operating room. In our experience, pericardiocentesis is seldom helpful in the acutely traumatized patient. Needle aspiration of the pericardium is unreliable (5) and difficult to perform in the setting of trauma resuscitation, risks needle laceration of the heart, and is therefore rarely indicated.

Air embolism occasionally complicates penetrating thoracic injuries as gas in the pleural space enters a branch of the pulmonary vein. Intubation and institution of mechanical positive-pressure ventilation can contribute to a rapid adverse course. Aspiration of an unexpectedly foamy arterial blood sample should suggest the diagnosis, as should direct observation of gas in the coronary vessels during emergent surgery. It is usually not possible to reposition the shock patient "head down, left side up" to keep the gas away from the right ventricular outflow tract. At the very least, attempts should be made to aspirate gas via the CVP line and consideration given to instituting cardiopulmonary bypass if immediately available. Hyperbaric oxygen therapy is of benefit if available (6).

Penetrating wounds that injure or transect the spinal cord cause traumatic paraplegia, distal sympathectomy, and vasodilation with consequent spinal shock. Physical examination is diagnostic based on findings, including bradycardia out of proportion to the hypotension, warm feet despite cold hands, absent rectal tone, and (in males) priapism. Initial treatment is rapid administration of volume followed by infusion of a vasoconstrictor such as phenylephrine.

Thoracic injuries that traverse the diaphragm obviously involve the abdomen and often cause exsanguinating abdominal hemorrhage (Fig. 15.2).

Tube Thoracostomy

Even the suspicion of a tension pneumothorax or hemothorax warrants immediate treatment by needle thoracostomy to convert it to an open pneumothorax or hemothorax. The largest available needle, often a 14- or 16-gauge intravenous cannula, is inserted into the second intercostal space anteriorly in the midclavicular line. Time should not be wasted trying to connect the needle to a water-filled syringe. Needle thoracostomy is followed by immediate tube thoracostomy on the same side.

Insertion of a chest tube in the trauma setting is somewhat different from an elective tube thoracostomy. Speed is paramount, and hence the risk of complications such as splenic or hepatic injury is proportionately higher. The procedure described below is safe and very fast, using a single tube to drain both air and blood from the pleural space.

The patient is positioned supine with the ipsilateral hand placed behind the head. The chest wall is quickly doused with antibacterial solution and prepped. Local infiltration with lidocaine (0.5–1%) is adequate to minimize pain. In males, the preferred site of incision is the intersection of the lower margin of the pectoralis major with the midaxillary line. In females, the site of incision is the intersection of the inframammary crease with the midaxillary line (Fig. 15.3). A 3-cm incision is made parallel to the top of the rib closest to the area specified. A blunt-tipped instrument (such as a Kelly clamp) is used to penetrate the chest wall directly, without the creation of a "tunnel." The clamp is spread and withdrawn with the jaws held widely apart. The

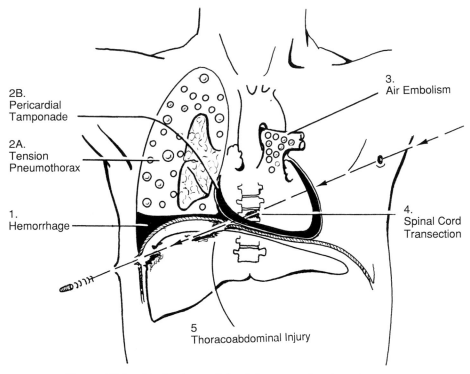

Figure 15.2.   Mechanisms of shock in penetrating thoracic trauma.

wound is explored digitally to confirm the intrathoracic anatomy. A no. 32 or no. 36 French chest tube is inserted and directed posteriorly through the wound. A heavy nylon suture secures the chest tube to the chest wall. Each connection is taped.

In thoracic trauma, large amounts of blood are often evacuated. Immediate drainage greater than 1500 ml of blood indicates major injury. In this *(and only this)* instance, the chest tube is briefly clamped to tamponade the injury and the patient is

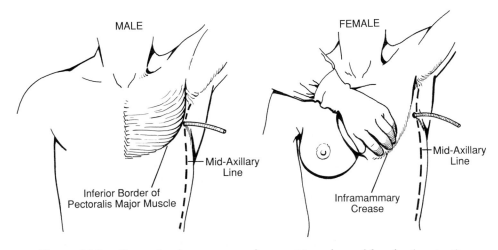

Figure 15.3.   Chest tube thoracostomy placement in males and females (see text).

transferred to the operating room for an immediate emergency thoracotomy. Otherwise, the chest tube should be connected to a collecting system that can provide 20 cm of water suction via an underwater seal. The collection system should provide for autotransfusion of the shed blood.

TRIAGE DECISION

Once the primary survey has been completed and resuscitation has been initiated, an important triage decision must be made: does this patient require emergency surgery and, if so, does he/she require emergency department thoracotomy? This decision must be made with an understanding of the potential benefits and risks in the particular therapeutic setting, which, in our case, is a level I trauma center with cardiopulmonary bypass capability.

If there is no sign of life prior to or during the prehospital phase of more than 10-min duration, and if the patient fails to respond to intubation, mechanical ventilation, tube thoracostomy, and volume infusion, there is less than a 1% chance for survival. To continue resuscitative efforts is as much an ethical decision as a medical one. We favor emergency department thoracotomy in this setting for four reasons: *(a)* a particular patient has a small but measurable chance for recovery, particularly if the arrest was also precipitated by hypothermia or intoxicants, both of which are common in our populations; *(b)* trauma teams must be well versed in the procedure if salvage rates are to be optimized; *(c)* internal cardiac massage with a cross-clamped aorta is more effective than closed-chest massage with respect to restoring cerebral and coronary blood flow; and *(d)* the actual cost reflects the disposables on the tray plus the cost of instrument sterilization and cleaning, as opposed to the charges that are used to discourage an often-futile procedure.

A patient with signs of life lost during the prehospital phase or primary survey requires immediate emergency department thoracotomy.

Emergency Department Thoracotomy

The patient should already have an adequate airway provided either by the translaryngeal route or a surgical cricothyroidotomy. The patient should also have at least one large-bore intravenous catheter above and one below the diaphragm. Simultaneous volume and chemical resuscitation should be continued throughout the procedure. Arterial blood should be sampled periodically for determination of oxygenation as well as acid-base abnormality to guide the patient's chemical resuscitation.

Position the supine patient's right and left hands behind the head. Douse the axillae, chest, and shoulder areas as well as the midabdomen with antibacterial solution: the right chest is also prepared to allow for extension of the incision, which is commonly required. For males, begin a transverse incision just below the left nipple, and incise from the sternum to the anterior axillary line and then extend it in an oblique fashion towards the axilla to the posterior axillary fold. For females, elevate the breast and incise the inframammary crease following the tail of the breast to the axilla. Incise the skin and underlying soft tissues to reach the underlying rib (usually the sixth). The pleural space is then entered just above that rib at the anterior axillary line. A partially opened pair of blunt-tipped, heavy scissors should then be pushed along the top of that rib to complete division of the pleura and intercostal muscles. The lower sternum can also be divided with heavy scissors to improve exposure of the heart. The internal mammary arteries will need to be clamped. A right thoracostomy tube, if not already present, should be inserted by an assistant to prevent an occult pneumothorax. On entering the left pleural cavity, insert a chest retractor and open it to expose the thoracic contents. Blood and clots should be evacuated quickly with pads and towels; rapid assessment should follow.

The first priority is to inspect the heart and exclude embarrassment of venous return. Hemopericardium means pericardial tamponade, so the presence of hemopericardium prompts a longitudinal pericardiotomy anterior to the phrenic nerve with evacuation of blood and digital control of the wound. If the patient is asystolic, bimanual compressions are performed.

The second priority is occlusion of the descending thoracic aorta to direct the marginal cardiac output to heart and brain. An assistant should retract the lung anteriorly and medially. The descending thoracic aorta may be deceptively small, particularly in a patient who is asystolic with no blood pressure. It can be palpated against the spine. The pleura overlying the aorta should be incised with scissors or digitally. A large vascular (atraumatic) clamp is then used to occlude the descending aorta.

The third priority should be identification and control of hemorrhage. Manual compression is used initially. If the lung injury is diffuse and bleeding rapidly, control is obtained by clamping the pulmonary hilum. The endotracheal tube should be palpated first to ensure that it is not positioned within the main stem bronchus. Bleeding secondary to injury of the great vessels in the thoracic inlet should be controlled temporarily by compression against the chest wall or the bony structures of the thoracic inlet if possible. Not infrequently, the patient's blood pressure will improve sufficiently after control of the hemorrhage for rapid transport to the operating room. During transport, monitor the patient's blood pressure by palpation of the proximal aorta within the chest.

SYSTOLIC BLOOD PRESSURE < 60 TORR

A patient who remains in profound shock despite the initial resuscitative maneuvers requires immediate additional therapy. To reiterate, persistent shock (with or without elevated CVP) warrants reconsideration of tension pneumothorax and pericardial tamponade as causes. Infuse additional fluid, perform bilateral tube thoracostomies (if not already done), and evaluate possible sites of extrathoracic blood loss. Continued shock requires an immediate operation—either relief of the tamponade by immediate emergency department thoracotomy or operating room control of intrathoracic and extrathoracic bleeding. Thoracic wounds often traverse the diaphragm to injure critical abdominal structures and result in intraabdominal exsanguination. Although rapid infusion of blood will create a "steady-state" situation with apparent hemodynamic improvement, such patients are nevertheless unstable. Potentially preventable deaths can occur because of hesitation to transfer such "stabilizing" patients to the operating room for definitive control of bleeding.

SYSTOLIC BLOOD PRESSURE > 60 TORR

Many patients who arrive in the emergency department in shock will respond favorably to initial stabilization, tube thoracostomy, and fluid therapy; they require different management strategies. The rate of blood loss will determine the subsequent sequence of investigation and further therapy. Ongoing thoracic bleeding is a threat to life, and rates greater than 200 ml/hr or a total of more than 1500 ml warrant prompt thoracotomy and repair. If urgent *thoracic* operative intervention appears unnecessary (slow bleeding and *no* evidence of mediastinal injuries), next exclude extrathoracic threats to life and limb. Again, a favorable response to resuscitation does not imply that the shock-causing process has been reversed, but only that intensive therapy is capable of at least temporarily "keeping up" with the patient. The priority in this subgroup of initial responders, therefore, is the exclusion of abdominal penetration, either with associated hemorrhage or visceral perforation. Abdominal involvement is equivalent to a separate abdominal injury, and the surgeon should follow a protocol to exclude or manage such injuries. Our preference is to perform celiotomy for juxtadiaphragmatic gunshot wounds. Stab wounds are evaluated by physical exam, local wound exploration, and diagnostic peritoneal lavage.

Secondary Survey

Following the primary survey and initial resuscitation, a meticulous head-to-toe examination should be carried out during the secondary survey. Penetrating wounds in the midneck and thoracic inlet should raise the suspicion of thoracic involvement associated with a downward trajectory. Ipsilateral hemothorax, hematoma, bruit, thrill, or evidence of neurovascular compromise (unilateral decrease in blood pressure or diminished motor function of the ipsilateral upper extremity) raises the specter of major vascular injury. If the patient is hemodynamically stable, an arch aortogram should be performed to exclude a subclavian or an innominate vascular injury; selective digital views may be useful. Penetrating wounds in the axilla are easily overlooked, particularly if caused by a knife or bullet that has already traversed the adjacent arm or shoulder. Meticulous inspection is necessary to identify the entrance wounds of small-caliber missiles, particularly ice picks. Anatomic considerations in this area are similar to those in the thoracic inlet with regard to the possibility of subclavian or axillary vascular injury. Again, emergency arch aortogram is indicated on the bases of hematoma, bruit, or neurovascular compromise on the ipsilateral upper extremity. Although proximity alone does not mandate a vascular imaging procedure, consider the study if the patient has an associated pneumothorax or hemothorax, particularly if the patient cannot be continuously observed (e.g., under anesthesia and drapes for an anatomically unrelated injury).

Secondary survey of the thoracic torso should include identification of all wounds. We number each wound with a radiopaque marker. Careful inspection may suggest the trajectory of the missile or weapon.

The thorax extends to the 12th rib posteriorly; complete examination includes logrolling the patient to examine the entire posterior torso. Anterior wounds at or below the nipple line may involve structures in both the thoracic cavity as well as the abdomen. Anterior wounds between the midclavicular lines, below the clavicle, and above the costal margins are penetrating cardiac wounds until proven otherwise. Probing of wounds with a cotton swab or metal instrument to determine track and depth is frequently unreliable, potentially dangerous, and not recommended.

The Chest X-ray in Penetrating Thoracic Trauma

Assuming the patient remains hemodynamically stable, a hypererect ($+105°$) chest x-ray is performed. Radiopaque markers are used to identify the wounds. If the clinical setting does not allow the safe performance of an erect chest x-ray, supine chest x-rays may be substituted but must be interpreted with special care. In a spine chest x-ray, a hemothorax may appear as a diffuse haziness or increased opacification. A pneumothorax in a supine anteroposterior projection may appear as increased lucency in the anterior costophrenic area. Both expiration and lateral decubitus films may be helpful to confirm or exclude a pneumothorax. Lateral chest films are helpful to localize a retained missile.

Contrast Radiography

Contrast radiography is used to diagnose/exclude esophageal injuries and vascular thoracic injuries. Although penetrating esophageal injuries are rare, the life-threatening consequences of an undiagnosed injury demand a high index of suspicion. Where the trajectory of the penetrating wound suggests even the possibility of esophageal injury, either a contrast esophagram or esophagoscopy (7, 8) should be performed to exclude esophageal perforation. Awake and cooperative patients should be evaluated with a water-soluble contrast study, followed by a barium swallow, since small injuries can be missed with the water-soluble contrast. Esophagoscopy requires sedation or even general anesthesia and is therefore most often used for patients with altered mental status, patients under anesthesia for another reason, or patients who cannot for other reasons cooperate with a radiologic study. Both contrast esophagography and esophagoscopy can overlook small perforations; close observation and serial chest x-rays are mandatory even in patients with "negative" studies.

Vascular imaging is essential to the evaluation and operative management of injuries to the thoracic inlet. Optimal operative exposure (particularly of injuries involving the left subclavian artery) depends on precise knowledge of the vascular anatomy. Arch aortography is the procedure of choice, supplemented with selective views so long as the patient is stable enough to tolerate an operative delay. A serious error related to contrast radiography in the thoracic trauma patient is the decision to delay surgery in an unstable or marginally stable patient in favor of such diagnostic studies.

Is Suspicion of Cardiac Injury an Indication for Echocardiography?

Even moderate suspicion of cardiac injury requires immediate subxiphoid pericardial exploration. Only if the trajectory suggests that the likelihood of cardiac injury is very low can two-dimensional echocardiography be considered to evaluate the pericardium. Patients with simple penetrating wounds of the thorax who require thoracostomy tubes for pneumothorax and/or hemothorax and who are *not* suspected of having *any* mediastinal injuries are simply observed for further blood loss in an intensive care setting.

Many penetrating wounds of the chest initially appear superficial and initial chest x-rays show no lesions. A patient with such a wound should be observed and a repeat expiration chest x-ray performed 6 hr later to exclude an occult pneumothorax (9).

The emergency department phase is summarized in Flow Chart 15.1.

OPERATING ROOM PHASE

Advanced planning is essential and begins with an evaluation of resources. The occasional need for cardiopulmonary bypass and a cardiothoracic surgeon for repair of complex cardiac injuries should be anticipated even if seldom required. In most institutions, a cardiopulmonary bypass team requires half an hour or more to assemble. Specialized equipment (such as a rapid warming infusion device, "cell saver," and sternal saw) are also commonly required. A plan for notification of the blood bank of an anticipated demand not only for packed red cells but also for other blood components, including fresh frozen plasma and platelet packs, is often crucial to operative success.

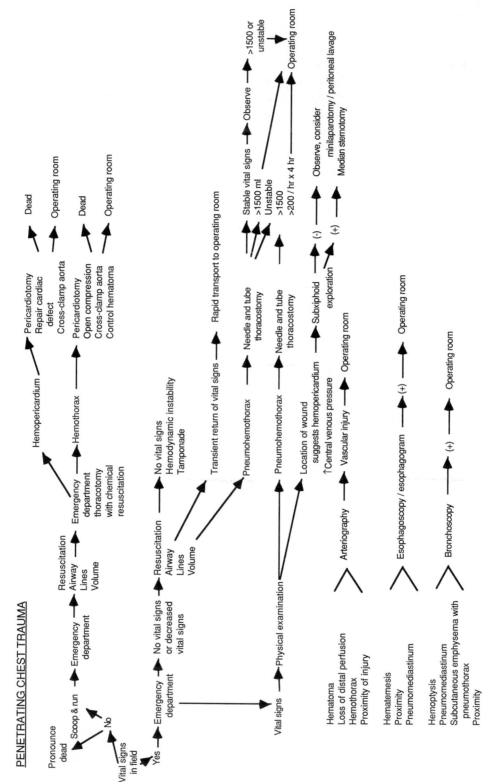

Flow Chart 15.1. Overview of the management of penetrating thoracic trauma.

Incision Decision

Perhaps the most important decision in the operative management of thoracic injuries is the choice of incision (Figs. 15.4–15.9). Positioning of the patient requires careful consideration of trajectory and access to the various potential internal injuries. Patients with central chest wounds, in whom subxiphoid exploration or median sternotomy is indicated, should be initially positioned supine. Penetrating cardiac injuries and injuries to the proximal innominate artery and the right subclavian artery as well as to the right and left common carotid arteries are also optimally managed via a median sternotomy, as are major venous injuries involving the innominate vein, superior vena cava, and inferior vena cava.

Patients with isolated right pulmonary injuries, azygos vein injuries, and injuries to the carina and middle third of the esophagus are best managed in the left lateral decubitus position via a right posterolateral thoracotomy.

Proximal left subclavian arterial injury, left pulmonary injury, and combined left pulmonary and cardiac injuries as well as upper or lower third esophageal injuries are best managed in the right lateral decubitus position via a left posterolateral thoracotomy.

Patients who arrive in deep shock (systolic blood pressure < 60 torr) should probably be positioned supine; *turning usually causes further decompensation.* The supine position will permit access to all major vascular structures as well as optimal exposure of the heart. Many pulmonary injuries may also be handled via a median sternotomy. In patients with high, left-side injuries where there is concern that the proximal descending aorta or left subclavian vessels may also have been injured, a

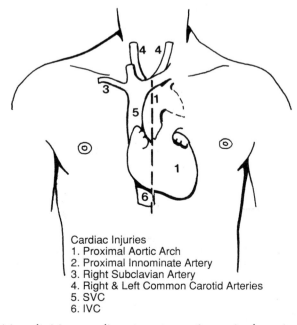

Cardiac Injuries
1. Proximal Aortic Arch
2. Proximal Innominate Artery
3. Right Subclavian Artery
4. Right & Left Common Carotid Arteries
5. SVC
6. IVC

Figure 15.4. Incision decision: median sternotomy. *1,* proximal aortic arch; *2,* proximal innominate artery; *3,* right subclavian artery; *4,* right and left common carotid arteries; *5,* superior vena cava; *6,* inferior vena cava.

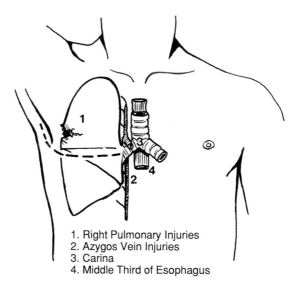

1. Right Pulmonary Injuries
2. Azygos Vein Injuries
3. Carina
4. Middle Third of Esophagus

Figure 15.5.   Incision decision: right anterolateral thoracotomy. *1,* right pulmonary injuries; *2,* azygos vein injuries; *3,* carina; *4,* middle third of esophagus.

modified "extended battle" position allows for reasonable exposure. This position is achieved by initially positioning the patient flat and then rotating the left chest and shoulder up to approximately 30–45° on a roll. The left arm is then draped anteriorly along an ether screen or other operative support.

Preparation of the patient includes clipping or shaving the groin and axilla. A wide prep is always used, beginning proximally from the midneck, with inclusion of thoracic outlet and the sternal notch. Inferiorly, it extends to include the entire abdomen and both inguinal areas to allow for femoral–femoral cardiopulmonary bypass and access for saphenous vein harvest should an autogenous graft be necessary for vascular reconstruction. Laterally, the prep should extend all the way to the operating table. A bladder catheter should be secured carefully and, in the supine patient, routed under

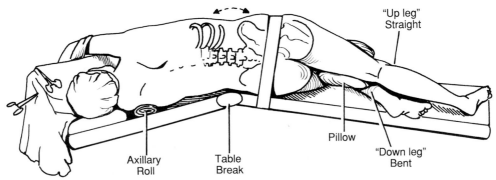

"Up leg"
Straight

Pillow

"Down leg"
Bent

Axillary
Roll

Table
Break

Figure 15.6.   Incision decision: position for right posterolateral thoracotomy.

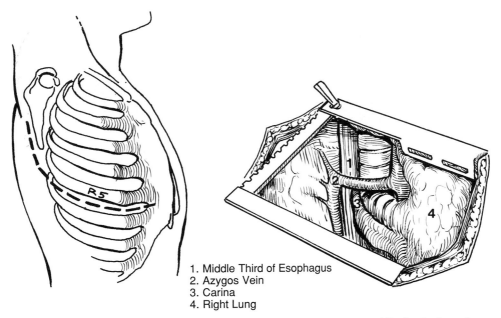

1. Middle Third of Esophagus
2. Azygos Vein
3. Carina
4. Right Lung

Figure 15.7.   Incision decision: right posterolateral thoracotomy. *1,* middle third of esophagus; *2,* azygos vein; *3,* carina; *1,* right lung.

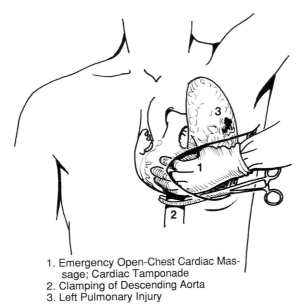

1. Emergency Open-Chest Cardiac Massage; Cardiac Tamponade
2. Clamping of Descending Aorta
3. Left Pulmonary Injury

Figure 15.8.   Incision decision: left anterolateral thoracotomy. *1,* emergency open-chest cardiac massage; cardiac tamponade; *2,* clamping of descending aorta; *3,* left pulmonary injury.

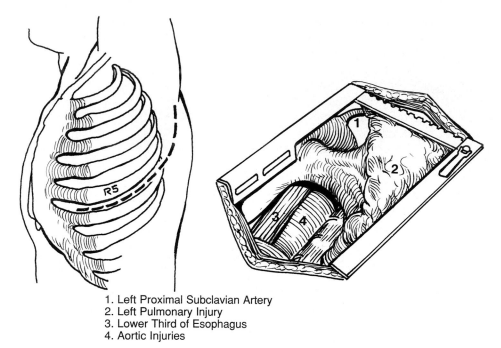

1. Left Proximal Subclavian Artery
2. Left Pulmonary Injury
3. Lower Third of Esophagus
4. Aortic Injuries

Figure 15.9. Incision decision: left posterolateral thoracotomy. *1,* left proximal subclavian artery; *2,* left pulmonary injury; *3,* lower third of esophagus; *4,* aortic injuries.

the thigh to facilitate access to the inguinal areas. Femoral catheters are subject to inadvertent dislodgement and disconnection under drapes; special attention should be paid to connecting tubing and stopcocks, ensuring that these connections are tight and taped.

Technical Considerations

A subxiphoid exploration is most often indicated in the stable patient with suspected hemopericardium, whether it is suggested by an elevated CVP or simply the proximity of injury to the heart. Position and prep the patient as for median sternotomy with possible abdominal extension, since the possibility of associated intraabdominal injury always exists. Make a midline incision measuring approximately 15 cm over the distal 5 cm of the sternum and extend it to the upper abdomen. If particularly prominent, excise the xiphoid process with electrocautery. Retraction of a small xiphoid process is also possible and may allow for adequate exposure. Dissect the soft tissue just posterior to the sternum bluntly, separating the anterior pericardium from the posterior aspect of the sternum. The pericardium is often visible as it falls away from the sternum. Next, apply two long clamps or traction sutures to either side of the planned site of pericardiotomy. Retraction on the clamps or sutures will stabilize and facilitate opening of the pericardium. It will also simplify closure of the pericardium in the event of a negative exploration. Hemostasis must be meticulous, so that the presence of even minor hemopericardium is obvious on opening of the pericardium. In the event of a negative subxiphoid exploration, close the pericardiotomy with a continuous 3–0 absorbable suture.

Often the next consideration is exclusion or identification of intraabdominal injury. Assessment can be either by performing a peritoneal lavage or by simply extending the incision and performing a limited exploratory laparotomy. The latter approach is much faster and is our choice in the already anesthetized patient.

In unstable patients with a high likelihood of cardiac and/or central vascular injuries (and those patients with hemopericardium demonstrated by a positive subxiphoid exploration), immediate median sternotomy is indicated (refer to Flow Chart 15.2). The skin incision should begin at the jugular notch and extend just below the xiphoid process. Special attention should be paid to the proximal extent of the incision, since it may subsequently interfere with a surgical airway. After the skin incision is made, electrocautery is used to deepen the incision onto the periosteum. Isolate the xiphoid process from the adherent muscle and fascia by sharp dissection. Blunt digital dissection behind the caudal sternum will separate the pericardium from the posterior periosteum. Next, excise the xiphoid process with cautery. At the cranial extent of the incision, dissect bluntly behind the manubrium. Sharply divide the constant heavy band of connective tissue just posterior and superior to the manubrium. Incomplete division of these fibers will make sternotomy difficult, whereas overzealous dissection can injure the underlying innominate vein. After completing the dissections, palpate both sternal borders to identify and mark the midline using electrocautery. An electric or air-driven sternal saw is preferred, but the Lebsche knife may be used to divide the sternum. A right-handed surgeon operates most easily from the right side of the patient, applying the saw from bottom to top of the sternum, simultaneously lifting the sternum to minimize risk to the heart and innominate vein. The first assistant retracts the skin of the jugular notch area to allow complete division of the sternum. Wax is helpful to achieve rapid bone hemostasis. The sternum is gradually but forcibly spread apart by the surgeon and first assistant. Electrocautery can be used for hemostasis of the surrounding fibromuscular tissue. A mechanical retractor is inserted and the sternum is gradually spread open.

Inspect the pleura immediately to exclude pneumothorax; if in doubt, make a nick in the pleura to evacuate any gas. If a question of pericardial tamponade exists, the pericardium should be opened vertically in the midline. Check the internal mammary vessels to ascertain that they were not injured.

Exposure of extracardiac great vessel injuries frequently requires an oblique extension of the median sternotomy. Right carotid and innominate arterial injuries are rapidly controlled with a large vascular clamp, with one jaw positioned inside the right pleura and the other outside, across the soft-tissue connection of this "flap." This gives immediate proximal control not only of the innominate artery but also of the superior vena cava. A right supraclavicular extension may be required to expose the more distal subclavian artery for inflow/outflow control.

To secure the common carotid artery, an oblique neck extension anterior to the sternocleidomastoid muscle is helpful. If the injury involves the innominate artery (and thus demands control of the proximal right common carotid artery), the approach can be made via the previously mentioned right supraclavicular "T" extension from the median sternotomy, avoiding the oblique neck extension. Injury to either proximal jugular vein is also handled via oblique neck extension.

Injuries to the jugular and larger intrathoracic veins are initially controlled with direct pressure. With additional exposure and suction, Allis or Babcock clamps are applied directly to the vein to prevent troublesome "ripping" as repair is attempted (Fig.

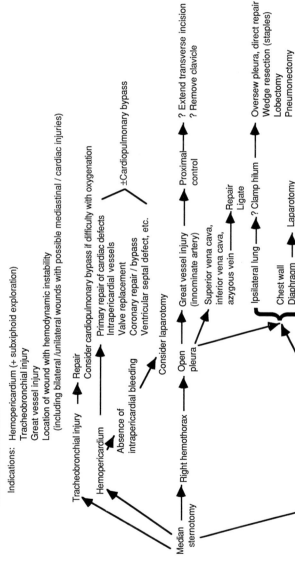

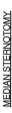

Flow Chart 15.2.   Indications for and applications of median sternotomy.

15.10). The pericardium can also be opened to gain additional length for proximal control.

Direct suture repair (lateral venography) of venous injuries is ideal. If it is necessary to even temporarily occlude the superior or inferior vena cava in the process of repair, venous return to the nonoccluded vein must be substantially augmented by rapid infusion to prevent severe hypotension.

Aortic arch injuries are initially controlled using direct pressure. If a simple laceration is encountered, repair it directly using polypropylene sutures with polytetrafluoroethylene pledgets. This can be facilitated by using controlled nitroprusside-induced hypotension for brief (<3-min) periods. Complex aortic arch injuries require cardiopulmonary bypass and possibly hypothermic circulatory arrest (10).

Most cardiac injuries are amenable to simple suture repair, particularly the more common anterior injuries involving the "right" side of the heart. After initial digital control of hemorrhage, place sutures with polytetrafluoroethylene pledgets. Injuries either adjacent to or actually involving either the right coronary artery and its branches or the left anterior descending artery require cardiopulmonary bypass for optimal repair and may even require the creation of an aortocoronary interposition graft.

Posterolateral injuries to the left heart are less accessible and involve a high-pressure system. Appropriate exposure and definitive repair requires at least "picking up" the heart to expose the posterior aspect, often with such compromise of venous return that cardiopulmonary bypass offers safer repair, particularly if hemorrhage can be at least temporarily controlled with digital pressure.

Failure to obtain normal hemodynamics following a superficial suture repair of the right heart suggests a deeper valvular or septal injury. In addition to direct examination of the heart to detect significant intracardiac shunting, pulmonary arterial catheter pressures and oxygen saturations may be helpful in confirming the presence of a left-to-right shunt. Esophageal echocardiography (11) is a promising but yet untested diagnostic tool for cardiac trauma management.

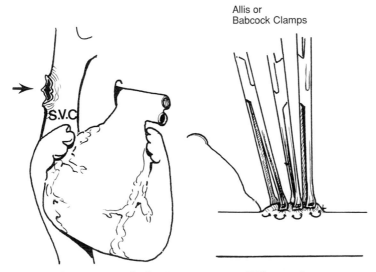

Figure 15.10.   Control of major venous tear. *SVC,* superior vena cava.

After repair of central vascular and/or cardiac injuries, hemostasis can be problematic. Coagulopathy in trauma patients is common. Multiple transfusions of fresh frozen plasma and platelets along with correction of acidosis, hypocalcemia, and hypothermia are essential.

At least one (and often both) pleura(e) is opened widely to prevent pericardial tamponade after sternotomy closure. Two large-bore (no. 32 or no. 36 French) mediastinal tubes are used. A right-angle tube is inserted into each open pleura, with a straight tube draining the mediastinum itself. The pericardium is left open. Heavy (no. 6) stainless steel wire sutures are used to close the sternum, generally with two through-and-through sutures closing the manubrium and four additional sutures for the remainder of the sternum. A continuous 2–0 absorbable suture is then used to close muscle and fascia, followed by a second continuous layer in the subcutaneous tissue. The skin is then closed either with skin staples or a subcuticular closure with an absorbable suture.

RIGHT THORACOTOMY

Patients with isolated right pulmonary injuries, injury to the carina, and/or injury to the middle third of the esophagus are managed through a right posterolateral thoracotomy (Flow Chart 15.3). The patient should be positioned initially so that the chest is perpendicular to and adjacent to the right edge of the operating table. A roll is inserted under the patient's left axilla to avoid compression of the brachial plexus and adjacent vasculature. Perhaps the easiest and quickest way to secure the patient in this position is a "bean bag": on application of suction, it molds itself to the patient, simultaneously providing support and immobilization. Alternatively, another (larger) roll is used to support the patient's anterior chest and abdomen. After double-checking that the patient's kidney area is located over the operating table break, the operating table should be "flexed," lowering both head and feet to "open up" the region between the costal margin and the wing of the ilium. Wide adhesive tape is pulled tight across the buttocks and secured to both sides of the operating table. The patient's legs are placed so that the left ("down") leg is flexed at both the hip and knee. The right ("up") leg is positioned straight and supported by two or three pillows. Next, the right ("up") arm should be either secured to the anesthetic screen or rested on a cushioned instrument stand.

Following wide prep and draping, a standard posterolateral thoracotomy incision is made. In women, the inframammary fold is the desired location, whereas the infrapectoral incision is used for males. For both, carry the incision around the tip of the scapula in a gentle curve, ending midway between the medial border of the scapula and the posterior spinous processes. Divide the underlying connective tissue with cautery. Following partial division of the trapezius, complete division of the latissimus dorsi and serratus anterior muscles, and upward retraction of the scapula, the desired interspace is identified. Right thoracotomy for trauma is generally best performed through the fifth or sixth interspace. The first rib may be identified by palpation as a short, broad rib at the apex of the thorax. The intercostal muscles at the appropriate interspace are divided using electrocautery, exposing the underlying parietal pleura in the middle of the incision. Sharply divide the pleura to allow the insertion of a finger. After ensuring that no adhesions are present, divide the remaining intercostal muscle and pleura simultaneously with the electrocautery. pushing the underlying lung away from the cautery with a gauze dissector or similar instrument. The two ribs immediately adjacent to the chest wall incision can be "notched" or a small posterior segment resected to

RIGHT POSTEROLATERAL THORACOTOMY

Indications: 1. Isolated right chest trauma without anterior mediastinal / cardiac involvement
>1500 ml of initial thoracostomy drainage or
>200 ml / hr x 4 hr
2. Posterior mediastinal injury — middle third of esophagus
3. Carina

Left lateral decubitus
Standard right posterolateral
thoracotomy incision, 4th-6th
intercostal space

<u>Vascular</u>   Superior vena cava, azygous vein, inferior vena cava
Subclavian, innominate arteries and veins
-Primary repair
-Interposition graft } ±Cardiopulmonary
-Ligation   bypass

<u>Pulmonary</u>   Pulmonary artery, pulmonary vein, parenchyma—
consider cross-clamp hilum
- Expose: "finger fracture"
- Primary repair
- Ligation
- Wedge resection, segmentectomy,
lobectomy, pneumonectomy

<u>Esophageal</u> - Primary repair, pleural flap resection ±
esophagus substitute ± proximal diversion

<u>Chest Wall</u> - Debride
- Close primarily

<u>Diaphragm</u> - Laparotomy

<u>Vertebral column</u> - Orthopedic stabilization

Anterior and
posterior
chest tubes
Continuous closure

Flow Chart 15.3.   Indications for and applications of right posterolateral thoracotomy.

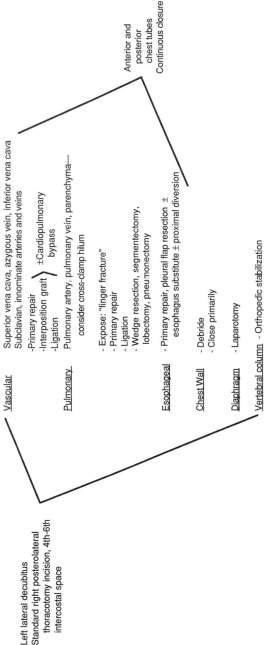

facilitate exposure while avoiding inadvertent fracture during retraction. Insert a mechanical chest retractor and gradually open it. Blood clots are most rapidly evacuated with pads. Obvious chest-wall or great-vessel bleeders should be compressed. Divide the inferior pulmonary ligament to mobilize the lower lobe. If massive bleeding is evident from the lung, either digital compression or application of a large atraumatic vascular clamp (such as a Satinsky clamp) across the hilum will give temporary hemostasis. Peripheral pulmonary parenchymal injuries are most expeditiously controlled by resection with a 90-mm stapler using 3.2-mm staples. Rapidly immobilize the area with lung clamps. Application of the stapler itself (even without firing of the staples) compresses the lung and therefore will immediately control strictly parenchymal bleeding. Either segmental resections or formal lobectomy can be performed to definitively manage parenchymal injuries and associated hemorrhage. Extreme cases require pneumonectomy.

Injuries to the azygos vein are most easily exposed using caudal/anterior retraction of the lung. Ligation is safe but venography may be faster.

The carina is exposed by sharp dissection away from the adjacent esophagus and vena cava *after ligation and division of the azygos vein,* which arcs over the right mainstem bronchus. The endotracheal tube can be advanced into the left mainstem bronchus to deflate the right lung and facilitate a repair. Simple interrupted fine absorbable sutures are used, reinforcing the repair with a vascular pleural or omental flap. It is important to identify and eliminate any air leaks that appear on application of a moderate amount (30 cm of H_2O) of airway pressure.

Injuries to the middle third of the esophagus are also exposed through a right posterolateral thoracotomy. The area of injury is identified and debrided as necessary, preserving the vagus nerves if they are uninjured. Two layers of interrupted suture are used for the repair. Ideally, a Maloney dilator is used as a stent during the repair to avoid compromise of the esophageal lumen. A vascular pleural flap is mobilized to reinforce the repair. A leak should be anticipated and a thoracostomy tube should be placed adjacent to *(but not on)* the repair. A feeding jejunostomy is always a desirable adjunct to postoperative care of most patients with esophageal injuries since leaks can be managed without long-term parenteral nutrition.

LEFT THORACOTOMY

With isolated left pulmonary parenchymal injury, injury to the upper or lower third of the esophagus, or documented injury to the descending thoracic aorta or left subclavian artery, a left posterolateral thoracotomy (Flow Chart 15.4) is indicated.

Procedure

The patient should be positioned in a right lateral decubitus position (left side up). The skin incision mirrors that for the right posterolateral thoracotomy. Left subclavian arterial injuries should be approached through a third or fourth interspace incision; otherwise, the fifth or sixth interspace incision is used. The pericardium should always be inspected and a longitudinal pericardiotomy (anterior to the phrenic nerve) performed if hemopericardium is present.

Divide the inferior pulmonary ligament up to the inferior pulmonary vein, which resides in its apex. Management of upper- or lower-third esophageal injuries is similar to that of middle-third esophageal injuries with one exception. In addition to a pleural flap, distal esophageal repairs are also effectively buttressed with a gastric fundus patch rolled up as in a Belsey Mark IV hiatal hernia repair.

LEFT POSTEROLATERAL THORACOTOMY

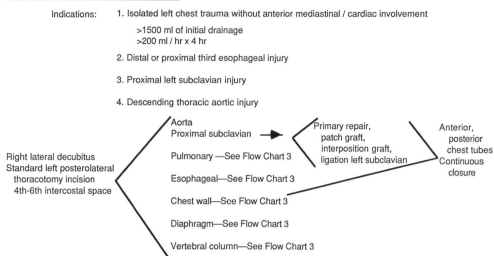

Indications:
1. Isolated left chest trauma without anterior mediastinal / cardiac involvement

>1500 ml of initial drainage
>200 ml / hr x 4 hr

2. Distal or proximal third esophageal injury

3. Proximal left subclavian injury

4. Descending thoracic aortic injury

Right lateral decubitus
Standard left posterolateral
thoracotomy incision
4th-6th intercostal space

Aorta
Proximal subclavian →

Pulmonary —See Flow Chart 3

Esophageal—See Flow Chart 3

Chest wall—See Flow Chart 3

Diaphragm—See Flow Chart 3

Vertebral column—See Flow Chart 3

Primary repair,
patch graft,
interposition graft,
ligation left subclavian

Anterior,
posterior
chest tubes
Continuous
closure

Flow Chart 15.4. Indications for and applications of left posterolateral thoracotomy.

Management of descending thoracic aortic injuries requires clamping of the distal aortic arch and the left subclavian artery for proximal control. Primary repair is desirable and sometimes feasible; otherwise, a low-porosity prosthetic interposition graft is used. Extreme caution should be exercised with respect to the duration of descending aortic occlusion: spinal artery hypoperfusion may result in paraplegia from even brief (20-min) periods of occlusion. The use of a heparin-bonded shunt from aortic arch to beyond the distal vascular clamp should be considered for all potentially prolonged repairs. If available, femoral–femoral or left atrial–femoral cardiopulmonary bypass can provide continuous flow to the lower portion of the body while the aorta is clamped.

Although the proximal left subclavian artery is directly accessible through a high left posterolateral thoracotomy, more distal control of the subclavian (or in some instances the axillary) artery often requires a separate infraclavicular incision. Dissection around the distal aortic arch at the origin of the left subclavian requires care to avoid injury to the recurrent laryngeal nerve. Repair options include primary repair with or without the use of an autogenous vein graft patch; more often, an interposition saphenous vein graft is used, particularly if there is substantial tissue loss.

Anterior and posterior chest tubes are inserted prior to closure of all posterolateral thoracotomies. Postoperatively, these tubes are attached to a collecting system that provides 20 cm of H_2O suction via underwater seal. Chest tubes, however, are generally not used for pneumonectomies because of the consequent mediastinal shift that occurs with application of suction to an empty hemithorax.

Just prior to the closure of the incision, infiltrate 0.5 or 0.25% bupivacaine in the area of neurovascular bundles to give intercostal blocks extending at least one rib above and below the incision. After all bleeding has been controlled, we irrigate with a warm antibiotic solution. Double strands of heavy absorbable suture are used for pericostal closure. Reapproximate the divided intercostal muscle using continuous absorbable suture to minimize the possibility of postoperative bleeding from a divided intercostal vessel and also to act as an infection barrier. The remaining layers of chest wall musculature are reconstructed using continuous absorbable suture. The subcutaneous space is also obliterated with a lighter continuous absorbable suture. The skin is closed using skin staples. Entrance and exit wounds are debrided, irrigated, and closed with as much reconstruction of the chest wall musculature as possible.

Postoperative Management

The postoperative management of patients with penetrating thoracic trauma resembles that of patients after elective thoracotomy. Several points warrant emphasis.

The first point concerns positive end-expiratory pressure. Although beneficial in improving oxygenation and preventing alveolar collapse, the increased airway pressure may also jeopardize the bronchial stump or pulmonary repair. In patients with major tracheobronchial reconstructions, high-frequency (jet) ventilation can minimize pressure on the repair.

Second, the common complications of intrathoracic bleeding and tension pneumothorax should be suspected in all trauma victims; the latter often presents several days following emergency thoracotomy. Immediate postoperative and 6-hr postoperative chest x-rays are essential to safe care.

Third, coagulopathic bleeding is not infrequent in patients with major cardiovascular and pulmonary trauma; there are often several causes, including hypothermia, transfusion of multiple units of blood (with loss of clotting factors), thrombocytopenia, and hypocalcemia. Meticulous correction of these multiple metabolic abnormalities is required to reverse the process. All patients should receive parenteral vitamin K. In the early postoperative period, we consider fresh frozen plasma and blood as the volume expanders of choice, avoiding crystalloids entirely.

Fourth, regional analgesia is helpful. As previously mentioned, intercostal blocks are given prior to closure of the thoracotomy incision. Morphine administered intrathecally or, even better, fentanyl administered via an epidural catheter is extremely effective in promoting posttraumatic pulmonary toilet (12). Alternatively, systemic analgesics can be administered in a continuous infusion system, preferably with some patient control.

Antibiotic Therapy

The use of antibiotics in penetrating chest trauma remains controversial. For simple injuries adequately managed by tube thoracostomy alone, studies support both the omission (13) and use (14) of prophylactic antibiotics. For complex injuries, the issue is not *whether* but rather *which* antibiotic to use. These controversies exist because infection in thoracic surgical wounds is comparatively infrequent and probably more related to accumulation of blood and nonviable tissue than to the injury or surgery itself. We use a first-generation cephalosporin directed primarily against skin flora, recognizing that seriously compromised patients who require a long stay in the intensive care unit are at particular risk for Gram-negative pneumonia. This latter risk cannot be mitigated, in our opinion, with prophylactic antibiotics but rather only by vigorous mechanical pulmonary toilet. Therapeutic antibiotics are chosen on the basis of known or suspected pathogens and their expected sensitivities to specific drugs.

CARDIOPULMONARY BYPASS

The majority of penetrating cardiac wounds have been, and continue to be, managed without the use of cardiopulmonary bypass. Nevertheless, the proliferation of open-heart surgical suites and the recent manufacture of free-standing cardiopulmonary support (15) devices (e.g., CPS, Bard Inc.) prompts review of the indications and the contraindications for this technique in the setting of penetrating thoracic trauma.

It has been impossible to design a cardiopulmonary bypass system that is nonthrombogenic. The major limitation on the use of such a device in the management of trauma is, therefore, the need for complete anticoagulation. Intracranial injuries and injuries to and adjacent to the spinal cord absolutely contraindicate anticoagulation and therefore cardiopulmonary bypass. There are, nevertheless, distinct advantages to the selective use of the technique. The first advantage relates to control of hemorrhage. With isolated thoracic injuries, cardiopulmonary bypass will stop both venous and arterial bleeding and allow a controlled if not leisurely repair of the injuries. Even if the injuries are thoracoabdominal, the negative pressure exerted through the venous cannula is so forceful that often even major venous injuries are rapidly identified and controlled once the blood is diverted into the cardiopulmonary bypass circuit.

The third and more conventional advantage of the technique is that it allows for cardioplegia and repair of injuries in a stilled heart.

In general, cardiopulmonary bypass is required when complex cardiac injuries involve the coronary arteries, valvular injuries, traumatic ventricular septal defects associated with hemodynamic instability, and extensive ventricular wall injuries. Foreign bodies within the left heart should be recovered while the patient is on cardiopulmonary bypass. We have found it difficult to repair posterior cardiac injuries without cardiopulmonary bypass because "lifting" the heart impairs venous return and often causes unacceptable falls in blood pressure. Although few victims of ascending and arch aortic injuries survive to reach a trauma center, those who do often require cardiopulmonary bypass for reconstruction. Indeed, arch reconstructions demanding prolonged occlusion of cerebral vessels may require not only cardiopulmonary bypass but also deep hypothermia and even circulatory arrest. Although some surgeons report successful management of the descending thoracic aorta without the use of either a heparin-bonded shunt or femoral–femoral cardiopulmonary bypass, the latter technique is particularly attractive because it permits leisurely inspection, dissection, and repair of the injured aorta while assuring adequate flow to the caudal structures maintained by femoral–femoral access to cardiopulmonary bypass. By sustaining adequate perfusion of the distal aorta throughout the repair, the chances of spinal cord ischemia may be reduced.

We have managed two patients with combined cardiac-abdominal injuries using cardiopulmonary bypass. In each case, complex cardiac injury required cardiopulmonary bypass for repair. Inspection of the missile tract suggested abdominal penetration and a celiotomy was performed even while bypass was continued. In each case, it was possible to exclude a major vascular injury and, therefore, the bypass cannulae were removed, anticoagulation was reversed, and the operation continued. Although the classic indications for the use of cardiopulmonary bypass in penetrating trauma are limited, cardiopulmonary bypass can probably be used safely if potential bleeding sites can be visualized and surgically controlled and even used to advantage in cases of exsanguinating hemorrhage from thoracic or even combined thoracoabdominal injuries. The benefits of stable hemodynamics may well outweigh the increased risks associated with anticoagulation until wounds can be repaired and the anticoagulation reversed.

CLINICAL EXPERIENCE

To examine the efficacy of the protocols described, we recently reviewed our experience with victims of penetrating cardiac trauma who presented to the trauma center with a sign of life—an electrocardiogram rhythm, pulse, or blood pressure.

During a 39-month interval, we managed 16 such patients, each of whom ultimately was determined as having a penetrating cardiac wound. There were 15 survivors. Demographics are given in Table 15.1. Two observations are particularly noteworthy. First, half of the patients presented with unremarkable hemodynamics—blood pressure > 100 and pulse < 120. The importance of treating every penetrating thoracic injury as possible penetrating cardiac injury is apparent. Based on the location of the wound, subxiphoid exploration was planned and performed in six of eight patients; the other two patients required sternotomy without subxiphoid exploration when they went into shock. The second observation relates to multiple organ injury: 9 of the 16 patients had combined thoracoabdominal injuries, and 2 of these were managed successfully with cardiopulmonary bypass. The goal must not be to treat the penetrating thoracic injury but rather to treat all of the injuries sustained by the trauma victim in an efficient and comprehensive plan. Irrespective of the complexity of the patient, the fundamental priorities of airway, breathing, circulation, and a thorough inventory of all wounds must be met if the victim of penetrating thoracic trauma is to survive.

SUMMARY/CONCLUSIONS

Successful management of penetrating thoracic trauma hinges on multiple critical decisions that often must be made within seconds and minutes of the victim's presentation to the trauma center. The basic protocols presented in the Advanced Trauma Life Support (1) course are particularly useful in initiating trauma resuscitation.

In penetrating thoracic trauma, the two most common mechanisms underlying circulatory shock are hypovolemia and embarrassment of venous return to the heart associated either with tension hemopneumothorax or with pericardial tamponade. Airway protection, mechanical ventilation, tube thoracostomy, and volume expansion are mainstays of emergency department therapy. *Persistent* unexplained shock indicates either occult (abdominal) bleeding or pericardial effusion with tamponade. In either case, the patient should be explored promptly.

Table 15.1.
Sixteen Penetrating Cardiac Trauma Victims Who Presented with a Sign of Life[a]

Characteristic	Range	Median
Age (years)	15–54	28
Presentation systolic blood pressure (torr)[b]	0–142	100
Presentation pulse (min^{-1})	48–172	109
Emergency/operating room (min)	15–170	40
Fluids (24)[c,d]		
Crystalloid (liters)	6–24	11
Blood (U)	0–41	9
LOS/ICU[e] (days)	1–11	3.5
LOS/total[e] (days)	6–38	12

[a]15/16 patients survived.
[b]Half of the patients presented with vital signs that belied their serious injury.
[c]Rapid volume infusion and prompt diagnostic subxiphoid exploration are essential even when the diagnosis is in doubt.
[d]2/9 patients with combined cardiac and abdominal injuries required and were successfully managed with cardiopulmonary bypass.
[e]Lengths of stay (LOS) were injury-related and not associated with multiple organ failure.

Although the need for operative management of penetrating thoracic trauma is rare, it is usually emergent. The most critical decision relates to selection of an incision that will provide adequate exposure. Operative priorities are hemostasis, visceral and vascular repair, and drainage.

Acknowledgements

Supported in part by grants from the National Institutes of Health (GM39756) and the American Heart Association (88-0710). TGB is a research fellowship awardee of the American College of Surgeons.

REFERENCES

1. Committee on Trauma, American College advanced trauma life-support course for physicians. Chicago: American College of Surgeons, 1989.
2. Salem MR, Sellick BA, Elam JO. The historical background of cricoid pressure in anesthesia and resuscitation. Anesth Analg 1974;53:230–232.
3. Moore FA, Haenel JB. Advances in oxygen monitoring of trauma patients. Med Instrum 1988;22:135–142.
4. Mangiante EC, Hoots AV, Fabian TC. The percutaneous common femoral vein catheter for volume replacement in critically injured patients. J Trauma 1988;28:1644–1649.
5. Trinkle JK, Franz J, Grover FL, et al. Affairs of the wounded heart: penetrating cardiac wounds. J Trauma 1979;19:467–472.
6. Murphy BP, Harford FJ, Cramer FS. Cerebral air embolism resulting from invasive medical procedures: treatment with hyperbaric oxygen. Ann Surg 1985;201:242–245.
7. Weigelt JA, Thal ER, Snyder WH, Fry RE, Meier DE, Kliman WJ. Diagnosis of penetrating cervical esophageal injuries. Am J Surg 1987;145:619–622.
8. Triggiani E, Belsey R. Oesophageal trauma: incidence, diagnosis and management. Thorax 1977;32:241–249.
9. Kerr TM, Sood R, Buckman RF, Gelman J. Prospective trial of the six hour rule in stab wounds of the chest. Surg Gynecol Obstet 1989;169:248–250.
10. Schmidt CA, Smith DC. Traumatic avulsion of arch vessels in a child: primary repair using hypothermic circulatory arrest. J Trauma 1989;29:248–250.
11. Sold M, Silber R, Hopp H, Meesmann M, Ertl G. Erfolgreiches vorgehen bei Mitralklappenruptur mit Papillarmuskel und Sehnenfadenausriss nach Mehrfachverletzung und stumpfen Thoraxtrauma. Anaesthestist 1989;38:262–265.
12. Diffman M, Keller R, Wolff G. A rationale for epidural analgesia in the treatment of multiple rib fractures. Intensive Care Med 1978;4:193–197.
13. LeBlanc KA, Tucker WY. Prophylactic antibiotics and closed tube thoracostomy. Surg Gynecol Obstet 1985;160:259–263.
14. LoCurto JJ, Tischler CD, Swan KG, et al. Tube thoracostomy and trauma—antibiotics or not? J Trauma 1986;26:1067–1072.
15. Mattox KL, Beall AC. Resuscitation of the moribund patient using portable cardiopulmonary bypass. Ann Thorac Surg 1976;22:436–442.

16 Penetrating Cardiac Trauma

Rao R. Ivatury, MD
Michael Rohman, MD

The incidence and severity of thoracic injuries are increasing because of recent escalations of civilian violence and motor vehicle accidents. It is a sad reflection on modern times that one leading trauma center amassed an experience with more than 400 cardiovascular injuries in a period of 1 yr (1). Drug-related violence in inner-city areas has reached proportions that are reminiscent of wartime. Apparently, this rise in civilian trauma is not limited to this country. For instance, a recent series from Bogotá, Colombia (2) dealt with 320 cardiac injuries accumulated over 8 yr. With improvements in prehospital care and rapid transport of trauma victims to emergency rooms, there has been a real increase in the number of patients arriving at the hospital with some chance of survival, even with injuries that formerly were lethal (3–11). The most dramatic among these are the penetrating cardiac wounds with or without cardiac tamponade. Prompt recognition and expeditious treatment of these injuries are crucial to achieve optimal survival.

HISTORICAL BACKGROUND

According to Karrel et al. (12), the first successful repair of a stab wound of the heart was performed in dogs by deVecchio in 1895 and, shortly thereafter, Rehn carried out the first successful human cardiorrhaphy. As quoted by these authors, the first cardiorrhaphy in the United States was achieved by Hill in 1902. In 1943, Blalock and Ravitch (13) recommended pericardiocentesis and observation as a method of management of penetrating cardiac wounds. However, thoracotomy and cardiorrhaphy gradually gained favorable attention as the preferred approach to these lesions as support systems such as transfusion, anesthesia, and antibiotics improved. In 1959, Isaacs (14) reported a remarkable series of 60 patients with cardiac injuries with a survival of 89% for stab wounds and 43% for gunshot wounds.

INCIDENCE AND ETIOLOGY

Cardiac penetration in civilian trauma most often is related to stab wounds by knives or ice picks and to firearm injuries. In rare instances it may result from a fractured sternum or rib. Iatrogenic penetrating wounds of the heart from intracardiac injections or central venous catheters have been recorded (12). Other unusual, but fascinating, causes of cardiac injury are migrating needles or pins (12), migrating staples (15), and forcibly

311

ejected sharp objects such as coat hangers (11). A case of cardiac tamponade following impalement on a wrought-iron fence was reported by McGill et al. (16.)

The prehospital mortality rate for penetrating cardiac trauma in the 1960s and the 1970s ranged from 50 to 85% (17–20). In 1980, Baker et al. (21) reported that 51% of their patients were dead on arrival at the hospital. In a more recent report from South Africa, Demetriades and VanderVeen (22) analyzed 532 cases of penetrating cardiac injuries collected in a 2-year period; 407 (76.5%) died before reaching medical attention. More recently, a significant number of patients arrive at the hospital alive, many in extremis, allowing a few moments in which resuscitation is still possible. In our own analysis of 228 cases of penetrating cardiac trauma (1963–1983), 50.8% of the patients either were clinically dead or in extremis on arrival at the emergency center (5). Furthermore, a higher number of patients presented in extremis in the later years of the study. These data point to a changing pattern of presentation of cardiac injuries, especially in inner-city trauma centers. This change probably is related to increasingly rapid transport of injured patients, who, in former years, would have died at the scene of injury.

The relative frequency of involvement of cardiac chambers depends on their anatomic location. The right ventricle, with its maximal anterior exposure, is the most commonly injured. In a collective review of 1802 patients, Karrel et al (12) found right ventricular involvement in 42.5% and left ventricular injury in 33%. The right atrium (15.4%) and left atrium (5.8%) were injured less frequently. The intrapericardial great vessels were penetrated in only 3.3% of the patients. Injury to the coronary vessels was infrequent.

PATHOPHYSIOLOGY

The clinical presentation of cardiac penetration is related to the relative predominance of pericardial tamponade or severe hemorrhage. Less commonly, valvular or septal defects and myocardial ischemia caused by coronary vessel injury or coincidental infarction may contribute to the overall clinical picture of hypotension and diminished cardiac output. The degree of pericardial tamponade is determined by the size of the rent in the pericardium, the rate of bleeding from the cardiac wound, and the chamber of the heart involved. With knife wounds, a small pericardial laceration may be sealed rapidly by clot and/or adjacent fat (19, 20). Consequently, 80–90% of patients with stab wounds present primarily with tamponade. On occasion, a small ventricular wound may seal before a significant amount of blood can accumulate in the pericardial sac; if the hemorrhage ceases, there may be an absence of the usual signs of tamponade (12). In the series reported by Demetriades and VanderVeen (22), 92.7% of patients with right ventricular wounds had tamponade as opposed to only 42.9% of patients with lacerated left ventricles.

When the pericardial laceration seals or is very small relative to the amount of hemorrhage, or the hemorrhage is very rapid, blood in the pericardial sac clots rather than undergoes defibrination—an important concept that contradicts classic teaching and explains the limitations of pericardiocentesis as a diagnostic and therapeutic modality. As little as 60–100 ml of blood and clots in the pericardium may produce the clinical picture of tamponade. This degree of tamponade, however, can be overcome easily by raising the cardiac filling pressure by rapid volume infusion: the stage of compensated tamponade. When the limits of distensibility of the pericardium are reached, however, further accumulation of even a small amount of blood causes a significant impairment of cardiac contractility, atrial filling, and cardiac output. A sudden and profound systemic hypotension ensues. Unrelieved, the tamponade causes a progressive decrease in coronary and cerebral perfusion and a rapid demise. The experimental work of Wechsler et al. (23) demonstrated that cardiac tamponade of any degree was detrimental; in the initial stages it affects the viability of the endocardium and later causes both epicardial and endocardial ischemia. These considerations are fundamental to the appreciation of the sense of urgency that should attend the relief of tamponade of any degree.

In contrast to stab wounds, gunshot wounds of the pericardium and cardiac chambers are large. Thus, pericardial tamponade is less likely to occur and the ensuing hemorrhage dominates the clinical presentation. Major associated injuries in the thorax and abdomen contribute to the blood loss and hypovolemia. Interestingly, tamponade, when it does occur, appears to be a favorable prognostic factor. Carasquilla et al. (24) noted that 2 of 14 patients died when tamponade was present as opposed to 5 of 13 patients without cardiac tamponade. Similar findings were recorded by Tassi and Davies (25). Moreno et al. (26) observed that the presence of tamponade improved survival for patients with stab and gunshot wounds of the right as well as the left ventricles. These investigators went on to suggest that tamponade may be more influential in predicting outcome than the presenting vital signs.

DIAGNOSIS

Cardiac penetration should be suspected in any patient who has anterior thoracic trauma with hemodynamic instability. The "danger zone" described by Sauer and Murdock, as quoted by Karrel et al. (12), includes the area of the precordium, epigastrium, and superior mediastinum. Penetrating wounds within this area associated with hypotension suggest a cardiac injury. Siemens et al. (27), for instance, found that 65% of their patients who required cardiorrhaphy had upper mediastinal wounds. DeGennaro et al. (28) analyzed 53 patients with penetrating wounds within the cardiac silhouette and found that 85% had thoracic injuries that required operative control, including 62% with cardiac injuries.

The symptoms and signs of cardiac tamponade vary, depending upon the amount of intrapericardiac blood and clot. Agitation, air-hunger, and obtundation rapidly progress to coma as the tamponade increases (19, 20). The classic Beck's triad (distended neck veins, muffled heart sounds, and hypotension) was noted to be present in less than 10% of cases in one series (22) and in less than 40% in several reports (19, 29, 30). Elevation of central venous pressure (CVP) with distension of neck veins, although strongly suggestive of tamponade, may also result from tension pneumothorax or raised intrathoracic pressure as in shivering or straining. Erroneous measurements of the CVP can occur in all of these situations as well as by a catheter malposition. Clinical signs, such as pulsus paradoxus, are seldom helpful in the diagnosis (12). Unfortunately, there are no roentgenographic findings specific for cardiac injury. On occasion, pneumopericardium has been mentioned as evidence of pericardial penetration (31). Fluoroscopy of the chest to demonstrate decreased cardiac motion and echocardiography to visualize pericardial fluid may be helpful (20). However, these investigations should not be relied upon except in the rare patient who is extremely stable. They require professional expertise that generally is not available in the acute setting and serve only to delay treatment in the majority of patients with cardiac penetration.

Pericardiocentesis by a paraxiphoid approach, carefully performed with electrocardiographic monitoring, often is described and advocated as a diagnostic modality. However, false results are common. Trinkle et al. (32), for example, noted three false-positives and nine false-negatives in a group of 47 patients who had pericardiocentesis. The pitfalls and occasional benefits of this procedure are discussed in a subsequent section.

We have presented an algorithm in Figure 16.1 that may facilitate the early diagnosis of cardiac tamponade in stable patients with precordial penetrating wounds. Hemodynamically stable patients with a potential for cardiac tamponade should be transported immediately to the operating room for continued observation and diagnosis. In such patients, a pericardiocentesis or, preferably, a subxiphoid pericardial window is indicated to confirm the diagnosis (33).

The technique of subxiphoid pericardial window is described and illustrated in

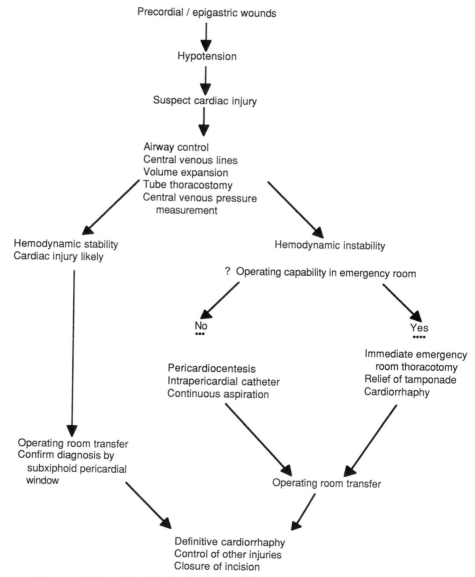

Figure 16.1. Algorithm for the management of penetrating cardiac injuries.

chapter 14 (Blunt Injuries of the Heart and Pericardium). Since direct visualization of the pericardial sac is possible, the technique is consistent in its accuracy. It has been our practice to add the subxiphoid pericardial exploration to the laparotomy in all upper abdominal/epigastric wounds with a potential for cardiac injury. In a recent series reported from Bogotá by Londono-Schimmer et al. (2), the subxiphoid exploration was positive in 65.5% of patients with suspected tamponade. Furthermore, it was positive in 35% when carried out solely on the basis of precordial external wound. Similar results were noted by Duncan et al. (34).

TREATMENT
Prehospital Management

The prehospital management of trauma victims is a matter of considerable discussion at the current time. Controversy continues in favor of and against stabilization in the field (35–37): Can and should patients be stabilized in the field before attempting to transport them to the hospital? Can the status of moribund patients (Trauma Score 1–3) be improved by advanced life support (ALS) maneuvers in the field?

Mattox and Feliciano (38) found no survivors when they analyzed 100 trauma patients who had external cardiac compression for more than 3 min in the prehospital period. Jacobs et al. (39) did not observe any benefit from prehospital ALS intervention in patients with a low Trauma Score. In a group of "potentially salvageable" patients with cardiac injuries, Gervin and Fischer (40) noted that there were no survivors in the group stabilized in the field, whereas the survival rate for patients who had no such delay was 83%.

Ivatury et al. (4) analyzed 100 consecutive patients with penetrating thoracic injuries who were in extremis and who had resuscitative thoracotomy in the emergency room. The physiologic and anatomic severity of injury as well as the results of field stabilization and prompt transport were compared. Interestingly, the average field time in 96% of the patients was 12.2 min, whereas the trauma center was located only 8 min away. Attempts at stabilization in the field, including endotracheal intubation, did not improve the Trauma Scores or the Physiologic Index in any patient. Ten patients survived; 9 of them had cardiac injuries. Furthermore, 6 of the 10 survivors were transported by police vehicles or private automobiles and did not receive resuscitative intervention in the prehospital period. These six survivors had the benefit of a lack of delay that inevitably would ensue had the emergency medical services been called and dispatched to the scene. Three other survivors received only basic life support care by the emergency medical services en route.

These data suggest that prompt transport to the hospital of the patient with penetrating thoracic trauma is crucial. Since the physiologic disruption may be a result of cardiac tamponade, these patients need to be in an emergency room where tamponade can be relieved immediately. None of the ALS procedures performed in the field, with the possible exception of airway control, can benefit this group of potentially moribund patients. An efficient patient transport system with proper medical control should optimize the prehospital management of these critically injured patients.

In-hospital Management

As with all trauma victims, the treatment of those with penetrating cardiac wounds begins with a rapid initial assessment and control of the ABCs of resuscitation (airway, breathing, and circulation). The airway should be maintained, ventilation ensured, and rapid volume infusion begun through large-bore intravenous lines. Early in the resuscitation, a central venous catheter should be placed and the CVP monitored frequently. Many of these patients have an associated pneumothorax and/or hemothorax, and early evacuation of the pleural space by a tube thoracostomy will improve ventilation and oxygenation. It will also permit a more meaningful assessment of the CVP.

As emphasized earlier, the subsequent management of these patients is determined by their hemodynamic stability (Fig. 16.1). Stable patients or those who can be stabilized easily by rapid volume infusion (initially by crystalloids and subsequently by type-specific blood) should be transported immediately to the operating room for observation, confirmation of the diagnosis by subxiphoid pericardial window, and/or median sternotomy or thoracotomy. Borderline stability is an indication for emergency room thoracotomy, relief of cardiac tamponade, and cardiorrhaphy. Pericardiocentesis and placement of an intrapericardiac catheter and aspiration of pericardial blood is an acceptable substitute only when operating capabilities are not available immediately.

The Role of Pericardiocentesis

In the modern era, pericardiocentesis is no longer an option in the definitive treatment of cardiac penetration with tamponade. It may, however, have a role in the initial stabilization of the patient, especially in centers that are not equipped to perform major operations in the receiving area of the hospital. Moreno et al. (26) advocated pericardiocentesis as a prelude to transfer of the patient to the operating room for a thoracotomy and recorded success in 12 of 16 patients. Breaux et al. (41) noted, however, that 35 of 85 patients who underwent pericardiocentesis had recurrent tamponade with deterioration of vital signs. The morality rate in these patients was 23% as opposed to 16% in those without recurrent tamponade. Sugg et al. (18) recorded a 23% incidence of false-negative results with pericardial aspiration. At thoracotomy, these patients had 100–650 ml of blood in the pericardial sac. These results illustrate some of the pitfalls associated with pericardiocentesis and are related to the frequent presence of clotted blood in the pericardial sac, which may not lend itself to aspiration. The false-negative tests provide an inappropriate sense of security that could end disastrously. The potential for cardiac and coronary artery injury by repeated attempts at pericardial aspiration is appreciable. In addition, the time wasted while performing the procedure and the consequent delay in the relief of tamponade may jeopardize an optimal outcome. Despite these considerations, pericardiocentesis, when performed appropriately, may be helpful in institutions where there are unavoidable delays in providing definitive operative management. An indwelling catheter in the pericardial sac and repeated aspirations may provide temporary hemodynamic stability while organizing for a thoracotomy.

The technical details of pericardiocentesis have been described in detail (13, 26, 40, 42, 43). It is generally agreed that the subxiphoid approach (Fig. 16.2) is the best and that the needle should be advanced under electrocardiographic monitoring. Tate and Horan (44) described a modification of this traditional method. The needle is advanced at a 45° angle to the frontal plane toward the right shoulder, thus placing the needle parallel, rather than at right angles, to the apex of the ventricles, and decreasing the possibility of myocardial injury.

The Role of Subxiphoid Pericardial Window

As discussed previously, this method has been advocated as a prelude to thoracotomy in stable patients to confirm the diagnosis of cardiac tamponade. Even though some

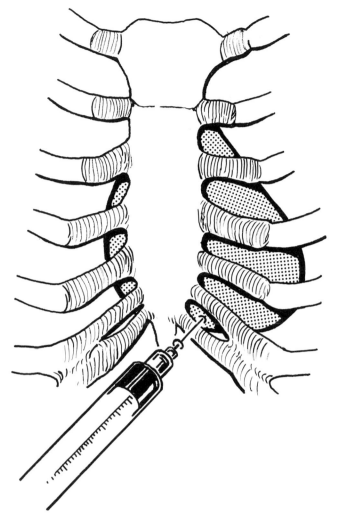

Figure 16.2.   Pericardiocentesis by a paraxiphoid approach with the needle advanced in a 45° plane.

authors recommend the procedure as a routine step prior to thoracotomy (26, 32, 45, 46), in our opinion and that of others (10, 11, 47, 48), the procedure is unnecessary in stable patients when the diagnosis of tamponade is definite. For patients who are unstable, the procedure of choice is an immediate thoracotomy without further delay.

Definitive Management
The definitive management of cardiac injuries is cardiorrhaphy through a thoracotomy or sternotomy. The surgical relief of tamponade and repair of cardiac lacerations should be performed as expeditiously as possible. Traditionally, a left anterior or anterolateral thoracotomy has been the incision of choice and is carried out through the fifth intercostal space. Further exposure, if necessary, is obtained by transsternal extension into the right chest. The pericardium is opened anterior to the phrenic nerve and the tamponade is relieved. The bleeding heart is controlled by digital occlusion and the laceration is sutured with horizontal mattress sutures of 3-0 Tevdck over Teflon

pledgets or strips of pericardium. Occasionally, a prosthetic mesh has been used to close a large defect caused by a missile (19, 20). Lacerations in proximity to the coronary vessels need special attention. Horizontal mattress sutures placed underneath the vessels avoid obstructing the coronary flow. Injury to major coronary vessels may be repaired primarily with or without cardioplumonary bypass. Penetrated and bleeding coronary branches may be ligated.

Wounds in the atria, cavae, or aorta can be controlled by placement of vascular clamps followed by running sutures. Larger wounds occasionally may require temporary in-flow occlusion by compression of the right atrium at the superior vena cava, placement of lateral vascular clamps, and repair.

Median sternotomy has been used in some centers for these lesions. The incision provides superb exposure of the heart and great vessels, facilitates access to the pulmonary hila, and permits extension to the abdomen for excellent exposure of the dome of the liver and other upper abdominal organs. This approach does have disadvantages: sternal infection is a rare but serious complication and posterior mediastinal structures such as the aorta and the esophagus are difficult to reach. In addition, rotating the heart to repair posterior wounds may be complicated by arrhythmias, which may result in a fatality. Consequently, this approach is avoided when the trajectory of the missile suggests a posterior injury.

Helpful ancillary techniques include autotransfusion, fine-screen filtration of blood, and cardiopulmonary bypass (10, 11, 43, 47, 48). Successful resuscitation of a heart in arrhythmia or fibrillation requires careful attention to detail. Defibrillation of an empty, acidotic, and hypoxic heart seldom is successful. Prompt volume expansion, correction of acidosis, maintenance of coronary perfusion by effective massage of the heart, and avoidance of hypothermia are crucial prerequisites for successful cardioversion. These conditions should be optimized before attempting defibrillation, since repeated attempts at defibrillation cause significant heat build-up and myocardial damage and minimize the chances for success.

These management concepts have yielded satisfactory results in penetrating cardiac trauma. The prognosis for patients who are stable and who can be transported to the operating room for definitive treatment is excellent. In our own experience with 228 patients with cardiac injuries (5), the survival for this subset of patients was 96.8% for stab wounds and 71.4% for gunshot wounds. Similar survival patterns were recorded by other authors (11, 12, 19, 20, 25, 27, 42–44, 49–58).

The Concept of Emergency Room Thoracotomy

Many patients who, in former years, would have died at the scene now arrive in extremis at the emergency center and require immediate and definitive management. They cannot tolerate further delay in the relief of cardiac tamponade while they are transported to an operating room located elsewhere in the hospital. Thus, the concept of emergency room thoracotomy (ERT) in well-equipped resuscitation rooms in the receiving area of the hospital was born. Steichen et al. (58), from our institution, were among the first proponents of this concept for penetrating cardiac trauma. Mattox and associates (10, 11, 47, 48) popularized the approach, which has now been extended to cardiac as well as noncardiac injuries, both blunt and penetrating. The procedure has been reported in community hospitals as well (59). Several critical reviews have analyzed the indications, patient selection, and the results of the procedure (3, 7, 21, 60–73). It is now apparent that the most pressing indication for ERT is the patient in extremis from cardiac tamponade due to penetrating chest trauma (4, 5, 8, 10, 11, 47, 48, 74).

INDICATIONS AND PATIENT SELECTION FOR ERT

As indicated in Figure 16.1, the absence of prompt stabilization after initial resuscitative efforts in a patient in extremis from penetrating chest trauma should prompt an immediate ERT. More specific indications for ERT can be defined by a patient classification of a graded severity of physiologic abnormality, based on the presenting clinical status (Table 16.1) (4–8, 67, 68). Patients who do not exhibit any signs of life in the prehospital phase usually are unsalvageable, and ERT or other attempts at resuscitation are futile. Patients in the "fatal" and "agonal" groups need immediate ERT for any chance of survival. Patients presenting in "profound shock" with a systolic blood pressure of less than 80 mm Hg can be managed initially by volume expansion. But lack of stabilization should prompt an immediate ERT. Deviation from this protocol results in increased mortality. For instance, five of our patients in the agonal group were transported to the operating room for a thoracotomy, and all of them died despite having potentially reparable cardiac and associated injuries (5). In each instance, tense tamponade was found at thoracotomy and would have been decompressed by an ERT. The technical details of ERT and the precautions and the pitfalls of the procedure have been described in an excellent review by Feliciano and Mattox (75) and should be studied by physicians interested in the procedure.

RESULTS OF ERT IN PATIENTS WITH NO VITAL SIGNS ON ADMISSION

In this group of patients, ERT yields the best results in the presence of definite cardiac trauma (Table 16.2). A considerable chance for survival is still possible even in the absence of cardiac activity or pupillary reactivity. Hence, ERT is indicated for patients who present "clinically dead" as long as there were some signs of life in the immediate prehospital phase.

The results of ERT for penetrating cardiac injuries in different series are difficult to analyze. As is apparent from Table 16.3, the terms employed to describe these patients are not uniform. The considerable variation in salvage rates may also be related to the relative number of stab wounds versus gunshot wounds in different series. For instance, Schwab et al. (69) documented survival of 13 of 14 patients in an agonal state, all with stab wounds. The results with gunshot wounds are much less favorable. Our classification of the patients undergoing ERT is described in Table 16.1 and correlates well with prognosis. The approximate survival in these four groups is 0, 30, 40 and 50%, respectively.

Table 16.1.
Classification of Patients Based on Presenting Vital Signs

Classification	Vital Signs
Dead on arrival	None on admission or in the prehospital phase
Fatal	None on admission but vital signs in transit to hospital
Agonal	Semiconscious, no palpable blood pressure, gasping respiration
Profound shock	Systolic blood pressure <80 mm Hg, alert

Table 16.2.
Results of Emergency Room Thoracotomy in Patients without Vital Signs on Admission after Penetrating Cardiac Trauma

Study	n	Survival
Steichen et al., 1971 (58)	21	33%
Mattox et al., 1974 (47, 48)	11	0
DeGennaro et al., 1980 (28)	13	15
Baker et al., 1980 (21)	29	17
Ivatury et al., 1981 (4)	22	36
Rohman et al., 1983 (68)	53	32
Demetriades, 1984 (53)	11	9
Tavares et al., 1984 (70)	13	23
Ivatury et al., 1987 (5–9)	63	30

QUANTIFYING THE SEVERITY OF ANATOMIC AND PHYSIOLOGIC INJURY FROM PENETRATING CARDIAC TRAUMA

The preceding discussion and a consideration of Table 16.2 establish the difficulty in evaluating and comparing different series of penetrating cardiac injuries. Trinkle (76) recently pointed out the difficulties in making patient and outcome comparisons between different clinical series. Invatury et al. (6) recently have proposed a severity index scheme for cardiac and thoracic injuries to quantify cardiac trauma in terms of its anatomic and physiologic injury severity. Since the magnitude of the associated injuries

Table 16.3.
Results of Emergency Room Thoracotomy in Penetrating Cardiac Injuries

Study	Total n	Survival		Clinical Status
		n	%	
Steichen et al., 1971 (58)	21	7	33	Lifeless
Beall et al., 1971 (29)	18	5	28	Cardiac arrest
Mattox et al., 1974 (47, 48)	37	25	68	Minimal signs
Sherman et al., 1978 (57)	41	9	22	Terminal
Breaux et al., 1979 (41)	44	5	11	No vital signs
Oparah and Mandal, 1979 (56)	14	2	14	Cardiac arrest
Baker et al., 1980 (21)	29	5	17	No vital signs
Ivatury et al., 1981 (4)	22	8	36	Fatal
Rohman et al., 1983 (68)	73	24	33	In extremis
Vij et al., 1983 (71)	25	4	16	Cardiac arrest
Demetriades, 1984 (53)	11	1	9	No vital signs
Danne et al., 1984 (3)	33	?	40	Extremis
Tavares et al., 1984 (70)	37	21	57	Pulseless, no blood pressure
Roberge et al., 1986 (67)	31	6	20	Extremis
Schwab et al., 1986 (69)	18	13	72	Agonal
Ivatury et al., 1981, 1987 (4–9)	91	28	31	In extremis[a]

[a]Majority of the patients without signs of life at the scene.

Table 16.4.
Quantifying Penetrating Cardiac Injury

Anatomic
    Organ risk factor: 5
    Injury severity estimate
        1. Tangential, involving pericardium or wall up to but not through the endocardium
        2. Single right-side chamber
        3. Comminuted tears of single chamber
        4. Multiple chambers, isolated left atrial or ventricular injury
        5. Coronary vessel injury, major intracardiac defects
Cardiac trauma index: 5 × injury severity estimate
Total thoracic trauma index: sum of the indices of all thoracic organs
Penetrating trauma index: thoracic trauma index + abdominal trauma index

Physiologic: physiologic index
    Fatal[a]   20
    Agonal   15
    Profound shock[a]   10
    Stable   5

[a]Clinical description as in Table 16.1.

plays a role in prognosis, the scheme supplements the Abdominal Trauma Index described by Moore et al. (77). As with the Abdominal Trauma Index, the Thoracic Trauma Index is based on an analysis of the organ risk factor and the severity of organ injury. Table 16.4 depicts the risk factors and organ severity index for thoracic organs and the calculation of the total Penetrating Trauma Index.

Cardiac tamponade produces a physiologic disruption that is out of proportion to its anatomic injury. Therefore, an evaluation of the resulting physiologic derangement is particularly important. For this reason, the physiologic injury severity should also be quantified and taken into account, as demonstrated in Table 16.4. An analysis of 112 patients with penetrating cardiac injuries (6) revealed these indices to have an excellent correlation with survival. Such a scheme of description of injury severity in future reports on cardiac trauma will allow a more scientific analysis of the therapeutic results.

PROGNOSTIC FACTORS IN PENETRATING CARDIAC TRAUMA

The favorable prognostic factors in cardiac trauma are single chamber injuries, stab wounds, and absence of significant intracardiac defects (19, 20). Hemodynamic stability on arrival or rapid stabilization by initial resuscitation resulting in transportation to the operating room for a thoracotomy is associated with a significantly higher survival (5). Moreno et al. (26) demonstrated that pericardial tamponade may have a protective effect by forestalling exsanguination; 73% of their patients with tamponade survived as opposed to 11% without tamponade.

The presence of significant associated injuries, gunshot wounds, coronary vessel lacerations, and multiple chamber injuries, as well as delayed diagnosis and treatment, are unfavorable prognostic factors. Since delay of definitive therapy by thoracotomy and cardiorrhaphy is an important prognostic consideration, the prehospital care of these patients must be optimized and time delay minimized.

"RESIDUAL AND DELAYED SEQUELAE" OF PENETRATING CARDIAC TRAUMA

Recent advances in noninvasive and invasive evaluation of cardiac hemodynamics have led to the discovery of an increasing number of intracardiac complications ("residual and delayed sequelae" (78)) in the survivors of penetrating cardiac trauma. Symbas et al. (78) were among the first authors to define this problem and presented their follow-up data in 56 patients with cardiac trauma. Fourteen patients had 16 instances of delayed sequelae: intracardiac shunts in five patients, valvular lesions in three patients, ventricular aneurysms in five patients, and retained foreign bodies in three patients. Fallahnejad et al. (79, 80) followed 29 of their survivors for 2 weeks to 15 yr. Secondary complications developed in 15 patients (50%) and included ventricular septal defect in four patients and aortocaval and aortopulmonary fistulae in two patients. Interestingly, routine postoperative cardiac evaluation in seven of nine patients in the later half of the study period revealed significant, unsuspected cardiac lesions in six. Based on these data, an aggressive, detailed evaluation was recommended for all survivors of penetrating cardiac injuries. Mattox et al. (81) followed all of their survivors of penetrating cardiac trauma with physical examination, cardiac enzyme determination, and electrocardiography. Symptomatic patients and patients with abnormal physical signs underwent further evaluation by two-dimensional and pulsed-Doppler echocardiography and/or cardiac catheterization. The echocardiogram was abnormal in 30 of the 37 symptomatic patients. Right ventricular turbulence from fistulae or a ventricular septal defect was detected in five patients, all of whom had secondary surgery for these conditions. Based on their observations, they recommended a scheme of evaluation of the postcardiorraphy patient (81), which is summarized in Fig 16.3. Such an evaluation should be a part of the management of penetrating cardiac trauma.

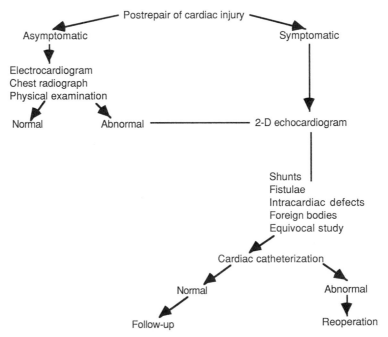

Figure 16.3. Cardiac evaluation after repair of penetrating heart wounds. (After Mattox KL, Limacher MC, Feliciano DV, et al. J Trauma 1985;25:758–765.)

Missile embolization from the heart to the systemic vessels is a potential complication after cardiac gunshot wounds. It is described in detail by Symbas and Harlaftis (82), Mattox et al. (83), and Graham and Mattox (84).

LINCOLN HOSPITAL SERIES

We recently analyzed a 20-year experience at our institution with 228 patients with penetrating cardiac injuries (5). Of 112 patients who arrived *with* vital signs, 82 survived (including 78.7% of 89 patients with knife wounds and 52.2% of 23 with gunshot wounds). Eighty-nine patients arrived "in extremis," 61.8% of whom could be stabilized by ERT and transported to the operating room for definitive cardiorrhaphy. Twenty-six patients (29.2%) in this subset eventually were discharged from the hospital. Twenty-seven patients were dead on arrival and had no vital signs in the prehospital period—the truly "dead-on-arrival" group; none of these patients could be resuscitated. Furthermore, the ratio of patients who were moribund on arrival to those with vital signs was 1:1.5 in the first 7 yr of the study as opposed to 1:0.5 in the last 7 yr. Interestingly, the survival rate for patients with stab wounds arriving with vital signs on admission increased from 76.7% in the first 7 yr to 95.8% in the last 7 yr of the study. However, in these two periods, the salvage rate for "in extremis" patients decreased from 41.2 to 22.7%. In addition, there was a yearly increase of gunshot wounds of the heart as well as an increase in the incidence of patients presenting without vital signs. A survival of 33.3% was achieved for these moribund patients in the last 7 yr of the study.

SUMMARY

These data (Figs. 16.4 and 16.5) substantiate a changing pattern of clinical presentation of penetrating cardiac injuries. In addition to an observed increase in gunshot wounds,

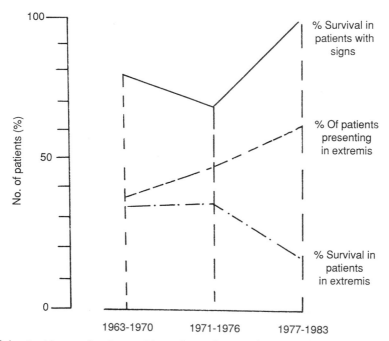

Figure 16.4. Incidence of patients with cardiac stab wounds presenting in extremis and their survival rates.

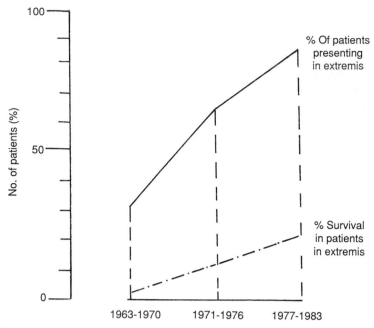

Figure 16.5. Incidence of patients with cardiac gunshot wounds presenting in extremis and their survival rates.

it appears that the patients with cardiac penetration are undergoing a process of self-selection. The more stable patients are reaching the hospital sooner and are being transported to the operating room with a significant survival rate (approximately 95% for stab wounds and 50% for missile wounds). Patients who would have died at the scene in former years are arriving at the emergency center with a few moments left for possible resuscitation. This group currently constitutes approximately 50% of the patients with penetrating cardiac trauma at this institution; they need desperate attempts, such as ERT, for resuscitation. Our current salvage has reached a plateau around 25–30% on a yearly basis for this group. Improved transport to the hospital of very severely injured patients in this desperate physiologic status may account for the improvement as well as a leveling off of our results. These data also point to the importance of ERT in urban trauma centers, which probably should be equipped with operating facilities in their receiving bays.

REFERENCES

1. Feliciano DV, Bitondo CG, Mattox KL, et al. Civilian trauma in the 1980's: a 1-year experience with 456 vascular and cardiac injuries. Ann Surg 1984;199:717–724.
2. Londono-Schimmer E, Ospinio-Londono J, De-La-Hoz J. Penetrating cardiac injuries. Presented at the 1st Pan American Trauma Society Congress, Puerto Rico, 1988.
3. Danne PD, Finelli F, Champion HR. Emergency bay thoracotomy. J Trauma 1984;24:796–802.
4. Ivatury RR, Shah PM, Ito K, et al. Emergency room thoracotomy for the resuscitation of patients with "fatal" penetrating injuries of the heart. Ann Thorac Surg 1981;32:377–385.
5. Ivatury RR, Rohman M, Steichen FM, et al. Penetrating cardiac injuries: twenty year experience. Am Surg 1987;53:310–317.
6. Ivatury RR, Nallathambi M, Rohman M, et al. Penetrating cardiac trauma: quantifying anatomic and physiologic injury severity. Ann Surg 1987;205:61–66.
7. Ivatury RR, Nallathambi M, Rohman M, et al. Penetrating thoracic injuries: in-field stabilization vs immediate transport. J Trauma 1987;27:1066–1073.

8. Ivatury RR, Rohman M. Emergency department thoracotomy for trauma: a collective review. Resuscitation 1987;15:23–35.

9. Ivatury RR, Rohman M, Nallathambi MN, Stahl W. Management of penetrating wounds of the heart. Surg Rounds 1987;12:39–47.

10. Mattox KL. Emergency department thoracotomy. J Am Coll Emerg Phys 1978;7:455.

11. Mattox KL, VonKoch L, Beall AC Jr, et al. Logistic and technical considerations in the treatment of the wounded heart. Circulation 1975;52:210–214

12. Karrel R, Shaffer MA, Franaszek JB. Emergency diagnosis, resuscitation, and treatment of acute penetrating cardiac trauma. Ann Emerg Med 1982;11:504–517.

13. Blalock A, Ravitch MM. A consideration of the nonoperative treatment of cardiac tamponade resulting from wounds of the heart. Surgery 1943;14:157–162.

14. Isaacs JP. Sixty penetrating wounds of the heart: clinical and experimental observations. Surgery 1959;45:696–708.

15. Wolfson HH, Moore EE, VanWay C. Delayed staple perforation of the heart: transthoracic migration with late tamponade. J Trauma 1986;26:293–294.

16. McGill JW, Moore EE, Marx JA, et al. Successful management of cardiac impalement: the result of an integrated EMS-trauma system. J Trauma 1986;26:702–705.

17. Cooley DA, Dunn RJ, Brockman ML, et al. Treatment of pericardial wounds of the heart: experimental and clinical observations. Surgery 1955;37:882–889.

18. Sugg WL, Rea WJ, Ecker RR, et al. Penetrating wounds of the heart: an analysis of 459 cases. J Thorac Cardiovasc Surg 1968;56:531–543.

19. Symbas PN. Cardiac trauma. Am Heart J 1976;92:387–396.

20. Symbas PN. Traumatic heart disease. Curr Prob Cardiol 1982;7:3–35.

21. Baker CC, Thomas AN, Trunkey DD. The role of emergency thoracotomy in trauma. J Trauma 1980;20:848–855.

22. Demetriades D, VanderVeen PW. Penetrating injuries of the heart: experience over two years in South Africa. J Trauma 1983;23:1034–1041.

23. Wechsler AS, Auerbach BJ, Graham TC, et al. Distribution of intramyocardial blood flow during pericardial tamponade. J Thorac Cardiovasc Surg 1984;68:847–856.

24. Carasquilla C, Wilson RF, Walt AJ, et al. Gunshot wounds of the heart. Ann Thorac Surg 1972;13:208–213.

25. Tassi A, Davies AL. Pericardial tamponade due to penetrating fragment wounds of the heart. Am J Surg 1977;118:535–538.

26. Moreno C, Moore EE, Majure JA, et al. Pericardial tamponade: a critical determinant for survival following penetrating cardiac wounds. J Tauama 1986;26:821–825.

27. Siemens R, Polk HC, Gray LA, et al. Indications for thoracotomy following penetrating thoracic injury. J Trauma 1977;17:493–500.

28. DeGennaro VA, Bonfils-Roberts EA, Ching N, et al. Aggressive management of potential penetrating cardiac injuries. J Thorac Cardiovasc Surg 1980;79:833–837.

29. Beall AC Jr, Gasior RM, Bricker DL. Gunshot wounds of the heart: changing patterns of surgical management. Ann Thorac Surg 1971;11:523–531.

30. Beall AC Jr, Patrick TA, Okies JE, et al. Penetrating wounds of the heart: changing patterns of surgical management. J Trauma 1972;12:468–473.

31. Michelow BJ, Bremmer CG. Penetrating cardiac injuries: selective conservatism—favorable or foolish? J Trauma 1987;27:398–401.

32. Trinkle JK, Marcos J, Grover FL, et al. Management of the wounded heart. Ann Thorac Surg 1974;17:230–236.

33. Fulda G. Rodriguez A, Turney SZ, Cowley RA. Blunt traumatic pericardial rupture: a 10-year experience (1979 to 1989). Presented at the XIX World Congress of the International Society for Cardiovascular Surgery, Toronto, 1989.

34. Duncan A, Scalea T, Phillips T, et al. Evaluation of occult cardiac injuries using subxiphoid pericardial window. Presented at the American Association for the Surgery of Trauma meeting, New Port Beach, California, 1988.

35. Border JR, Lewis FR, Aprahamian CA, et al. Pre-hospital care: stabilize or scoop and run [Panel]. J Trauma 1983;23:708–711.

36. Coppas MK, Oreskovich MR, Bladergroen MR, et al. Prehospital cardiopulmonary resuscitation of the critically injured patient. Am J Surg 1984;148:20–26.

37. Smith JP, Bodai BI, Hill AS, et al. Prehospital stabilization of critically injured patients: a failed concept. J Trauma 1985;25:65–70.

38. Mattox KL, Feliciano DV. Role of external cardiac compression in truncal trauma. J Trauma 1982;22:934–936.

39. Jacobs LM, Sinclair A, Beiser A, et al. Prehospital advanced life support: benefits in trauma. J Trauma 1984;24:8–13.

40. Gervin AS, Fischer RP. The importance of prompt transport in salvage of patients with penetrating heart wounds. J Trauma 1982;22:443–448.

41. Breaux ED, Dupont BJ Jr, Albert HM, et al. Cardiac tamponade following penetrating mediastinal injuries. J Trauma 1979;19:461–466.

42. Evans J, Gray LA, Rayner A, et al. Principles for the management of penetrating cardiac wounds. Ann Surg 1979;189:777–784.

43. Levitsky S. New insights in cardiac trauma. Surg Clin North Am 1975;55:43–55.

44. Tate JS, Horan PD. Penetrating injuries of the heart. Surg Gynecol Obstet 1983;157:57–63.

45. Arom KV, Richardson JD, Webb G, et al. Subxiphoid pericardial window in patients with suspected traumatic pericardial tamponade. Ann Thorac Surg 1977;23:545–549.

46. Trinkle JK, Toon RS, Franc JL, et al. Affairs of the wounded heart: penetrating cardiac wounds. J Trauma 1979;19:467–472.

47. Mattox KL, Espada R, Beall AC Jr. Performing thoracotomy in the emergency center. J Am Coll Emerg Phys 1974;3:13–17.

48. Mattox KL, Beall AC Jr, Jordan GL Jr, et al. Cardiorrhaphy in the emergency center. J Thorac Cardiovasc Surg 1974;68:886–895.

49. Beach PM Jr, Bognolo D, Hutchinson JE. Penetrating cardiac trauma. Am J Surg 1976;131:411–414.

50. Bolanowski PJ, Swaminathan AP, Neville WE. Aggressive surgical management of penetrating cardiac injuries. J Thorac Cardiovasc Surg 1973;66:52.

51. Borja AR, Lansing AM, Ransdell HT Jr. Immediate operative treatment for stab wounds of the heart. J Thorac Cardiovasc Surg 1970;50:662–667.

52. Boyd TS, Streider JW. Immediate surgery for traumatic heart disease. J Thorac Cardiovasc Surg 1973;50:305–315.

53. Demetriades D. Cardiac penetrating injuries: personal experience of 45 cases. Br J Surg 1984;71:95–97.

54. Kish G, Kozloff L, Joseph W, et al. Indications for early thoracotomy in the management of chest trauma. Ann Thorac Surg 1976;22:23–28.

55. Maynard ADI, Cordice JW, Naclerio EA. Penetrating wounds of the heart: report of 81 cases. Surg Gynecol Obstet 1952;94:605–618.

56. Oparah SS, Mandal AK. Operative management of penetrating wounds of the chest in civilian practice: review of indications in 125 consecutive cases. J Thorac Cardiovasc Surg 1979;68:886–895.

57. Sherman MM, Saini YK, Yarnoz MD, et al. Management of penetrating heart wounds. Am J Surg 1978;135:553–558.

58. Steichen FM, Dargan EL, Efron G, et al. A graded approach to the management of penetrating wounds of the heart. Arch Surg 1971;103:574–580.

59. MacDonald JR, McDowell RM. Emergency department thoracotomies in a community hospital. J Am Coll Emerg Physicians 1978;7:423–428.

60. Bodai BI, Smith JP, Blaisdell FW. The role of emergency thoracotomy in blunt trauma. J Trauma 1982;22:487–491.

61. Bodai BI, Smith JP, Ward RE, et al. Emergency thoracotomy in the management of trauma: a review. JAMA 1983;249:1891–1896.

62. Cogbill TH, Moore EE, Millikan JS, et al. Rationale for selective application of emergency department thoracotomy in trauma. J Trauma 1983;23:453–460.

63. Feliciano DV, Bitondo CG, Cruise PA, et al. Liberal use of emergency center thoracotomy. Am J Surg 1986;152:654–659.

64. Flynn TC, Ward RE, Miller PW. Emergency room thoracotomy. Ann Emerg Med 1982;11:413–416.

65. Hoffman JR. Emergency department thoracotomy. Ann Emerg Med 1981;10:275–278.

66. Moore EE, Moore JB, Galloway AC, et al. Post-injury thoracotomy in the emergency department: a critical evaluation. Surgery 1979;86:590–598.

67. Roberge RJ, Ivatury RR, Stahl WM, et al. Emergency department thoracotomy for penetrating injuries: predictive value of patient classification. Am J Emerg Med 1986;4:129–135.

68. Rohman M, Ivatury RR, Steichen FM, et al. Emergency room thoracotomy for penetrating cardiac injuries. J Trauma 1983;23:570–576.

69. Schwab CW, Adcock OT, Max MH. Emergency department thoracotomy (EDT): a 26-month experience using an "agonal" protocol. Am Surg 1986;52:20–29.

70. Tavares S, Hankins JR, Moulton AL, et al. Management of penetrating cardiac injuries: the role of emergency room thoracotomy. Ann Surg 1984;38:183–187.

71. Vij D, Simoni E, Smith E, et al. Resuscitative thoracotomy for patients with traumatic injury. Surgery 1983;94:554–561.

72. Washington BW, Wilson RF, Steiger Z, et al. Emergency thoracotomy: a four-year review. Ann Thorac Surg 1985;40:188–191.

73. Wahlstrom HE, Carroll BJ, Phillips EH. Emergency thoracotomy: indications and technique. Surg Rounds 1986;11:23–34.

74. Shimazu S, Shatney CH. Outcome of trauma patients with no vital signs on hospital admission. J Trauma 1983;23:213–217.

75. Feliciano DV, Mattox KL. Indications, techniques and pitfalls of emergency center thoracotomy. Surg Rounds 1981;12:32–40.

76. Trinkle JK. Penetrating heart wounds: difficulty in evaluating clinical series. Ann Thorac Surg 1984;38:181–182.

77. Moore EE, Dunn EL, Moore JB, et al. Penetrating abdominal trauma index. J Trauma 1981;21:439–445.

78. Symbas PN, DiOrio DA, Tyras DH, et al. Penetrating cardiac wounds: significant residual and delayed sequelae. J Thorac Cardiovasc Surg 1973;66:526–532.

79. Fallahnejad M, Wallace HW, Su CC, et al. Unusual manifestations of penetrating cardiac injuries. Arch Surg 1975;110:1357–1362.

80. Fallahnejad M, Kutty ACK, Wallace HW. Secondary lesions of penetrating cardiac injuries. A frequent complication. Ann Surg 1980;191:228–233.

81. Mattox KL, Limacher MC, Feliciano DV, et al. Cardiac evaluation following heart injury. J Trauma 1985;25:758–765.

82. Symbas PN, Harlaftis N. Bullet emboli in the pulmonary and systemic arteries. Ann Surg 1977;185:318–320.

83. Mattox KL, Beall AC Jr, Ennix CL, et al. Intravascular migratory bullets. Am J Surg 1979;137:192–195.

84. Graham JM, Mattox KL. Right ventricular embolectomy without cardiopulmonary bypass. J Thorac Cardiovasc Surg 1981;82:310–313.

17 The Child with Thoracic Trauma

Kurt D. Newman, MD
Martin R. Eichelberger, MD

The care of the child who sustains cardiothoracic trauma is a major challenge. At the Children's National Medical Center (CNMC) in Washington, DC, of 2400 (4.5%) trauma admissions in 36 months, 104 children manifested injury to the chest; the median age was 5 yr, 20% were under the age of 2, and the overall mortality rate was 25%, an astounding fact (1). Most children demonstrate multisystem organ injury. If the child sustains an isolated thoracic injury, the mortality rate is 5%; however, if other organ systems are involved, the mortality rate reaches up to 47% for combined injury to the head, chest, and abdomen. Principles fundamental to maintaining ventilation and perfusion require understanding of the special differences in anatomy, physiology, and mechanism of injury unique to children.

Although once rare, cardiothoracic trauma is now seen more frequently at pediatric trauma centers. This trend is due not only to an increased incidence, but also to improved methods of field triage and resuscitation that increase the likelihood of successful transport to the trauma center. The mechanisms of injury are grouped in three main categories: pedestrian/vehicular, passenger/vehicular, and penetrating injury. The most common mechanism is a pedestrian being struck by a car (37% in our series), followed by injuries sustained as a passenger in a motor vehicle crash (31%). In large metropolitan areas, penetrating trauma is more frequent than in rural areas, accounting for 10% of thoracic injuries; burns also cause injury to the thorax.

Children are different from adults in more than just age. The differences in anatomy and physiology alter the response of a child to thoracic injury and necessitate modifications in management. The anatomic differences of a child's airway, for example, are critical (2). The tongue is quite large relative to the smaller oropharynx and obstructs easily. The epiglottis is floppy and difficult to displace during intubation. The larynx is more anterior and cephalad than in the adult, making esophageal intubation a hazard. The cartilaginous and distensible vocal cords are more prone to damage. The narrowest part of the airway of a child is at the cricoid ring; subglottic stenosis is a result of prolonged intubation, and enlargement of the tonsils or adenoids makes vocal cord visualization difficult. Uncuffed endotracheal tubes are used to avoid edema and pressure necrosis. The trachea of infants and young children is short, requiring careful placement of endotracheal tubes to avoid bronchial intubation or perforation. Successful management of the airway of a child with thoracic trauma requires knowledge of these differences.

The chest structure of a child is also quite different from that of an adult (3). The thorax is extremely compliant because of the greater elasticity of the bones and greater cartilage content. The anterior/posterior diameter of the chest cavity is smaller. With blunt trauma, the child may incur severe internal injury without trauma to the skeletal structures of the chest. The mediastinum is more freely moveable, especially in infants and young children. Tension pneumothorax causes wide displacement of the heart, resulting in angulation of the great vessels, reduction of venous return to the right side of the heart, and resultant decrease in cardiac output, impairing adequate peripheral perfusion. Mediastinal displacement also compresses the lung and angulates the trachea, further compromising the child.

A child's small size makes providing intravenous access and maintaining thermoregulation difficult (4). Percutaneous venous cannulation is possible but not absolutely reliable; rapid access is via the surgical, cut-down technique of the saphenous vein at the ankle and groin; the cephalic vein at the elbow is used less frequently. Unnecessary central venous access lines should be avoided since pneumothorax or subclavian artery laceration is possible. Resuscitation with fluid is safe and effective through a peripheral intravenous cannula. Intraosseus infusion is useful for small children when venous access is difficult.

Because a child's blood volume is small (80 ml/kg), the loss of a relatively small amount leads to hypovolemia and shock (5). The child's larger body surface area relative to weight, combined with less skin and fat insulation, creates a propensity for hypothermia and metabolic acidosis. Overhead heaters, warming blankets, and blood warmers prevent heat loss.

The psychology and behavior of a child create unique challenges for the trauma team (6). Natural behavior patterns and curiosity may lead to foreign body aspiration, toxin ingestion, or burns. Altered family dynamics result in child abuse, which leads to "battered" children and potential thoracic trauma. Children may be unable to express themselves, leading to difficulty in localizing pain and injury.

A common response to injury by the child is aerophagia and tachypnea. The resulting gastric dilatation reduces diaphragmatic excursion that compromises ventilation. Reflex ileus exacerbates the situation, so nasogastric tube placement is necessary to relieve the gastric distension and prevent aspiration. Pneumoperitoneum from a perforation of the stomach or small bowel can also impede diaphragmatic excursion; needle aspiration is lifesaving (7).

Unlike adults, children rarely have preexisting disease of the lungs and heart. However, neonates excrete sodium with less efficiency and are unable to concentrate urine as well as older children and adults; care must be taken to avoid sodium overload during and after resuscitation (8). Newborns are also more susceptible to infection because their immune defense system is immature. Trauma produces greater depression of the immune system in children than in adults (9). Adequate nutrition is of prime importance to children recovering from trauma; 19% of patients in the pediatric intensive care unit at CNMC were found to have acute protein calorie malnutrition (10). Although children are generally healthy, the surgeon caring for children with chest trauma must pay special attention to the nuances of the immature and developing physiologic systems.

RESUSCITATION

Resuscitation of the child with cardiothoracic trauma begins with airway management followed by evaluation of the mechanics of breathing and restoration of adequate circulation. Assume the presence of a cervical spine injury in all children. Initially, protect the cervical spine with in-line stabilization of the neck or a rigid collar while providing 100% oxygen. Suction the oropharynx to remove all secretions and any foreign body that may be present. Next, use the chin lift or jaw thrust to displace the tongue forward and open the upper airway. Frequently, mask-assisted ventilation improves oxygenation and ventilation. Any doubt concerning patency of the upper airway requires orotracheal intubation, which also prevents aspiration when a head injury or altered consciousness is present. Upper airway obstruction, manifested by stridor, either from direct tracheal injury or edema, is an indication for needle cricothyroidotomy or tracheostomy to provide airway access.

Once the airway is secure, the adequacy of ventilation or breathing requires evaluation. If pneumothorax is present, a needle thoracocentesis in the midaxillary line and the fourth intercostal space evacuates the air efficiently. A chest tube directed to the apex of the lung is imperative. In a small infant, use a no. 12 French tube; in a larger child, use a no. 20 to 24 French tube. Ensure intravenous access and resuscitate the child with fluid prior to insertion of the thoracostomy tube if there is lack of ventilation due to hemothorax. If the respirations are compromised by open pneumothorax, cover the defect with Vaseline-impregnated gauze and a sterile dressing and place a chest tube through a separate site. Flail chest is rare in children but is treated with positive end-expiratory pressure. Evaluate the adequacy of ventilation by serial blood gas analysis.

After establishment of an airway and ventilation, management of the circulation and prevention of shock are essential. First, apply direct pressure to sites of external bleeding and establish venous access. Begin external cardiac massage if the child is in cardiac arrest. The initial treatment of shock is resuscitation with crystalloid fluid infusion: 20 ml/kg of Ringer's lactate. If the signs of perfusion (capillary refill, pulse rate, blood pressure) do not improve, repeat the 20 ml/kg fluid infusion. If the response is inadequate, the child should be given packed red blood cells (10 ml/kg) to help improve the circulation (11). Children unresponsive to rapid volume infusion who manifest a decrease in pulse pressure, neck vein distension, or pulsus paradoxus require pericardiocentesis to treat cardiac tamponade.

The indications for emergency room thoracotomy are a penetrating wound of the heart, continuous intrapleural hemorrhage, or an open pneumothorax with a major defect of the chest. Usually, delay thoracotomy until transfer to the operating room. Urgent indications are an aortic laceration, a ruptured esophagus, a massive pleural air leak suggestive of a ruptured bronchus, or a traumatic diaphragmatic hernia.

INJURY PROFILE

The severity of injury depends upon the specific mechanism of injury, the force applied, and the response of the organs of the injured child. Mortality relates directly to the number and type of organ systems injured. When only the chest is injured, the mortality rate is 5%; the rate rises to 15% for chest and abdominal injuries, to 32% for chest and head injuries, and to 47% when injuries occur to the chest, head, and abdomen. Within the thoracic trauma category, there is a broad spectrum of injury.

Chest Wall Injury

Chest wall injury can be as minor as a contusion or as severe as a flail chest. The chest wall and supporting structures of the young child are very compliant and often diffuse the kinetic energy. Soft-tissue hemorrhage may result from a blunt injury producing a contusion; but do not overlook significant blood loss from a superficial laceration.

Chest trauma can fracture a child's ribs (12); at CNMC, 38% of children admitted with chest trauma have sustained rib fractures. Many of the fractures are painful and lead to splinting; however, respiratory compromise from atelectasis is rare. Analgesics provide effective pain control, but persistent severe pain is best managed by an intercostal nerve block with bupivacaine hydrochloride (Marcaine). A rib fracture can secondarily produce a pneumothorax that requires thoracostomy tube placement for treatment, life-threatening hemorrhage from a pleural tear, or intercostal vessel injury from ragged bone edges (13). Rib fractures usually heal in 6 weeks.

Although more common in adults, sternal fracture is rare in children since steering-wheel impact is an infrequent mechanism of injury. Rib fracture in children is an indicator of severe injury; in our series, 47% of children with rib fractures died from associated severe injuries.

Flail Chest

Although the chest wall of a child is flexible, severe blunt trauma can produce a free floating segment of the chest wall known as flail chest. Injury to multiple ribs destroys the integrity of the chest wall and the muscles of breathing, producing an asynchronous flail segment (14). Although quite rare in childhood, flail chest is suspected when the mechanism of injury is blunt trauma from a motor vehicle crash or child abuse. A contusion or ecchymosis in the soft tissue often leads to the recognition of the fractured ribs. The most characteristic sign is paradoxical movement of the flail segment with breathing. Since the flail segment is no longer in continuity with the rest of the chest wall, changes in intrathoracic pressure govern its movement. Upon inspiration, the flail segment collapses inward, while the rest of the thorax is expanding. On expiration the opposite occurs as the flail segment moves outward with positive intrathoracic pressure. Insufficient ventilation caused by the impairment of chest wall integrity produces respiratory compromise. The thorax cannot generate the pressures necessary to move air well. A child's mediastinum swings back and forth with the pressure changes, impairing venous return to the right side of the heart and compressing the contralateral lung. Associated pneumothorax worsens an already tenuous ventilation. Pulmonary contusion produced by the blunt trauma leads to further impairment of gas exchange.

Treatment is directed at reducing the edema and hemorrhage from the underlying pulmonary contusion (15). The child is most often intubated and placed on positive end-expiratory pressure. Chest tube placement evacuates air and blood from the pleural space, and careful control of fluid administration prevents excess alveolar interstitial edema formation. Flail chest is rarely an isolated injury, and mortality relates to the associated injuries (16).

Pneumothorax

Both blunt and penetrating trauma produce pneumothorax. Blunt trauma to the chest wall creates a pneumothorax when a rib is fractured; the sharp fragments puncture the pleura, allowing air into the pleural space. Penetrating trauma produces pneumothorax when air is introduced into the pleural space either from outside through the laceration or when the lung is injured by a missile or blade. Simple pneumothorax is created when air in the pleural space accumulates, causing the lung to collapse on that side. Suspect pneumothorax in all gunshot wounds to the chest, flank, or abdomen since the actual trajectory of a bullet is difficult to gauge.

The child with pneumothorax often displays signs of respiratory compromise with tachypnea, pallor, and hemoglobin desaturation. Physical examination reveals diminished or absent breath sounds on the involved side in association with increased resonance to percussion. Obtain a chest x-ray if the child is stable. Air in the pleural space and collapse of the ipsilateral lung are diagnostic. Chest tube insertion resolves the pneumothorax immediately. If the child is unstable, place a chest tube on the involved side without chest x-ray confirmation; morbidity is low and the maneuver is lifesaving. At CNMC, pneumothorax was present in 40% of children with cardiothoracic injuries. The mortality rate among children who sustained a pneumothorax as one of their injuries was 30%.

Ongoing accumulation of air in the pleural space from pulmonary parenchymal or bronchial injury produces tension pneumothorax. The increasing air cannot escape, creates pressure, and compresses the ipsilateral lung. The mediastinum then shifts away from the involved side. As the mediastinum shifts, compression of the contralateral lung and angulation of the great vessels increases. Venous return to the heart is diminished and hypotension and shock ensue if untreated. Since children have such flexible, moveable mediastinums, this scenario may occur very quickly. Suspect tension pneumothorax in any child with trauma to the chest, respiratory distress, and shock. Tension pneumothorax occasionally develops in a delayed fashion following intubation and positive pressure ventilation in children with injury to the lung parenchyma. Needle aspiration of the pleura followed by chest tube placement is lifesaving (Figs. 17.1–17.9). Chest tube placement will evacuate air and improve the mechanics of ventilation. A chest x-ray will confirm proper chest tube placement and the effectiveness of air evacuation.

Although rare, penetrating trauma can produce an open pneumothorax, a potentially lethal injury. The wound produces a hole through which air can enter the thorax. The chest wall no longer generates negative intrathoracic pressure, compromising ventilation and permitting air to rush into the pleural space, which produces a "sucking" chest wound. Initial treatment requires wound closure to restore chest wall

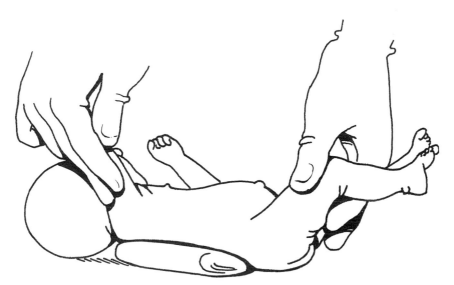

Figure 17.1. Assemble all equipment and tubes of appropriate size. Position the infant with the affected side elevated by a small roll.

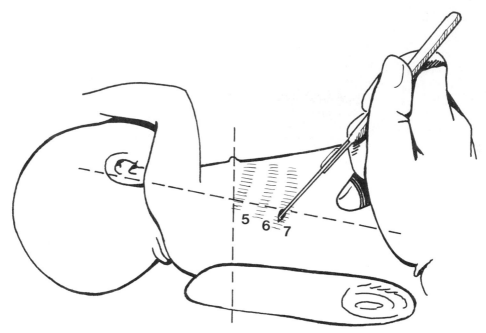

Figure 17.2. Using sterile technique and local anesthesia, make a small incision in the midaxillary line in the sixth (6) or seventh (7) intercostal space.

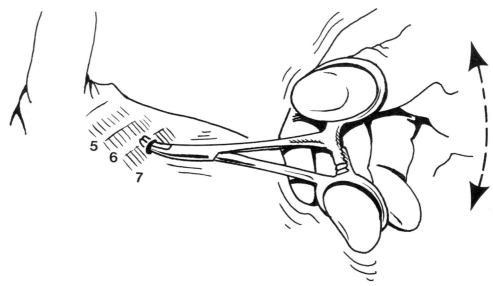

Figure 17.3. Make a subcutaneous tunnel using a small hemostat up to the fourth intercostal space.

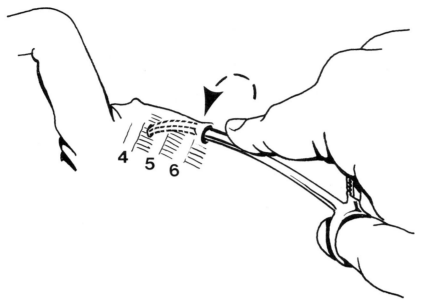

Figure 17.4. Push the closed hemostat gently but forcefully into the pleural space while listening for a rush of air to confirm pleural entry.

integrity and chest tube placement through a distant site. Antibiotic administration prevents the development of empyema.

Hemothorax

Chest trauma can produce bleeding into the pleural space from injury to the intercostal vessels, pulmonary parenchyma, or heart and great vessels. When a child becomes hypotensive without any obvious sign of blood loss, suspect hemothorax, which often

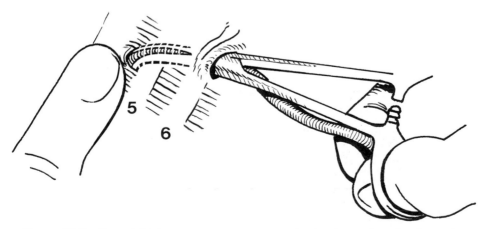

Figure 17.5. Spread the hemostat to create an opening just larger than the chest tube.

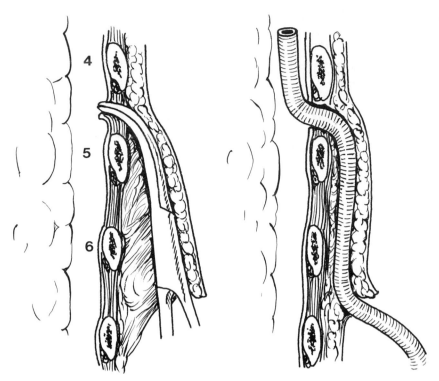

Figure 17.6.   *Left,* to prevent pulmonary parenchymal injury, avoid penetrating too deeply into the pleural space. *Right,* insert the tube into the pleural space with the hemostat left in place as a guide, or grasp the tip of the tube with the hemostat and place it directly.

coexists with pneumothorax. In children, hemothorax is an indicator of increased mortality; 67% of children with hemothorax at CNMC died.

Hemothorax can be life-threatening, producing shock with hypovolemia. As the blood accumulates, the lung is compressed and the mediastinum displaced, resulting in decreased cardiac output. Direct treatment toward restoring intravascular volume and evacuating the blood by thoracostomy tube placement. A bleeding rate of 1–2 ml/kg/hr from the thoracostomy tube suggests the need for thoracotomy to establish hemostasis.

Lung Contusion

Parenchymal damage creating a lung contusion is most often produced by blunt injury, although the explosive force of penetrating injury can create a similar pattern (17). With blunt trauma to the chest, the force of the blow is transmitted via the chest wall to the pulmonary parenchyma. Injury to the parenchyma results in transudation of fluid and hemorrhage into the alveoli, creating a ventilation-perfusion abnormality and poor oxygenation. Barotrauma occurs following attempts to improve ventilation by increasing inflation pressure, which can produce pulmonary fibrosis.

Initially, the child may appear well and then develop worsening signs of respiratory distress. The chest x-ray is often clear at first but, over the ensuing hours, fluffy infiltrates develop and progress to consolidation. The computerized axial tomography scan provides earlier evidence of parenchymal injury than does the plain x-ray. Devote treatment to enhancing respiratory efficiency while minimizing further parenchymal

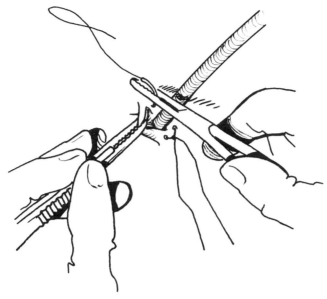

Figure 17.7. After making sure that all of the side holes are in the chest, secure the tube tightly with two skin sutures, which also make the incision airtight.

injury. Restricting fluid after resuscitation minimizes transudation from the capillary. A Swan-Ganz catheter is a useful monitor of pulmonary capillary wedge pressure to avoid fluid overload and further interstitial edema. Positive end-expiratory pressure with mechanical ventilation is the mainstay of treatment; steroids have little role in treatment.

At CNMC, pulmonary contusion was the most common thoracic injury, present in 52% of patients. The mortality rate for patients with pulmonary contusion of one lobe

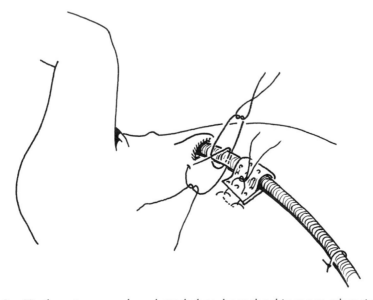

Figure 17.8. Tie the sutures snugly and attach the tube to the skin at one other site to prevent dislodgement.

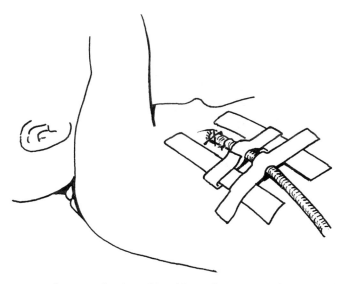

Figure 17.9.   A meticulous tape bridge adds additional security and prevents kinking. Obtain a chest radiograph to confirm proper tube position.

was 15%; however, if multiple lobes were involved, it was 43%. The development of pulmonary contusion is difficult to differentiate from respiratory distress syndrome produced by pancreatitis, sepsis, or head trauma. Pneumonia can supervene in the injured segment; prevention by careful technique of suctioning and physiotherapy reduces the morbidity. Identification of pathogenic bacteria with routine tracheal culture will allow early selection of antibiotics against susceptible organisms.

Tracheobronchial Injury

Injury to the tracheobronchial tree most often presents as respiratory distress. The degree of distress relates to the level of injury or obstruction; injury involving the larger airways produces more distress. A tear or shear of the bronchial tree produces dissection of air in the mediastinum and soft tissues of the neck and chest wall, manifested as crepitus of the skin.

Laryngotracheal trauma is uncommon in children; a bronchial tear or a tracheal injury is difficult to diagnose (18). Hoarseness, subcutaneous emphysema, or crepitus suggests the injury. Plain x-ray films may show little, but if air is present in the soft tissue or mediastinum, the diagnosis is possible. Employ bronchoscopy to make a definitive determination; fiberoptic bronchoscopy is useful in children if the patient is intubated, but rigid bronchoscopy under anesthesia is the procedure of choice. The trachea and bronchi are inspected as distally as possible; a tear is manifested by hematoma or separation of the wall. Care must be taken during the procedure to ensure adequate ventilation. Associated injuries to the cervical spine and other structures of the neck are common with laryngeal or tracheal trauma.

Small tears of the distal bronchi may heal spontaneously, but tears of the larger bronchi or trachea require operative intervention. Resection of the involved lung segment and direct suture anastomosis of the airway are useful techniques (19).

Aspiration of Foreign Bodies

TRACHEOBRONCHIAL

Children, especially toddlers, are particularly prone to foreign body aspiration. Taking a careful history is crucial; choking after placement of a toy, nut, or other small object in the mouth is enough to warrant further investigation. Physical examination often reveals a differential in breath sounds from one side of the chest to the other. X-ray films can show hyperinflation on the involved side, especially with expiration, since the object prevents egress of air. The mediastinum is often shifted away from the involved side; however, radiographs may show no abnormality.

The procedure of choice for diagnosis and treatment is rigid bronchoscopy under anesthesia (20). With the use of a ventilating fiberoptic endoscope, the foreign body is visualized and manipulated while adequate ventilation is provided. Grasping forceps placed through the bronchoscope allow removal of most foreign bodies. Peanuts are notorious for causing extensive reaction and are difficult to remove, especially if they have been in the bronchus for some time. Use of a Fogarty catheter and irrigation of the bronchus are helpful techniques. A missed foreign body results in bronchiectasis and may necessitate subsequent resection of the involved segment.

ESOPHAGEAL

When a child swallows a foreign object, it often obstructs the esophagus. The most common levels of obstruction are the cricopharyngeal muscle, the middle third of the esophagus, and the gastroesophageal junction. Drooling, pain, and airway obstruction are helpful signs (21).

Because of the potential for aspiration, obstruction, or perforation, the foreign body must be removed. X-rays will document the location of radiopaque objects. All objects are retrieved using endoscopy with anesthesia. Most objects that reach the stomach will pass without incident.

Burns

Burns are a significant cause of injury in children. Although most pediatric burns are caused by a scald from hot water, flame burns cause the highest mortality probably due to associated respiratory injury. There are three types of respiratory injury due to burn injury: smoke inhalation, direct burns of the upper airway, and carbon monoxide poisoning (22). Flame burns can produce respiratory distress through the actual burn wound. Edema of the neck or upper airway can progress to airway obstruction. The initial examination includes inspection of the mouth for erythema and blisters. Early intubation is lifesaving. Burn wounds involving the chest wall may produce a circumferential thick eschar, preventing chest wall expansion and reducing air exchange. Escharotomy releases the wound, permitting chest wall expansion.

Smoke inhalation is suspected in all children with flame burns. Singed nasal hairs, burned oral mucosa, or burns involving the face are clues to the diagnosis. Sputum showing charred material is also a lead. A history of being burned in a closed space suggests pulmonary injury. Arterial blood gas analysis that reveals a carbon monoxide level of greater than 10% provides evidence of injury. Plain x-rays are often initially normal despite severe injury.

The burn injury is produced not only by direct thermal contact but also by inhalation of noxious poisons produced by burning material. Smoke destroys the cells lining the bronchial airways and alters the surfactant. Direct treatment to providing respiratory support until healing can take place. With severe injury, use of positive end-expiratory pressure helps support ventilation. Though prophylactic antibiotics are not used, surveillance for bacterial colonization is imperative.

The third type of injury is carbon monoxide poisoning. The diagnosis is made by measuring the carboxyhemoglobin level in the blood gas. Carbon monoxide has a tremendous affinity for hemoglobin; levels of 30% or higher usually result in death. Central nervous system symptoms are the most common findings prior to coma and death. Provision of 100% oxygen helps displace the carbon monoxide from the hemoglobin molecule. The use of hyperbaric oxygenation is controversial, although there are multiple case reports of improvement, especially in children with neurologic symptoms following the inhalation.

Pericardial Tamponade

Penetrating injury to the chest can result in pericardial tamponade. Bleeding into the pericardial space produces compression of the heart, which reduces venous return of the right heart and decreases cardiac output, leading to hypotension and death. In children, relatively small amounts of blood produce tamponade. The classic picture of tamponade with pulsus paradoxus, distended neck veins, muffled heart sounds, and a chest x-ray showing a large heart is rare. More often, the child presents with a history of penetrating trauma and shock; if the child is stable, pericardiocentesis provides the diagnosis and often enough blood is aspirated to alleviate the cardiac compromise. Urgent transport to the operating room to control the bleeding is indicated. If the child is unstable, emergency room thoracotomy relieves the tamponade and the cardiac injury is controlled.

Infants are especially prone to pneumopericardium following initiation of high pressure ventilatory support. A small volume of air severely interferes with cardiac function. Infants are at risk for developing pericardial tamponade by erosion of catheters used for long-term venous support (23). The catheter erodes through the right atrium, allowing blood or intravenous solutions to surround the heart with subsequent tamponade (24).

Cardiac Injury

Cardiac lacerations by knife or gunshot are best controlled by suture ligation. Knowledge of cardiac anatomy is critical in order to avoid injury to the coronary arteries. The sutures should use felt pledgets to prevent myocardial tissue injury during closure of the wound, especially in a thin-walled atrium. The mortality rate from injuries to the heart and great vessels was more than 80% at CNMC, but the injury occurred in less than 6% of the children with thoracic injuries.

Myocardial Injury

Blunt trauma producing myocardial contusion is a rare injury in children. Myocardial contusion is a focal injury to the myocardium and usually resolves spontaneously (25). The electrocardiogram will show ST-T wave changes or conduction abnormalities; elevation in the creatinine phosphokinase–muscle-brain (CPK-MB) band is the most sensitive indicator of cardiac injury, but false-positives do occur. Echocardiography and radionuclide angiography have also been used to define the extent of injury. Although most contusions resolve, severe arrhythmias or cardiac failure can ensue. For these reasons, all children with suspected cardiac contusion are monitored for 24 hr with serial electrocardiogram and CPK isoenzyme measurement. Direct trauma to the heart can produce rupture of the myocardium, which usually results in instant death. Papillary muscle disruption and rupture of the ventricular septum are lethal injuries if not recognized early and treated promptly. Echocardiography is extremely useful in identifying these injuries in children (26).

Aortic Injury

Aortic rupture is rare in children. The mediastinal structures of children are extremely flexible and have little atherosclerosis, accounting for the decreased likelihood for shearing at the point of attachment of the ligamentum arteriosum. At CNMC, only one rupture has been seen in the evaluation of 104 thoracic injuries.

When arotic rupture does occur, the child survives to reach the emergency room in a small percentage of instances. The child is usually a passenger in a motor vehicle crash or has fallen from a great height. The child is hypotensive with mediastinal widening on a chest x-ray or computerized tomography scan. An aortogram is helpful in determining the extent of injury. Direct surgical repair is effective and prevents death from rupture of a pseudoaneurysm.

Esophageal Injury

Traumatic injury to the esophagus of a child is unusual. The most common source of injury is from iatrogenic manipulation, e.g., esophagoscopy or dilatation for stricture. Occasionally, a child's esophagus is injured by impalement of a sharp object in the hypopharynx.

One should consider the diagnosis of esophageal injury when the path of the penetrating object might involve the esophagus. Blunt injury produces a tear of the esophagus by the forceful ejection of air and stomach contents into the lower esophagus with a blow to the chest or abdomen. Crepitus in the neck often appears, and the x-ray will demonstrate air in the mediastinum. Esophagoscopy is often useful to define the injury but a metrizamide swallow enhances the accuracy of diagnosis.

Surgical treatment is tailored to the time since injury, severity of damage, and the quality of tissue (viable or necrotic) encountered. Wide drainage is the mainstay of treatment to prevent mediastinitis. If a small tear is identified and the esophagus is dissected back to good tissue margins, it should be closed in layers. If the wound cannot be safely closed, the esophagus should be diverted in the neck and the stomach drained by gastrostomy.

Caustic Ingestion

Injury to the esophagus from ingestion of a caustic substance affects up to 5000 children/yr in the United States. Most of the children are under the age of 5. Both alkaline and acidic agents can produce injury, although the corrosive alkali are the most common cause (80%). Disc batteries are an increasing source of injury.

The major determinants of injury are the amount of agent, concentration, time of contact, solubility, and type (acid or alkali) (27). A thorough investigation is warranted in all children with a suspicion of ingestion, since many of the historical details are unknown at the time of presentation. Even small amounts of caustic agent can produce major tissue injury.

At CNMC, evaluation begins with esophagoscopy under general anesthesia, after examining the mouth, hypopharynx, epiglottis, and vocal cords. Terminate the procedure at the level of the first significant burn to reduce the risk of perforation. If circumferential burns are present or a stricture is identified, a gastrostomy is placed for feeding and to provide a channel through which a silk guideline is placed for future dilatation. Serial x-ray examinations with contrast dye are used to define the development of stricture.

The immediate complications of caustic injury relate to aspiration or perforation. The major long-term complication is stricture formation, seen in approximately 15% of children. Although esophageal replacement may be necessary, serial dilatation is usually sufficient to maintain adequate esophageal patency.

Traumatic Asphyxia

Traumatic asphyxia is a rare injury; it is seen more commonly in children than adults. Although the clinical appearance is frightening, the injury is self-limited (28). The child demonstrates petechial hemorrhages in the sclera and skin of the upper body. The injury results from a forceful blow or compression of the chest that raises intrathoracic pressure enough to elevate postcapillary pressure and cause injury to the capillary. The significance of finding traumatic asphyxia relates to the association with other severe injuries from the impact: cardiac contusion, hepatic injury, and pulmonary trauma. Treatment is supportive and concentrated on associated injuries, since the manifestations of traumatic asphyxia will resolve with time.

Chylothorax

Chylothorax results from rupture of the thoracic duct with hyperextension injury. Penetrating trauma rarely severs the duct; however, iatrogenic injury to the thoracic duct during surgery is a common cause of chylothorax. Clinical recognition is often delayed, until the chyle accumulates and causes respiratory embarrassment. Lymphocytopenia and nutritional depletion are late consequences. Resolution may occur using medium-chain triglyceride solutions or total parenteral nutrition to minimize chyle production. Thoracentesis or a thoracostomy tube are employed to drain the chyle. Most traumatic or iatrogenic chylothoraces require early surgical intervention; spontaneous healing rarely occurs in these instances (29, 30).

Diaphragmatic Hernia

A forceful blow to the lower chest or abdomen may disrupt the diaphragm (31). The intraabdominal pressure rises high enough to tear the diaphragmatic muscle, forcing the abdominal organs into the chest cavity. X-rays showing a bowel pattern in the chest or auscultation of the chest revealing bowel sounds confirms the diagnosis. Recognition is often delayed until a complication occurs, such as intestinal strangulation. Operation to reduce the intraabdominal contents and repair the diaphragm is curative. Assessment of associated intraabdominal injury is best done through a laparotomy.

Stab and gunshot wounds to the chest can penetrate the diaphragm, creating intraabdominal hollow viscus injury.

SUMMARY

Pediatric thoracic trauma is rare; of 2400 trauma admissions to CNMC over a 36-month period, only 104 children sustained chest injury. Yet the mortality rate of 25% is unacceptably high. Programs stressing prevention are the best strategy to reduce the morbidity and mortality. Once a thoracic injury has occurred, the trauma team must possess knowledge of the unique anatomic and physiologic characteristics of children and pattern of injury to prevent loss of life.

REFERENCES

1. Peclet M, Newman KD, Eichelberger MR. Patterns of injury in children. J Pediatr Surg, 1990;25:85–92.
2. McGill WA. Airway management. In: Eichelberger MR, ed. Pediatric trauma care. Rockville, MD: Aspen Publishers, 1988:5–57.
3. Eichelberger MR, Randolph JG. Thoracic trauma in children. Surg Clin North Am 1981;6:1181–1197.
4. King DR. Trauma in infancy and childhood: initial evaluation and management. Pediatr Clin North Am 1985;32:1299–1310.
5. Shires GT, Conizaro PC. Fluid resuscitation in the severely injured child. Surg Clin North Am 1973;53:1341–1350.
6. O'Neill JA. Infants and children as accident victims. In: Welch KJ, Randolph JG, Ravitch MM, O'Neill JA, Rowe MI, eds. Pediatric surgery. Chicago: Year Book Medical Publishers, 1986:133–135.
7. Eichelberger MR. Pediatric trauma. In: Edlich R, ed. Current emergency medical therapy. New York: Appleton-Century-Crofts, 1984:676–690.
8. Spitzer A. The role of the kidney in sodium hemostasis during maturation. Kidney Int 1982;21:539–544.
9. Hauser GJ, Holbrook PR. Immune dysfunction in the critically ill infant and child. Crit Care Clin 1988;4:711–733.
10. Pollack MM, Wiley JS, Kanter R. Malnutrition in critically ill infants and children. JPEN 1982;6:20–26.
11. Committee on Trauma. Advanced trauma life support: course manual. Chicago: American College of Surgeons, 1989;215–231.
12. Schweich P, Fleisher G. Rib fractures in children. Pediatr Emerg Care 1985;1:187–189.
13. Meller JL, Little AG, Shermeta DW. Thoracic trauma in children. Pediatrics 1984;74:813–819.
14. Haller JA. Thoracic injuries. In: Welch KJ, Randolph JG, Ravitch MM, O'Neill JA, Rowe MI, eds. Pediatric surgery. Chicago: Year Book Medical Publishers, 1986:133–135.
15. Trinkle JK. Flail chest and pulmonary contusion. In: Trinkle JK, Grover FI, eds. Management of thoracic trauma victims. Philadelphia: Lippincott, 1980:39–50.
16. Blair E, Topuzlu C, Davis JH. Delayed or missed diagnosis in blunt chest trauma. J Trauma 1971;11:129–134.
17. Smyth BT. Chest trauma in children. J Pediatr Surg 1979;14:41–47.
18. Grover FI, Ellested C, Arom KU. Diagnosis and management of major tracheobronchial injuries. Ann Thorac Surg 1979;28:384–391.
19. Deslauriers J, Bussieres J. Bronchial rupture. In: Grillo HC, Austen WG, Wilkins EW, Mathisen DJ, Vlahakes GJ, eds. Current therapy in cardiothoracic surgery. Toronto: BC Decker, 1989:42–45.
20. Johnson DG. Bronchoscopy. In: Welch KJ, Randolph JG, Ravitch MM, O'Neill JA, Rowe MI, eds. Pediatric surgery. Chicago: Year Book Medical Publishers, 1986:619–622.
21. Sharp RJ. Esophageal foreign bodies. In: Ashcraft KW, Holder TM, eds. Pediatric esophageal surgery. Orlando, Grune & Stratton, 1986:137–150.
22. Moylan JA. Smoke inhalation and burn injury. Surg Clin North Am 1980;60:1533–1540.
23. Hall RT, Rhodes PG. Pneumothorax and pneumomediastinum in infants with idiopathic respiratory distress syndrome receiving continuous positive airway pressure. Pediatrics 1975;55:493–497.
24. Fisher GW, Scherz RG. Neck vein catheters and pericardial tamponade. Pediatrics 1973;52:868–870.
25. Golladay ES, Donahoo JS, Haller JA. Special problems of cardiac injuries in infants and children. J Trauma 1979;19:526–531.
26. Tellez DW, Hardin WD, Takahashi M, Miller J, Galuis AG, Mahour GH. Blunt cardiac injury in children. J Pediatr Surg 1987;22:1123–1128.
27. Tunell WP. Corrosive strictures of the esophagus. In: Welch KJ, Randolph JG, Ravitch MM, O'Neill JA, Rowe MI, eds. Pediatric Surgery. Chicago: Year Book Medical Publishers, 1986:698–703.
28. Haller JA, Donahoo JS. Traumatic asphyxia in children: pathophysiology and management. J Trauma 1971;11:453–457.
29. Bessone LN, Ferguson TB, Busford TH. Chylothorax. Ann Thorac Surg 1971;12:527–550.
30. Ramzy A, Rodriguez A, Cowley RA. Pitfalls in the management of chylothorax. J Trauma 1982;22:513–515.
31. Adeymi SD, Stephens CA. Traumatic diaphragmatic hernia in children. Can J Surg 1981;24:355–359.

18 Blunt Chest Trauma in the Elderly: The MIEMSS Experience

Robert M. Shorr, MD

In the United States, trauma is the leading cause of death in persons under the age of 40. Nevertheless, a rapidly growing and complex group of trauma patients is emerging in this country—the elderly. The United States Census Bureau estimates that the current population of persons 65 yrs of age or older will increase about 2.6-fold by the year 2050 and that the population of persons 75 yrs or older will increase 8 times (Table 18.1) (1). As rescue, transportation, and resuscitative techniques have continued to improve, the unique elderly trauma patient population has emerged.

The incidence of patients 65 yrs of age or older sustaining blunt chest trauma approaches 10% of all blunt chest trauma patients. Unlike the younger trauma patients, males do not predominate in the elderly trauma group. Males and females are equally affected. In our experience in the analysis of nonelderly patients, a male-to-female ratio of 2.7:1 was found. In the elderly population, females approached males in frequency, with a male-to-female ratio of 1.2:1 (1–2).

DIAGNOSIS

The diagnosis of blunt chest trauma in the elderly embraces the standard tenets of general trauma care. Because the elderly population generally has less of a hemodynamic reserve, they will frequently present with earlier instability and shock than younger patients. Blunt chest trauma victims, regardless of age, are subject to polytrauma. As in nonelderly patients, approximately 50% of elderly patients with chest trauma will have extrathoracic injury. Bony thorax fractures, followed by hemopneumothoraces and pneumothoraces, are the most common injuries involving elderly chest trauma patients (2).

Table 18.1.
Projections of the Population of the United States by Age[a]

Age Group	1950	1980	2000	2050
65 yr and over	12,397,000	25,145,000	34,921,000	67,412,000
75 yr and over	590,000	2,271,000	4,926,000	16,034,000
100 yr and over	NA[b]	25,000	108,000	1,029,000

[a]From United States Census Bureau. Projections of the population of the United States by age, sex, race: 1983–2080. Series T25, no. 952. Washington, DC: Government Printing Office, 1986.
[b]NA, not available.

Table 18.2.
Mortality in 515 Cases of Blunt Chest Trauma by Age Group

	Teens	20–40 yr	41–64 yr	Elderly
Deaths	18%	13%	12%	37%[a]
Survival	82	87	88	63

[a]$p = 0.0002$.

Like their younger counterparts (3), elderly patients can have significant chest injuries in the absence of bony thorax fractures. The most common mechanisms of injuries of blunt chest trauma in the elderly are motor vehicle, accidents, accidents in which the patient is a pedestrian struck by a motor vehicle, and falls. Predictably, in our experience and that of others, no motorcycle accidents occurred among the elderly; however, that trend may change in the future.

TREATMENT

The treatment for blunt chest trauma in elderly patients is essentially identical to the approach to their younger counterparts. The "ABCs" of initial resuscitation are the same. Recognition of the potential of a decreased cardiopulmonary reserve or significant underlying disease may temper overzealous fluid administration and prompt inotropic support earlier than in other patients. However, the basic trauma resuscitation guidelines should be applied to the elderly.

OUTCOME

The morbidity and mortality of such trauma in older patients are significant in our experience (Table 18.2). Major morbidity specifically related to chest trauma, including atelectasis, pneumonia, and acute respiratory distress syndrome, approaches almost 50% of elderly patients. Mortality rates generally are higher in elderly patients, both during the acute phase of their injury and later in their course of hospitalization.

MIEMSS EXPERIENCE

During a 3-year period, 515 patients were admitted with blunt chest trauma to the Shock Trauma Center of the Maryland Institute for Emergency Medical Services Systems (MIEMSS) (2). Within this group, there were 46 patients (9%) who were 65 yrs of age or older. The 469 nonelderly patients from the general blunt chest trauma group serve as a control for comparison.

Blunt chest trauma victims, regardless of age group, are subject to polytrauma (4). We found no difference in the numbers of extrathoracic injuries in the elderly and nonelderly groups—85 and 83.5%, respectively. Forty-six percent of elderly patients sustained two or more extrathoracic injuries, compared with 48% of the nonelderly group.

The mechanism of injury was similar in the two groups, with motor vehicle accidents and accidents in which the patient is a pedestrian struck by a motor vehicle predominating. Types of injuries were similar in the two groups, with bony thorax fractures most common, followed by hemopneumothoraces and pneumothoraces. The fact that significant chest injuries can occur in the absence of bony thorax fractures was apparent in both elderly and nonelderly populations.

However, in comparing our elderly and nonelderly chest trauma patients, significant differences were found. In addition to the nearly equal preponderance of males and females in the study group (mentioned earlier), admission vital signs were different between the elderly and nonelderly populations. Although similar percentages of elderly and nonelderly patients presented with initially stable vital signs, a small percentage of elderly patients presented in shock, and a statistically significant higher percentage of elderly patients presented with absent vital signs. This difference may be due to the much higher hemodynamic and cardiopulmonary reserve in nonelderly patients and a decreased ability of elderly patients to tolerate hypovolemia and shock.

The higher overall morbidity of 46% in the elderly group (although not statistically significant compared with the 35% morbidity in the nonelderly group) suggests an increased trend of complications. The specific complications were similar in both groups: atelectasis, pneumonia, and acute respiratory distress syndrome (ARDS) predominated.

The most striking difference between the two populations we studied is in the mortality rates (Table 18.2). The elderly group had 17 deaths, for a mortality rate of 37%; the rate in the nonelderly group was 13.4%. Eleven of the elderly deaths were either acute deaths complicated by severe associated injuries or fatal head injuries. These deaths are generally difficult to prevent, and therapeutic options are limited. Six deaths (35% of total deaths in the elderly group) were late deaths compared with 16% occurring in the nonelderly population. This difference is statistically significant ($p = 0.07$). Within this elderly late death group, several trends are apparent. All patients in this group had extrathoracic injuries; 41% of patients sustained two or more associated injuries. Five of six patients were involved in motor vehicle accidents, five were female, and five sustained more than three rib fractures. Admission vital signs did not have statistical significance: three patients had stable vital signs and three patients had unstable vital signs.

CONCLUSION

Since the morbidity and mortality associated with chest trauma are significantly higher in the elderly, the approach to these patients should include recognition of their high risk for morbidity and mortality, careful fluid management, aggressive pulmonary toilet, pulmonary embolus prevention, cardiac rhythm monitoring, and measurement of cardiac indices.

REFERENCES

1. United States Census Bureau. Projections of the population of the United States by age, sex, race: 1983–2080. Series T25, no. 952. Washington, DC: Government Printing Office, 1986.
2. Shorr RM, Rodriguez A, Indeck MC, Crittenden MD, Hartunian S, Cowley RA. Blunt chest trauma in the elderly. J Trauma 1989;29:234–237.
3. Shorr RM, Crittenden M, Indeck M, Hartunian SL, Rodriguez A. Blunt thoracic trauma: analysis of 515 patients. Ann Surg 1987;206:200–205.
4. Kirsh MM, Sloan H. Blunt chest trauma. Boston: Little, Brown, 1977.

Table 19.2.
Observations in 1992 Cardiothoracic Injuries

	Average or Number	Percent
Operations	1.2	
Blood units	4	
Intravenous liters	18	
Transport time (min)	10	
Transport distance (miles)	2	
Under age 40	1594	80
Male:female	3.6:1	
Surgery during active combat	438	22
Substandard surgical conditions	139	7

Cardiac injuries make up 14% of the total thoracic casualties. This compares with a 2.8% incidence reported from the Vietnam War (7) and 3.3% from World War II (4).

A second system-associated injury was noted in 456 patients. The distribution is as follows: abdominal, 251; orthopedic, 96; peripheral vascular, 41; spinal cord, 36; and cranial, 32.

Table 19.2 reflects averaged patient data, the proximity to hospital, and the rapid transportation of combat casualties. Associated with good field communication networks, these factors enhance early retrieval of the critically wounded, especially the cardiac casualties, and quick transport to a thoracic center.

Beirut, where a sophisticated medical referral center is located, received major educational input over the years from great American surgeons who taught at the American University of Beirut. These contributors included Whipple, McDonald, Wilson, Churchill, Simeone, and DeBakey. In this surgical tradition, the logistic establishment in 1977 of a modern cardiothoracic center in the combat zone area was important (11). Table 19.3 outlines the provisions of this unit, which raises the level and uniformity of specialty care in Beirut and allows clinical research and documentation.

The Miami Data

As popularity of the television show "Miami Vice" was peaking, a new protocol was initiated in 1984 by the division of thoracic surgery at the University of Miami's Jackson Memorial Hospital (12). The program adopted the early surgical approach to major penetrating thoracic injuries and was based on significant parallel combat studies from

Table 19.3.
Cardiothoracic Combat Zone Center Contributions

Around-the-clock thoracic team readiness
Cardiopulmonary bypass systems
Autotransfusion and modern blood bank facilities
Ventilatory systems
Radio communications
Underground emergency, operating, intensive suites
Auxiliary electric, water, medical supplies
Computerized documentation systems

Lebanon. Early results were impressive in that 9 of 10 consecutive patients with cardiac injuries managed in this way survived in 1985.

Table 19.4 summarizes pertinent observations in a series of 10 consecutive major civilian combat-like injuries in 1986. All 10 survived; one patient suffered spinal paralysis.

A recent review of 130 consecutive civilian combat injuries shows the mechanism to be penetrating in 119 and blunt in 11 (12a). Gunshot wounds are causative in 72, stabs in 47. Mean age is 27 years, mean casualty lag time until surgery is 100 min, and mean operating time is 3 hr.

Findings from these two broad-based sets of clinical data provide guidelines to the management of critical civilian combat casualties.

HIGH-VELOCITY MISSILE INJURIES

These injuries are caused by missiles with muzzle velocity over 500 m/sec. A clinical sample is noted in Table 19.5. Dramatic local and general damages result from thoracic injuries caused by high-velocity missiles (HVMs). The magnitude of injury is exponentially greater than in wounds due to classic low-velocity missiles. The deleterious effects of HVMs are summarized in Figure 19.1.

HVMs are so effective because they emit major kinetic energy into the target tissue (13). The transmitted energy is quantitated by the following equation:

$$\text{Kinetic energy} = (\text{mass} \times \text{velocity squared}) \div 2$$

This great quantity of transmitted kinetic energy into the chest causes local tissue disruption and extensive cavitation, which develops rapidly—in certain experimental trials, within 20 msec of injury (14). Because of varied pressures within the temporary cavity, it pulsates. Shock waves radiate outward, crushing tissue peripheral to the pathway of the missile. Experimental studies show peripheral crush effects to reach a

Table 19.4.
Ten Consecutive Major Cardiothoracic Injuries: Miami 1986

Patient	Main Site	Mode	Hours in Operating Room	Hospital Days	Survival
1	Right ventricle	GSW[a]	3	4	Yes
2	Right atrium, superior vena cava	Stab	3	17	Yes
3	Right ventricle	Stab	2	8	Yes
4	Right ventricle, pulmonary artery, lung	GSW	3	31	Yes (paralysis)
5	Thoracic aorta	Blunt	3	11	Yes
6	Thoracic aorta, lung	GSW	3	20	Yes
7	Thoracic aorta	Stab	3	18	Yes
8	Pericardium, right atrium, lung	GSW	3	19	Yes
9	Pericardium, right atrium	GSW	3.5	20	Yes
10	Pericardium, internal mammary artery	Stab	4	13	Yes

[a]GSW, gunshot wound

Table 19.5.
Popular High-velocity Weapons in the Lebanon Conflict

High-velocity rifles
   M-15 automatic
   M-16 automatic
   Kalashnikov
   Soviet AKM
Dynamite
   Trinitrotoluene (TNT)
   Advanced plastics
   Phosphorus
Rockets
   Katyusha
   Grad
   Antitank B7
   Air-to-land; sea-to-air
Cannons
   Bazooka
   155-mm
   120-mm

distance 30 times the diameter of the HVM (14). Evidence of major energy transfer is demonstrated from recordings of shock waves in the aorta following HVM trauma to the hind leg in dog experiments (15). Vital circulatory changes are also noted regionally and include loss of vasoconstrictor tone. Generalized circulatory and neurologic effects are also observed in these experiments.

As negative pressure develops at either end of the cavitation, contamination of the

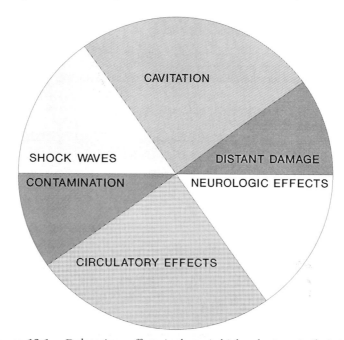

Figure 19.1. Deleterious effects in thoracic high-velocity missile impact.

devitalized tissue follows. Sources of infection are the missiles, skin, clothes, and external surfaces. Experimental studies show 76% of certain HVM wounds developing heavy bacterial growth within 6 hr after injury. Adequate surgical treatment within 6 hr controls the infection, while delay beyond 12 hr leads to poor infection control (16).

The extent of cavitation varies with the HVM velocity, the density of surrounding tissue, and the rotational behavior of the missile. Figure 19.2 demonstrates differences in injury potential of common weapons, based on energy transmission.

Enhanced absorption of kinetic energy, hence tissue damage, follows the deceleration, yaw, and tumble of HVMs. Secondary projectiles multiply the injury when HVMs pass through ribs and vertebrae. Injuries of the spinal cord and blood vessels can result from the pressure waves and the mechanothermal forces produced by the adjacent projectile (8).

Our clinical experience confirms these pertinent experimental observations. These findings dictate certain corollaries in surgical management that supersede classic approaches. These are reemphasized as follows:

1. The locus of maximal intrathoracic injury may not follow the pathway predicted by examination of the external wounds. X-ray findings and clinical evaluation are helpful; early exploration is at times essential.
2. Debridement of HVM wounds should encompass the full missile track and be performed at an early stage.
3. Diagnosis of secondary injuries from shock waves and from satellite projectiles is as important as evaluation of the primary injury.
4. Resuscitation should be fashioned to counter the generalized adverse effects on the circulatory and central nervous systems caused by HVMs.

Figure 19.3 illustrates the local impact of close range buckshot injury.

MANAGEMENT GUIDELINES FOR CIVILIAN COMBAT INJURIES
The thoracic surgeon plays a pivotal role as a charismatic team leader and decision maker who possesses the technical ability to achieve rapid intrathoracic exposure and

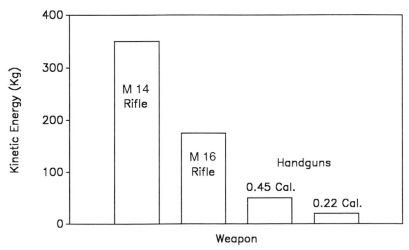

Figure 19.2.   Comparative kinetic energy emissions by popular weapons.

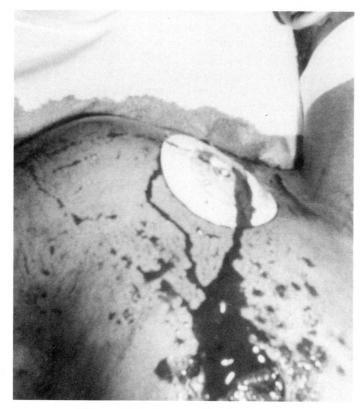

Figure 19.3.   Impact of buckshot injury.

corrective repairs. The hospital should dedicate significant facilities to care of patients with critical injuries during paroxysms of combat and catastrophic situations. A state of readiness, efficient streamlining of diagnostic and surgical services, and minimum administrative delays are basic requirements.

Special logistics must be considered for young casualties; arrival of critically injured patients who, under usual situations, would expire during transportation; major HVM wounds; and close-range intrathoracic missile trauma. Successful treatment demands strict adherence to certain principles. In critical civilian combat injuries there are three essential principles:

1. Effective resuscitation.
2. Early intrathoracic surgical control at the focus of the injury.
3. Early definitive surgical correction.

Resuscitation

The initial supportive measures are listed in Table 19.6. Rapid volume replacement is achieved via large-bore plastic catheters placed into the femoral veins, the preferred entry sites whenever injury to the subclavian veins or the superior vena cava is suspected. Errors in venous access choice are shown in Figures 19.4 and 19.5.

Precise total body examination must include a search for pulse deficits and

Table 19.6.
Emergency Steps in Critical Injuries

Airway control and ventilatory support
Multiple venous lines, blood sample
Rapid infusion crystalloids, blood
Clothes removal, wound identification
Foley catheter, nasogastric tube
Overhead x-rays, cardiac monitor
Thoracostomy
Operating room readiness

neurologic evaluation, especially for spinal cord injury. All entrance/exit missile sites should be located, and overhead chest radiographs taken.

Chest x-ray films can transmit valuable information and clues. Enlarging posterior mediastinal hematoma or widened mediastinum are suspicious of aortic injury. Figure 19.6 represents one of the initial x-ray views for a combat casualty who suffered high-velocity anterior chest wall injury. The clinical condition was stable, no pulse deficits existed, and computerized tomography (CT) scanning was nondiagnostic. The slightly widened mediastinum was further evaluated with aortography. Figure 19.7 reveals a false traumatic aneurysm localized at the ductus arteriosus level. An urgent left posterior thoracotomy was performed. The periaortic hematoma was holding solely by the undamaged layer of adventitia. The aorta was cross-clamped above and below the

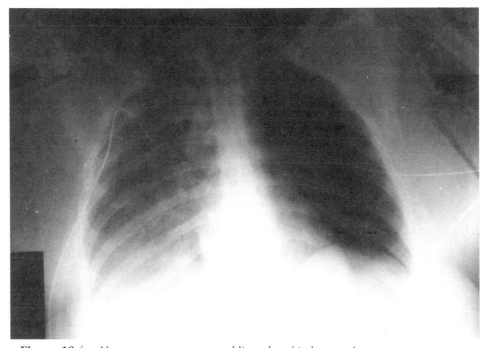

Figure 19.4.   Management error: central line placed in lacerated superior vena cava.

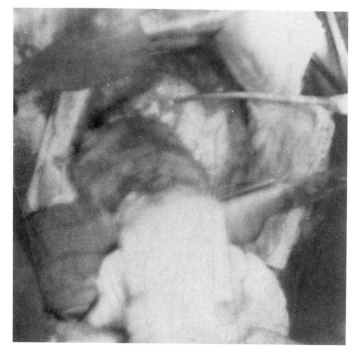

Figure 19.8. Suction tip points at completed aortic repair.

3. An esophagogram may delineate the location of the esophageal injury in approximately 50% of patients.

In the case presented in Figure 19.9, the bullet entered the left chest, crossed the posterior mediastinum, and lodged in the right posterior chest wall. A moderate left hemopneumothorax was drained by chest tube suction. There were no neurologic or vascular deficits and the patient was stable. An esophageal study was actively pursued.

Figure 19.10 shows barium leaking out of the upper esophageal wall. A right thoracotomy, promptly performed, revealed full-thickness entry/exit wounds in the upper esophagus, measuring 2 inches each. These were debrided and suture-repaired in two layers, the inner being continuous chromic catgut and the outer, interrupted silk.

An extensive broad-based parietal pleural flap was developed from the posterior and lateral chest wall. It was doubly folded, wrapped around the repaired esophagus, and sutured in place.

Postoperative chest x-ray studies (Fig. 19.11) and a barium swallow (Fig. 19.12) were satisfactory. A year later, upon the patient's insistence, the bullet was removed; he continues with excellent recovery 5 yr hence.

Tube thoracotomy is an essential diagnostic and therapeutic procedure. The following technical steps are recommended:

1. A fresh site distant from missile wounds and from the lines of potential thoracotomy incisions should be chosen. Sites of choice are the second midaxillary area for pneumothorax evacuation and the sixth interspace for hemothorax drainage. Two or more chest tubes may be required in patients with major air leaks and hemothorax.
2. A gloved finger should be used to first enter the pleural space and palpate for

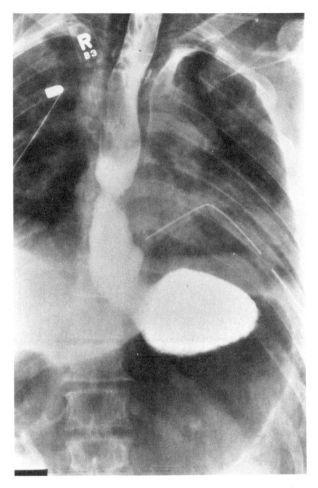

Figure 19.9.   Bullet crossing posterior mediastinum, causing two esophageal perforations.

pulmonary damage, lung collapse, diaphragmatic rupture, and herniation of abdominal viscera into the thoracic cavity.

3. Chest tube insertion by gentle pressure is recommended. Initial evacuation of hemothorax, when performed in an unstable patient, should be intermittent.

The degree and persistence of air leak into the underwater seal system are good indicators of the extent of bronchial injury.

Early Intrathoracic Surgical Control and Correction

Conventional approaches of limited surgical intervention, while applicable to some stab wounds and low-velocity injuries, are not as effective in high-velocity injuries or in closer range intrathoracic injuries of civilian combat. In these conditions, the presence of a significant intrathoracic wound should be assumed and early control at the level of the injured site is recommended.

In critical wounds, this step is performed concomitantly with active resuscitation (Fig. 19.13). An initial positive response to volume replacement and ventilatory support

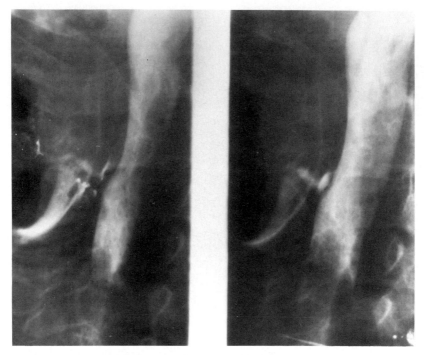

Figure 19.10.   Esophagogram shows site of upper perforation in esophagus.

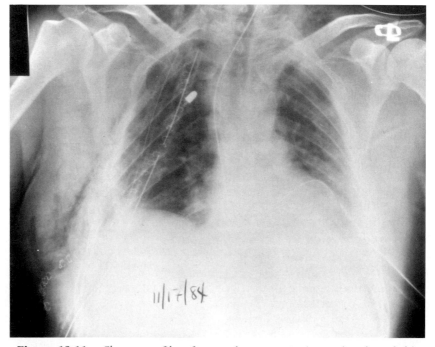

Figure 19.11.   Chest x-ray film after esophagus repair shows clear lung fields.

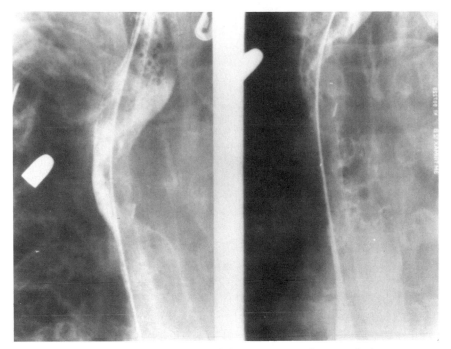

Figure 19.12.   Esophagogram 4 days postrepair shows no leakage.

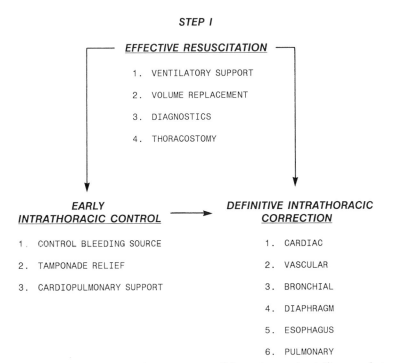

STEP I

EFFECTIVE RESUSCITATION

1. VENTILATORY SUPPORT

2. VOLUME REPLACEMENT

3. DIAGNOSTICS

4. THORACOSTOMY

*EARLY
INTRATHORACIC CONTROL*

1. CONTROL BLEEDING SOURCE

2. TAMPONADE RELIEF

3. CARDIOPULMONARY SUPPORT

*DEFINITIVE INTRATHORACIC
CORRECTION*

1. CARDIAC

2. VASCULAR

3. BRONCHIAL

4. DIAPHRAGM

5. ESOPHAGUS

6. PULMONARY

Figure 19.13.   Essential components of thoracic care in civilian combat.

is desirable in order to gain needed time but should not necessarily negate rapid intrathoracic exploration in the critically wounded.

The timing of thoracotomy and its indications require experience and proper decision making. Table 19.7 summarizes six criteria to be considered for urgent thoracotomy in the operating room (17–22). Rarely should urgent thoracotomy be performed in the emergency suite, and then only under the direct supervision of a thoracic surgeon.

Early thoracotomy is documented as contributing to life salvage in about one-third of casualties in our experience. In order of prevalence, the benefits of early thoracotomy are the following:

1. Early diagnosis and control of cardiac, thoracic, vascular, and pulmonary rupture.
2. Control of significant thoracic hemorrhage.
3. Tamponade relief.
4. Cardiac resuscitation.
5. Control of major air leaks.
6. Early diagnosis of esophageal and diaphragmatic wounds.
7. Early evacuation of foreign bodies (e.g., missiles).

Figure 19.14 shows the initial emergency room chest roentgenogram of a 40-year-old casualty, shot point-blank with a 22-mm handgun. The bullet entered the left neck and is shown lodged against the right inferior chest wall. Rapid endotracheal intubation and volume replacement with blood and Ringer's lactate solution were instituted. Based on his shock status and the x-ray film, he was rushed to the operating room, and a right anterolateral thoracotomy was performed within minutes. The surgical incision was through the fourth intercostal space. Brisk bleeding was noted from tears in the pulmonary hilar vessels, right ventricle, and upper lobe. Manual control of the hilum was followed by the placement of two curved vascular clamps.

The laceration of the ventricle was exposed by a longitudinal incision to the pericardium, preserving the phrenic nerve, and was repaired with pledgeted Prolene sutures. These technical steps at the locus of the injury controlled the life-threatening hemorrhage. At this stage, operative conditions were improved by suctioning secretions and blood from the bronchial tree, further blood volume restitution, correction of acidosis, and normal saline irrigation of the pericardial and pleural cavities. Corrective repair was next performed. The pulmonary vessels were anatomically dissected; the lacerations were debrided and repaired with polypropylene sutures. The pulmonary laceration was debrided, bronchial air leaks were repaired with sutures, and the bullet was removed prior to insertion of double thoracostomy drains.

The postoperative chest x-ray film (Fig. 19.15) shows residual pulmonary hematoma, which resorbed fully 2 weeks later (Fig. 19.16). This bullet also caused high

Table 19.7.
Guidelines in Urgent Thoracotomy for Critical Injuries

Presence of life signs
Transportation lag, level of shock
Resuscitation response
Wound sites, missile etiology
X-ray, thoracotomy findings
Logistic options

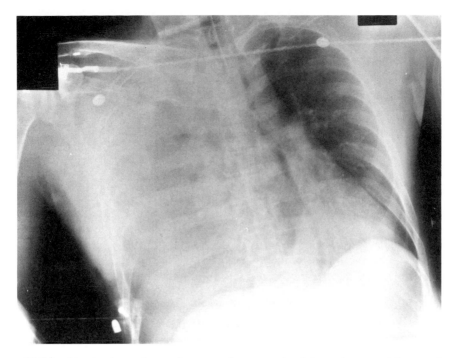

Figure 19.14. Massive hemothorax from gunshot wounds of the pulmonary hilum and right ventricle.

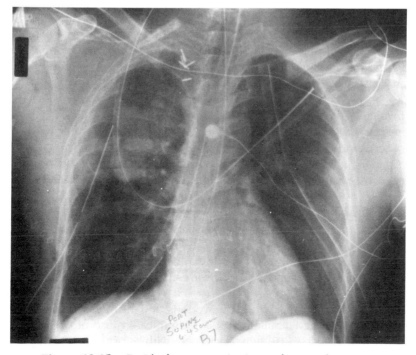

Figure 19.15. Residual postoperative intrapulmonary hematoma.

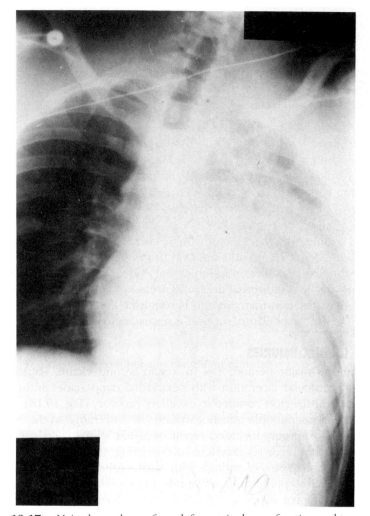

Figure 19.17.   Major hemothorax from left ventricular perforation and tamponade.

appears to result from the systemic effects of acidosis and shock, rather than the site or degree of cardiac injury. A cardiac site is related to better survival when injuries involve only the pericardium or the coronary vessels. Survival drops to 46% in left ventricular injury and is reflective of pump failure.

Early surgical correction includes the relief of tamponade and closure of cardiac perforations (23, 24). Pharmacologic support and volume replacement are important.

Exact diagnosis of internal cardiac injury is a major obstacle in the treatment of acute cardiac injuries. The repair of septal defects and valvular injuries with mild to moderate hemodynamic instability is generally delayed until the patient is stabilized and accurate diagnosis is made. Inflow occlusion with moderate hypothermia was used in 17 patients with acute cardiac injuries (10). Occlusive tourniquets are placed around the superior and inferior venae cavae. The aorta and pulmonary arteries are cross-clamped after blood is massaged out of the heart. Rapid repair of atrial and ventricular septal defects, as well as ventricular tears, and removal of foreign bodies can be accomplished. Survival was 82% in this group. The safe occlusion time is 6 min, and

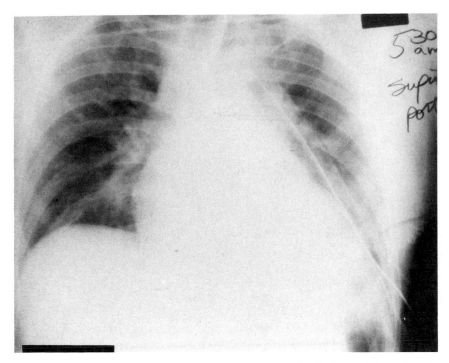

Figure 19.18.   Postoperative chest x-ray film upon repair of left ventricle perforation.

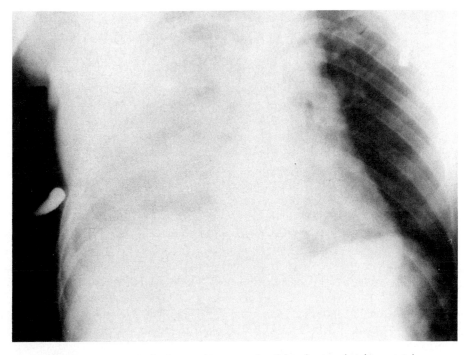

Figure 19.19.   Multiple gunshot wounds of the chest and right ventricle.

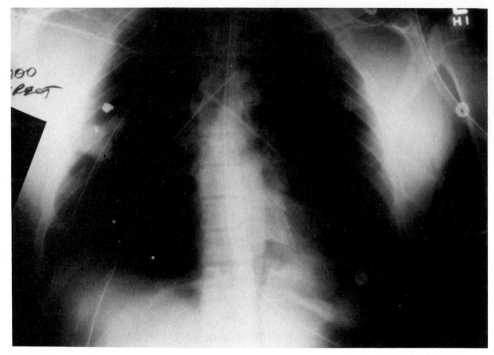

Figure 19.20. Chest x-ray film after repair of right ventricular injury using inflow occlusion technique.

inflow occlusion can be repeated if needed. In selected cases, inflow occlusion combines speed with simplicity and obviates the need for generalized heparinization in acute trauma.

Cardiopulmonary bypass was established in nine other casualties, with four survivals (10). Lack of bypass equipment and delay in bypass setup can be a handicap. The technique of femoral artery/femoral vein bypass (25) was not attempted. Because it is less time-consuming, it may prove to be a valuable method. Assist devices in acute cardiac injuries may also have potential, considering the young age of patients. In a recent review, the author could not identify reports of the use of an intraaortic balloon pump device in acute cardiac trauma (26). Cardiac hemorrhage, rupture, and arrhythmias accounted for 62% of the mortalities.

MAJOR PULMONARY INJURIES

Figure 19.21 shows a postoperative chest radiograph taken after a major buckshot wound to the left chest. The patient presented in profound shock with a gaping chest wall wound and profuse external bleeding. He was transported immediately to the operating room, where a left thoracotomy was performed. The left upper lobe was totally destroyed. There were six pellet tears of the descending aorta. The aorta was compressed manually and the lacerations sutured with pledgeted polypropylene sutures (Fig. 19.22) after debridement of the blackened edges. A left upper lobectomy was performed. The residual tears of the left lower lobe were debrided and repaired by suture. Pectoralis muscle rotation was employed to close the gap in the chest wall. His

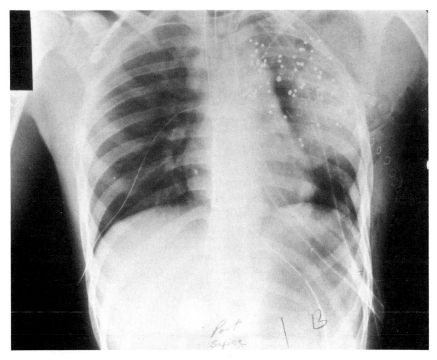

Figure 19.21. Postoperative chest x-ray film after upper lobectomy and aortic repair.

postoperative course was complicated by a recurrent left pneumothorax, which required chest tube suction (Fig. 19.23). This patient recovered and is well 4 yr hence.

Most penetrating and perforating wounds of the lung from HVMs should be explored by thoracotomy. Tube thoracotomy is an important early supportive and diagnostic measure. It is the definitive treatment in less than half of such major injuries.

In 1251 thoracic injuries in the Lebanon conflict, 54% required thoracotomy as the definitive procedure (8). This is a higher incidence than reported in standard civilian practices (27, 28) with low-velocity injuries. Wedge, segmental, and lobe resections were frequently required, in view of the severity of pulmonary destruction from HVM, in this group of young patients who survived transportation. There is growing evidence from the literature supporting early thoracotomy and pulmonary resection from HVM injury (13, 29, 30), as some patients treated with chest tubes alone and others treated with thoracotomy, but without resection, in HVM trauma later died (30, 31). The results in this series of patients are shown in Table 19.9.

There is no notable increase in mortality due to the thoracotomy itself. Effective control of hemorrhage, air leaks, pulmonary rupture, decortication, debridement, and the removal of foreign bodies are better performed via thoracotomy in patients with major penetrating wounds of the chest.

Injuries of the diaphragm (32, 33) and the esophagus (34, 35) should be repaired surgically before the onset of life-threatening complications. In 17 esophageal injuries from penetrating wounds, primary repair after debridement was possible in 5. This repair was reinforced by pleural wraps, doubly folded and sutured around the repaired esophagus. Gastric patch onlays were successful in the treatment of lower esophagus

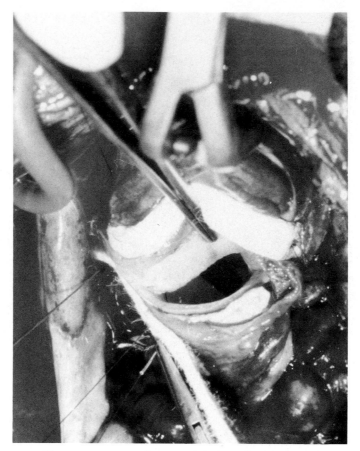

Figure 19.22. Technique of pledgeted aortic repair.

wounds (36). In one patient who was referred after empyema and mediastinitis had set in, conservative treatment with chest tube drainage, nasograstric suction, and other supportive measures failed. He was operated on via a right thoracotomy; total necrosis of the thoracic esophagus was found. The esophagus was totally resected along with the empyema cavity and necrotic pleura. Cervical esophagostomy was performed and the gastroesophageal junction was stapled. Dramatic clinical improvement followed. One

Table 19.9.
Mortality in Primarily Thoracic Casualties

Procedure/Organ	No. of Patients	Died	Percent
Tube thoracostomy	570	4	0.7
Resection	258	5	1.9
Pulmonary hemorrhage	140	2	1.4
Decortication	68	1	1.5
Air leak	61	2	3.3
Chest wall	52	0	0
Esophagus	8	0	0
Mammary/intercostals	40	0	0
Great vessels	54	7	13.0
Total	1251	21	1.7

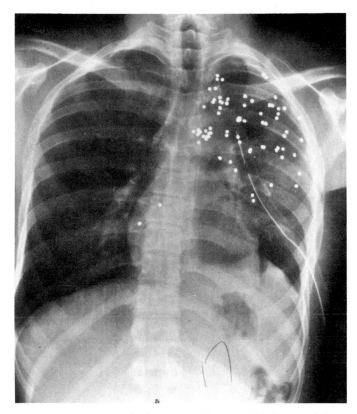

Figure 19.23.   One week after repair of aorta and left upper lobectomy.

month later, a substernal left colon interposition was performed, and the patient was subsequently discharged in satisfactory condition.

CONCLUSION

Most of the clinical case studies presented in this chapter are derived from American civilian casualties. Our experience in the treatment of 2000 cardiothoracic casualties in paramilitary combat and in a major United States civilian trauma zone demonstrates improved patient survival and fewer late complications when early open surgical treatment is implemented for penetrating cardiothoracic injuries, especially those from high-velocity missiles and similar major weaponry fired at close range. With the advent of modern resuscitation systems, early intrathoracic surgical control at the locus of the injury allows effective patient stabilization and safe correction of cardiothoracic structural injury.

REFERENCES

1. DeBakey ME, Simeone FA. Battle injuries of arteries in World War II: an analysis of 2,471 cases. Ann Surg 1946;123:534–579.
2. Elkin DC, DeBakey ME. Surgery in World War II, vascular surgery. Washington, DC: Office of the Surgeon General, Department of the Army, 1955.
3. Parmly LE, Mattingly TW, Marion WM. Penetrating wounds of the heart and aorta. Circulation 1958;17:953–973.
4. Berry EF. Surgery in World War II, thoracic surgery. Washington, DC: Office of the Surgeon General, Department of the Army, 1963.

5. Hughes CW. Acute vascular trauma in Korean War casualties: an analysis of 180 cases. Surg Gynecol Obstet 1970;99:91–100.
6. Rich NM, Baugh JH, Hughes CW. Acute arterial injuries in Vietnam: 1,000 cases. J Trauma 1970;10:359–368.
7. Gielchinski I, McNamara JJ. Cardiac wounds at a military evacuation hospital in Vietnam. J Thorac Cardiovasc Surg 1970;60:603–606.
8. Zakharia AT. Cardiovascular and thoracic battle injuries in the Lebanon War: analysis of 3,000 personal cases. J Thorac Cardiovasc Surg 1985;89:723–733.
9. Zakharia AT. Thoracic battle injuries in the Lebanon War: review of the early operative approach in 1,992 personal cases. Ann Thorac Surg 1985;40:209–214.
10. Zakharia AT. Analysis of 285 cardiac penetrating injuries in the Lebanon War. J Cardiovasc Surg 1987;28:380–383.
11. Zakharia AT. Cardiovascular and thoracic center. Beirut, Lebanon: Archives of the Arab Research Center for Injuries, 1977.
12. Zakharia AT, Kaiser G. An outline of basic trauma care protocol for the thoracic specialty. Miami, FL: University of Miami Division of Thoracic Surgery, 1985.
12a. Zakharia AT. Unpublished data, 1989.
13. Besson A, Vecerina S, Steichen FM. Penetrating and perforating wounds of the chest. In: Color atlas of chest trauma and associated injuries. Oradell, NJ: Medical Economics Co., 1983:123–152.
14. Rybeck B, Lewis DH, Sandegard J, Seeman T. The immediate circulatory response to high velocity missiles. J Trauma 1975;15:323–335.
15. Berlin R. Energy transfer and regional blood flow changes following missile trauma. J Trauma 1979;15:170–176.
16. Dahlgren B, Berlin R, Brandberg A, Rybeck B, Seeman T. Bacteriological findings in the first 12 hours following experimental missile trauma. Acta Chir Scand 1981;147:513–518.
17. Turney SZ, Attar S, Ayella R, Cowley RA, McLaughlin J. Traumatic rupture of the aorta: a five year experience. J Thorac Cardiovasc Surg 1976;72:727–734.
18. Mattox KL, Beall AC Jr, Jordan GL, DeBakey ME. Cardiorrhaphy in the emergency center. J Thorac Cardiovasc Surg 1974;68:886–895.
19. Bodai BI, Smith JP, Ward RE, et al. Emergency thoracotomy in the management of trauma. JAMA 1983;249:1891–1896.
20. Rohman M, Ivatury RR, Steichen FM. Emergency room thoracotomy for penetrating cardiac injuries. J Trauma 1983;23:570–576.
21. Baker CC, Thomas AN, Trunkey DD. The role of emergency room thoracotomy in trauma. J Trauma 1980;20:848–855.
22. Flynn TC, Ward RE, Miller PW. Emergency room thoracotomy. Ann Emerg Med 1982;11:413–416.
23. Mandal AK, Okpako A, Oparah SS. Experience in the management of 50 consecutive penetrating wounds of the heart. Br J Surg 1979;66:565–568.
24. Mattila S, Laustella E, Tala P. Penetrating and perforating thoracic injuries. Scand J Thorac Cardiovasc Surg 1981;15:105–110.
25. Cooley DA. Techniques in cardiac surgery. 2nd ed. Philadelphia: Saunders, 1984.
26. Zakharia AT, Kaiser GA. Intraaortic balloon pumping. In: Sprung CL, ed. Invasive procedures in critical care. New York: Churchill Livingstone, 1985:179–190.
27. Lewis FR. Thoracic trauma. Surg Clin North Am 1982;62:97–103.
28. Webb WR. Thoracic trauma. Surg Clin North Am 1974;54:1179–1192.
29. Grover FL. Treatment of thoracic battle injuries versus civilian injuries. Ann Thorac Surg 1985;40:207–208.
30. McNamara JJ, Messersmith JK, Dunn RA. Thoracic injuries in combat casualties in Vietnam. Ann Thorac Surg 1970;10:385–394.
31. Fischer RP, Geiger JP, Guernsey JM. Pulmonary resections for severe pulmonary contusions secondary to high velocity missile wounds. J Trauma 1974;14:293–296.
32. Estera AS, Plat MR, Mills LJ. Traumatic injuries of the diaphragm. Chest 1979;75:306–313.
33. Sterns LP, Kensen NK, Schmidt WR. Diaphragmatic disruption in major thoracic trauma: a review of 16 cases. Can J Surg 1969;12:426–431.
34. Urschel HC, Razzuk MA, Wood RE, Galbraith N, Puckey M, Paulson DL. Improved management of esophageal perforation: exclusion and diversion in continuity. Ann Surg 1974;179:587–591.
35. Symbas PN, Hatcher CR, Vlassis SE. Esophageal gunshot wound injuries. Ann Surg 1980;191:703–707.
36. Robinson JC, Isa SS, Specs EK. Substernal gastric bypass for palliation of esophageal carcinoma. Surgery 1982;91:305–311.

20 Tracheoinnominate Artery Fistula

DiAnne J. Leonard, MD
Aurelio Rodriguez, MD

Tracheoinnominate artery fistula resulting in rapid exsanguination is a rare but devastating complication of tracheostomy. Although reported to occur in 0.6–0.7% of all tracheostomies (1), its incidence may be decreasing due to the use of soft-cuffed, low-pressure tracheostomy tubes. The lethal nature of this complication, however, remains evident. In 1976, Jones et al. (1) reviewed the world literature and found only 10 long-term survivors out of 137 reported cases. Recent experience indicates that the survival rate after innominate artery erosion can be improved (2) if several basic concepts are applied: (*a*) prompt recognition of the significance of tracheostomy site bleeding, (*b*) rapid institution of maneuvers to control hemorrhage and maintain airway patency, and (*c*) definitive surgical treatment with innominate artery resection.

ETIOLOGY

Korte (3), in 1879, was probably the first to describe fatal rupture of the innominate artery after tracheostomy in a 5-year-old child with diphtheria. He suggested that this problem occurred only with low tracheostomies. Since that time, multiple etiologies have been implicated in the development of tracheoinnominate artery fistulas. Localized ischemic pressure necrosis of the innominate artery by the tracheostomy tube or cuff seems to be the common denominator (4). The injuries may be classified as extratracheal or endotracheal in origin (5).

Extratracheal injuries result from erosion of the innominate artery by the inferior surface of the tracheal cannula at the ostomy site—usually a consequence of tracheostomy placement below the fourth tracheal ring (Fig. 20.1, *left*). Neck hyperextension for exposure and tracheal evaluation by hooks may contribute to low airway entry. Accordingly, tracheostomies should be placed no lower than the third tracheal ring. Anatomic anomalies such as a high-lying innominate artery or aberrant origin of the carotid arteries may lead to arterial erosion by even a normally placed tracheostomy tube (6).

Endotracheal injuries result from direct pressure of the cuff or tip of the tracheostomy tube on the anterior tracheal wall (Fig. 20.1, *center, right*). Tracheal mucosa is intolerant of constant pressure and, after 48 hr, tracheal injury is universally present (7). Erosion into the contiguous innominate artery may occur with development of a true tracheoinnominate artery fistula. Although numerous studies have confirmed that low-pressure, high-volume cuffs reduce tracheal damage (8, 9), caution

373

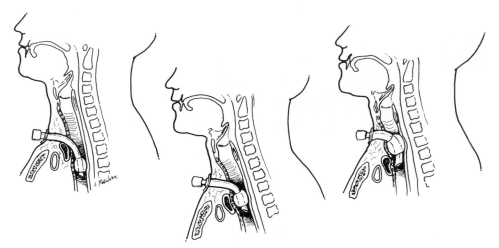

Figure 20.1. Mechanisms of development of tracheoinnominate artery fistula. *Left,* erosion of innominate artery by inferior surface of tracheal cannula. *Center,* pressure necrosis from inflated cuff. *Right,* direct pressure from tip of tracheostomy tube.

must be taken to avoid overinflation of these cuffs. Excessive motion of the tracheostomy tube in spastic, neurologic, and seizure patients should be avoided.

Factors that adversely affect wound healing have also been implicated in predisposing the patient to tracheal injury (1). Tracheal infection, steroid administration, sepsis, hypotension, and malnutrition may lower mucosal resistance, thereby increasing the risk of tracheoinnominate artery erosion.

DIAGNOSIS

The diagnosis of tracheoinnominate artery fistula should be considered in any patient who has arterial bleeding from a tracheostomy tube or stoma. In 50% of cases, a transient sentinel hemorrhage occurs several hours to several days prior to massive cataclysmic hemorrhage (10). Early hemorrhage occurring within hours of tracheostomy is usually due to inadequate hemostasis or coagulation defects. Half of the individuals with tracheostomy bleeding 48 hr or later after tracheostomy, however, will have tracheoinnominate erosions (1). Spontaneous cessation of the bleeding or easy control with packing must not be interpreted as an indication that a fistula does not exist (11).

TREATMENT
Emergency Maneuvers

Hemorrhage from a tracheoinnominate fistula may be rapidly fatal unless immediate measures are taken to secure the airway and control bleeding. The cuff of the tracheostomy tube should be hyperinflated and suprasternal pressure should be applied. If bleeding persists after cuff inflation, the innominate artery should be dissected off the trachea with the index finger and the posteromedial aspect of the artery occluded against the sternum (12) (Fig. 20.2). An oral or nasal endotracheal tube inserted proximal to the tracheostomy tube allows immediate removal of the latter tube and advancement of the endotracheal tube if airway patency is compromised. The patient should be transported rapidly to the operating room.

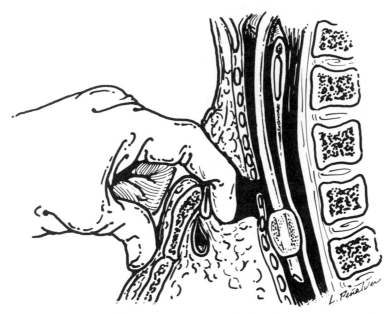

Figure 20.2.   Compression of the innominate artery by digital pressure against the sternum.

Surgical Technique

In the presence of massive hemorrhage, immediate median sternotomy is performed without any complementary investigations. If the situation has stabilized, the tracheostomy is removed and an oral or nasal endotracheal tube placed. Careful fiberoptic bronchoscopy is performed while deflating the cuff and gradually withdrawing the tube. The tracheal stoma wound is also explored. Alternative sites and etiologies for tracheostomy bleeding include granulation tissue at the stoma, subcutaneous vessels, tracheitis, coagulopathy, and tracheal erosion at the cuff site without fistula. Failure to find a clear explanation for the bleeding in a stable patient should prompt angiographic evaluation.

If erosion of the innominate artery is confirmed, exposure is accomplished by median sternotomy. The pericardium is entered and the proximal innominate artery identified and controlled (Fig. 20.3, *top*). The surgeon must be aware of possible anatomic variations of the great vessels arising from the aortic arch. In approximately 10% of Caucasians and 30% of Blacks, the left common carotid artery arises from the innominate artery rather than from the aortic arch (5). This anomaly must be carefully sought. In most cases, adequate exposure can be obtained by retracting the left innominate vein superiorly (Fig. 20.3, *bottom left*). Ligation of this vein may produce obstruction to venous return from the head and left upper extremity. Control of the innominate artery is then obtained distal to the fistula and proximal to the right carotid and subclavian vessels. Proximal and distal vascular clamps are applied, thereby isolating the fistula. The portion of innominate artery in contact with the tracheal erosion is then resected, and the arterial stumps are oversewn with 3–0 Prolene sutures (Fig. 20.3, *bottom right*). Vascularized flaps of sternocleidomastoid muscle or pericardium can be used to cover the exposed arterial stump. Vascular reconstruction through the infected operative field is unwarranted due to the high risk of anastomotic

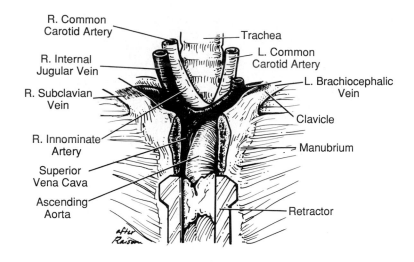

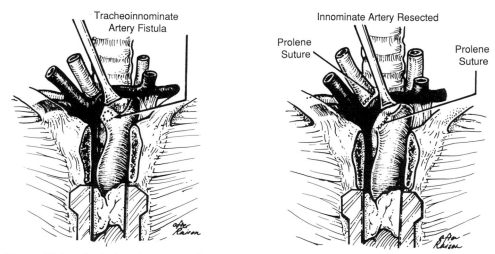

Figure 20.3.   Technique for repair of tracheoinnominate artery fistula. *Top,* exposure of vessels. *Bottom left,* elevation of left innominate vein to expose fistula. *Bottom right,* completed innominate artery resection. (From Courcy PA, Rodriguez A, Garrett HE. Operative technique for repair of tracheoinnominate artery fistula. J Vasc Surg 1985;2:332–334.)

breakdown with recurrent hemorrhage. Neurologic symptoms rarely occur with innominate artery ligation due to extensive collateral circulation (4, 6, 11, 13). The distal innominate artery stump pressure can be measured intraoperatively, however, and should be greater than one-third of the proximal pressure. In the event of negligible or very low pressures, reconstruction of the cerebral circulation should be considered. Alternatively, intraoperative electroencephalography can be used to monitor cerebral function (14–16). Should acute neurologic symptoms develop in the immediate perioperative period, a carotid–carotid or femoral axillary bypass can be performed.

The tracheal defect is not repaired primarily but is allowed to close by granulation. Necrotic trachea is debrided and wound cultures are obtained. Infection is controlled by mediastinal drainage and appropriate antibiotics. Postoperatively, the airway is maintained by a nasal or oral endotracheal tube with a balloon positioned below the tracheal defect.

In the postoperative period, nutrition should be optimized, any unnecessary steroid therapy discontinued, and early extubation achieved as soon as feasible. Bronchoscopy may be necessary to document tracheal healing and rule out the presence of significant tracheal stenosis.

CLINICAL EXPERIENCE AT THE MIEMSS SHOCK TRAUMA CENTER

Between July 1981 and July 1987, 796 tracheostomies and 35 cricothyroidotomies were performed at the Shock Trauma Center of the Maryland Institute for Emergency Medical Services Systems. During this period, three patients developed tracheoinnominate artery erosions and one patient developed a tracheocarotid artery fistula, for an incidence of 0.5%. In this subset of four patients, elective tracheostomies were performed the day of admission on three patients with complex facial fractures; the remaining tracheostomy was performed on day 13 for prolonged ventilatory support. All of the patients were critically ill and three had associated closed head injuries. One patient had an associated tracheoesophageal fistula.

The time between performance of the tracheostomy and manifestation of the fistula ranged from 4 to 15 days. Three patients presented with massive hemorrhage from the tracheostomy sites with associated hypotension. One thoracotomy was performed at bedside in the critical care unit with ligation of the innominate artery. Two patients were taken to the operating room for immediate median sternotomy. One innominate artery resection was performed; the other patient required ligation of the right carotid artery (tracheocarotid fistula).

The fourth patient presented with tracheostomy hemorrhage, which was easily controlled with cuff hyperinflation and suprasternal pressure. Bronchoscopy and local wound exploration revealed peristomal inflammation but no site of active bleeding. An angiogram demonstrated a pseudoaneurysm of the innominate artery; definitive treatment included median sternotomy with tracheoinnominate artery resection.

There were no intraoperative mortalities. Two of the four patients survived. One death occurred from intracranial hypertension during the immediate postoperative period in a patient with severe associated closed head injury. The other death occurred on the fourth postoperative day from adult respiratory distress syndrome. One survivor developed a mediastinal wound infection that required drainage, debridement, and flap coverage. The survivors had no neurologic sequelae after innominate artery interruption.

SUMMARY

A tracheoinnominate artery fistula is a true surgical emergency. Patient survival depends on the care-giver's prompt recognition of the significance of bleeding from a tracheostomy site and knowledge of how to obtain emergency control of hemorrhage. Definitive surgical repair then becomes a lifesaving possibility.

REFERENCES

1. Jones JM, Reynolds M, Hewit RI. Tracheo-innominate artery erosion: successful surgical management of a devastating complication. Ann Surg 1976;184:194–204.
2. Hafez A, Courard L, Velly JF, Bruneteau A. Late cataclysmic hemorrhage from the innominate artery after tracheostomy. Thorac Cardiovasc Surg 1984;32:315–319.

3. Korte W. Ueber einige seltenere Nachkrankheite nach der Tracheotomie wegen Diphtheritis. Arch Klin Chir 1879;24:238–264.

4. Cooley DA, Wukasch DC. Vascular injuries. In: Cooley DA, Wukasch DC, eds. Techniques in vascular surgery. Philadelphia: Saunders, 1979:188–198.

5. Carberry DM, Bethea MC. Intervention in tracheal fistula. Contemp Surg 1977;11:9–11.

6. Courcy PA, Rodriguez A, Garrett HE. Operative technique for repair of tracheoinnominate artery fistula. J Vasc Surg 1985;2:332–334.

7. Cooper JD, Grillo HC. The evolution of tracheal injury due to ventilatory assistance through cuffed tubes: a pathologic study. Ann Surg 1969;169:334–348.

8. Ching NPH, Ayra SM, Spina RC, Nealon TF. Endotracheal damage during continuous ventilatory support. Ann Surg 1974;179:123–127.

9. Shelly WM, Dawson RB, May IA. Cuffed tubes as a cause of tracheal stenosis. J Thorac Cardiovasc Surg 1969;57:623–627.

10. Tournigand P, Djurakdjian S, Jajah S, Morisset P. Successful surgical repair of a tracheo-innominate fistula: tactical consideration. J Cardiovasc Surg 1982;23:247–251.

11. Cooper JD. Tracheo-innominate artery fistula: successful management of 3 consecutive patients. Ann Thorac Surg 1977;24:439–447.

12. Utley JR, Singer MM, Roe BB, et al. Definitive management of innominate artery hemorrhage complicating tracheostomy. JAMA 1972;220:577–579.

13. Myers WO, Lawton BR, Sautter RD. An operation for tracheal-innominate artery fistula. Arch Surg 1972;105:269–273.

14. Bloss RS, Ward RE. Survival after tracheoinnominate artery fistula. Am J Surg 1980;140:251–253.

15. Brewster DC, Moncure AC, Darling RC, Ambrosino JJ, Abbott WM. Innominate artery lesions: problems encountered and lessons learned. J Vasc Surg 1985;2:99–112.

16. Nelems JM. Tracheoinnominate artery fistula. Am J Surg 1981;141:526–527.

21 Traumatic Asphyxia

Wendell A. Goins, MD
Aurelio Rodriguez, MD

Traumatic asphyxia (masque ecchymotique, compression cyanosis) is a syndrome that results from a crush injury to the chest, usually of short duration. A patient classically has the triad of subconjunctival hemorrhage, upper body and facial edema with a cyanotic hue, and petechiae. It was first described by Ollivier in 1837 following autopsy examination of crush victims (1). The true incidence of traumatic asphyxia is unknown, but the condition is rare (2). Only 10 cases were identified in a 12.5-yr period at the Shock Trauma Center of the Maryland Institute for Emergency Medical Services Systems (3). Over 253 cases have been reported (4, 5).

MECHANISM OF INJURY

Most crush injuries of the chest are the result of motor vehicle accidents in which the victims were either pinned between the car seat and steering wheel or ejected and rolled over by the vehicle. Four of six patients in Landercasper and Cogbill's series sustained injury secondary to vehicular accidents, three of which involved tractors (6). Forty percent of Sklar et al.'s 35 cases were the result of motor vehicle accidents; 64% of these patients were ejected and crushed as the vehicle rolled over them (4). They also reported that 26% of their cases were due to the slippage of cars from jacks and 20% were secondary to work-related accidents. Other causes of this syndrome include railway accidents, seizures, vomiting, asthma, and sea diving (7). Gorenstein et al. reported that motor vehicle accidents caused traumatic asphyxia in 68% of their pediatric series (8). Five of six children in Sklar et al.'s series were crushed by household objects (4).

PATHOPHYSIOLOGY

Although the exact pathophysiology of traumatic asphyxia is unknown, it has been related to an increase in superior and inferior vena caval pressure due to compressive forces on the thorax. The presence of a closed glottis at the time of injury appears to be essential in the process. The "fear response" produces a Valsalva maneuver, which may protect the lower torso from the effects of traumatic asphyxia by compressing the inferior vena cava (9). Blood is then forced from the right atrium and superior vena cava into the valveless veins of the head, neck, and upper torso. The increased pressure in the innominate, jugular, and cephalic veins is transmitted to small venules and capillaries, which dilate and may hemorrhage, producing petechiae.

Venous stagnation and subsequent desaturation produce the cyanotic discoloration of the skin. The skin changes may be strikingly absent where there is counterpressure by hats, head bands, and collars.

Changes in mental status are fairly common in patients with traumatic asphyxia—the presence of associated head injury, hypercarbia, or anoxia may be partially responsible. Autopsy studies most commonly show cerebral edema with congestion of the pial vessels, although the presence of intracerebral and petechial subarachnoid hemorrhage has been reported. The skull may exert enough counterpressure to prevent more extensive intracranial hemorrhage.

Motor paralysis has been suggested to occur as a result of increased pressure of the intervertebral venous plexus in the thoracic spine, proceeding to venous thrombosis, ischemia, and anoxia to those areas of the spinal cord. Minor fractures of the spine were seen in 40% of patients in Ectors et al.'s review (10).

DIAGNOSIS

Most patients with traumatic asphyxia present with cyanotic discoloration and edema of the face and upper torso with petechiae and subconjunctival hemorrhage. All three signs were present in 58% of cases in Sklar et al.'s autopsy series (4); two of the three signs were present in 88%. Subconjunctival hemorrhage is seen in as many as 80% of cases (6, 8). Altered mental status occurs in more than 50% of patients, with loss of consciousness present in 30% (4, 6, 10). Crepps and Rodriguez (3) reported that loss of consciousness was present in 66% of the 38 patients with traumatic asphyxia whom they reviewed. The presence of seizures, coma, aphasia, agitation, and decerebrate posturing has been reported. Ectors et al. (10) reviewed five cases of paraplegia or quadriplegia associated with traumatic asphyxia. Landercasper and Cogbill (6) reported that 30% of their patients sustained lacerations to the external auditory canal. Visual and ocular abnormalties such as pupillary inequalities, diplopia, proptosis, and loss of vision may be seen, especially in the pediatric population. Mucosal petechiae, hemoptysis, esophageal hemorrhage, rectal bleeding, hematuria, and proteinuria have been reported.

TREATMENT

Associated injuries are common with traumatic asphyxia. The initial management of these patients should be directed toward these injuries. Injuries to the chest wall are most common, but lung and liver injuries also occur frequently. Thoracic injuries have been reported in 58% of patients (3). Landercasper and Cogbill's patients (6) had a mean Injury Severity Score (ISS) of 14, while those of Crepps and Rodriguez (3) had a mean ISS of 25. Patients with traumatic asphyxia should undergo thorough neurologic and ophthalmologic examinations. Head elevation and supplemental oxygen administration should be instituted while these patients are monitored closely. For patients with more severe injuries, intubation and mechanical ventilation may be necessary.

MORBIDITY AND MORTALITY

The majority of patients with isolated traumatic asphyxia survive; Crepps and Rodriguez (3) reported a mortality rate of 13%. Death usually occurs at the scene or early in the hospital course. Morbidity and mortality are primarily related to associated injuries or cerebral anoxia. The duration and severity of compression are important factors in the outcome: when the duration of compression is greater than 5 min, the mortality rate may be as high as 26% (3). The loss of consciousness is transient and usually resolves within 48 hr. Spinal deficits require aggressive physiotherapy and commonly result in recovery. Resolution of cyanotic discoloration and subconjunctival hemorrhage may require as long as 2 and 5 weeks, respectively (10). Landercasper and Cogbill (5) reported resolution of cyanosis, edema, petechiae, and neurologic abnormalities in their series of long-term survivors.

REFERENCES

1. Ollivier D. Relation medicale des evenemements surveuus au Champ-de-Mars le 14 Juin 1837. Ann d'Hyg 1837;18:485–489.
2. Dwek J. Ecchymotic mask. J Int Coll Surg 1946;9:257–265.
3. Crepps JT Jr, Rodriguez A. Traumatic asphyxia: review and reappraisal. Trauma Q 1988;5:23–29.
4. Sklar DP, Baack B, McFeeley P, Osler T, Marder E, Demarest G. Traumatic asphyxia in New Mexico: a five-year experience. Am J Emerg Med 1988;6:219–223.
5. Haller JA, Donahoo JS. Traumatic asphyxia in children: pathophysiology and management. J Trauma 1971;11:453–457.
6. Landercasper J, Cogbill TH. Long-term follow-up after traumatic asphyxia. J Trauma 1985;25:838–841.
7. Hambeck W, Pueschel K. Death by railway accident: incidence of traumatic asphyxia. J Trauma 1981;21:28–31.
8. Gorenstein L, Blair GK, Shandling B. The prognosis of traumatic asphyxia in childhood. J Pediatr Surg 1986;21:753–756.
9. Thompson A, Illescas FF, Chin RCJ. Why is the lower torso protected in traumatic asphyxia? A new hypothesis. Ann Thorac Surg 1989;47:247–249.
10. Ectors P, Bosschaert T, Vincent G, Franken L. Traumatic asphyxia: an unusual cause of traumatic coma and paraplegia. J Neurosurg 1979;51:375–378.

22 Traumatic Chylothorax

Wendell A. Goins, MD
Aurelio Rodriguez, MD

Traumatic chylothorax, a rare complication of penetrating or blunt chest trauma, is caused by disruption of the thoracic duct.

ANATOMY

The thoracic duct arises from the cisterna chyli at the level of the first or second lumbar vertebra and accompanies the aorta through the diaphragmatic hiatus on the right of the midline. It crosses to the left side of the midline at the level of the fifth or sixth thoracic vertebra and continues to the base of the neck, where it passes along the medial edge of the scalenus anterior muscle to join the confluence of the left internal jugular and subclavian veins. Anatomic variations occur in approximately 40% of individuals, and an extensive collateral system is present (Fig. 22.1).

MECHANISM OF INJURY

Nonpenetrating trauma accounted for 62% of the cases in Goorwitch's 1955 series (1). Blunt trauma such as sustained in a crush or a fall may produce hyperextension of the spine, which can rupture the thoracic duct or major lymphatic collaterals in the thorax, especially when the duct is distended after a recent meal. It may be associated with spinal injuries. Traumatic chylothorax has also been associated with blunt injuries to the base of the neck related to the effects of shoulder straps during motor vehicle accidents (2, 3). Isolated penetrating injuries to the thoracic duct are also rare and may accompany injuries to nearby structures, which take precedence. Penetrating injuries to the base of the neck may involve the thoracic duct as it enters the subclavian vein on the left. Traumatic chylothorax has been reported after a traumatic amputation of the left upper extremity where thrombosis of the subclavian vein occurred (4).

CLINICAL PRESENTATION

Chylothorax may present anytime from the day of injury to months later. Patients will present with respiratory symptoms or with a pleural effusion, which is more common on the right side (1). The diagnosis of traumatic chylothorax may be challenging in multiply injured patients. The character of the pleural fluid may be serous or bloody initially; if the patient is fasting because of abdominal injuries, the flow of chyle is low, which may result in an insignificant leak. A "chyloma" (a collection of chyle in the posterior mediastinum) may eventually rupture into one or both pleural spaces. When

11. Milsom JW, Kron IL, Rheuban KS, Rodgers BM. Chylothorax: an assessment of current surgical management. J Thorac Cardiovasc Surg 1985;89:221–227.
12. Ngan H, Fok M, Wong J. The role of lymphography in chylothorax following thoracic surgery. Br J Radiol 1988;61:1032–1036.
13. Ramzy AI, Rodriguez A, Cowley RA. Pitfalls in the management of traumatic chylothorax. J Trauma 1982;22:513–515.
14. Little AG, Kadowaki MH, Ferguson MK, Staszek VM, Skinner DB. Pleuroperitoneal shunting. Ann Surg 1988;208:443–450.

23 Gas Embolism

Roy A. M. Myers, MD

DEFINITION OF GAS EMBOLISM

Gas embolism is defined as the passage of air into either the arterial or venous system of the body. The symptomatology varies greatly, depending on the site of entry, the amount of gas entering, and the speed of entry into the system. Classically, gas embolism enters the venous system, passes into the heart, and then passes into the pulmonary arteries; if a patent foramen ovale is present, the air passes directly into the systemic circulation. It may bypass the lungs through shunts in the pulmonary and systemic circulation or pass into the lung where most of the air is absorbed. The severity of the manifestations depends on which systemic arteries are obstructed, particularly those of the central nervous system or coronary circulation.

Major differences in symptomatology depend on the initial location of the air embolism (namely, venous or arterial) and also on the amount of air necessary to produce serious symptoms or death. Venous embolism occurs when air enters a systemic vein. In large enough quantities, it will result in an obstruction to the right ventricular outflow tract. Volumes of air from 100–150 ml or more may be necessary to produce death. Factors that will alter the amount injected include the pressure under which that gas is injected, the speed of the injection, and, most importantly, the position of the patient at the time the air entered the circulation. Venous air embolism occurs under many different circumstances in medical practice but, in all such incidences, it obstructs the pulmonary circulation and yields pulmonary clinical manifestations.

Venous air embolism occurs when air gains entrance into a pulmonary vein or an artery. The resultant clinical picture differs entirely from that of arterial air embolism. In arterial air embolism, the manifestations are due to obstruction of systemic arteries, including the major vessels of the central nervous system and the coronary vessels. This type of problem can develop with pneumothorax, thoracentesis, thoracic surgical procedures, or direct air access to an arterial line (arterial line pressure monitoring).

BACKGROUND

Morgagni (1) was the first to recognize and report postmortem findings of arterial air embolism; his observations and findings were translated into English in 1769. In 1878, Bert (2) reported the effects of cerebral embolism in dogs and prescribed a specific therapy. He pointed out that the volume of the gas bubble lodged in the vessels of the brain needed to be reduced immediately so that blood would drive the air out of the vessels.

The first actual iatrogenic incident of arterial air embolisms was most likely in the 1800s when empyema cavities were irrigated. According to Schlaepfer (3), a French physician, Roger, first called attention to these accidents in 1864; he described the condition as a pleural eclampsia or pleural epilepsy, thinking that the clinical syndrome was due to nervous origin. With the introduction of artificial pneumothorax by puncturing the chest as a treatment, more of these cases occurred. In 1912, Brandes (4) actually showed the mechanism of the injury: after bismuth paste was injected into a patient's empyema cavity, the patient started convulsing and died. At postmortem sectioning of the walls of the sinus and the pleural empyema cavity, Brandes showed that the catheter had open communication to the pulmonary veins, and bismuth was found in the smallest vessels of the cerebral cortex of both hemispheres. Brauer's (5) proposal that the accidents occurring in this type of treatment (pneumothorax production) were from air embolism, not pleural reflexes, was confirmed by Wever (6) with animal studies in 1913. However, it took another 30 yr for this etiology to be generally accepted (7, 8). The recognition and treatment of iatrogenic cerebral gas embolism have lagged far behind our medical knowledge of the condition even today, despite the fact that air emboli have been seen in the retinal vessels (9–12).

PATHOPHYSIOLOGY

Substantial morbidity and mortality occur from venous air embolism, which, however, is an uncommon problem and a most difficult one to diagnose and document. Small air emboli may pass undetected with the production of no clinical signs or symptoms. When clinical signs and symptoms are present, they may mimic acute cardiopulmonary and cerebrovascular events, thus obscuring the diagnosis. Like pulmonary thrombi embolism, venous air embolism is very often postulated but requires ventilation perfusion scans and angiography to document. Durant et al. (8) injected large air emboli into the central veins of open chests in dogs. They noted gross anatomic changes: immediate dilatation of the right atrium, ventricular, and pulmonary outflow tracts, followed by rapidly developing ischemia over the right ventricle. It was postulated that the pulmonary outflow tract of the right ventricle had been obstructed by the large air embolus.

Air embolism induced in animals demonstrated histologic and ultrastructural changes that support the hypothesis of lodgment and obstruction of blood flow in the heart and vasculature by the air emboli (13, 14). The air–blood interaction produces a network of air bubbles and fibrin strands interspersed with aggregates of platelets, red blood cells, and fat globules. The whipping action of the heart or the vortex flow of blood from the turbulence results in air bubbles partly occluding but not stopping the flow. With platelet aggregation and fibrin formation, a number of physiologic abnormalities develop, including increased airway resistance, pulmonary edema, decreased lung compliance, pulmonary hypertension, hypoxemia, and myocardial ischemia. Kahn et al. (15) studied the effects of various types of gas embolism on airway resistance. Oxygen and nitrogen increased the airway resistance, but carbon dioxide or inert gases (such as helium, argon, xenon, or neon) had no effect. The effects of the oxygen and nitrogen could be prevented by pretreating animals with heparin sodium or by administering an antiserotonin agent such as methysergide. Carbon dioxide, because it is very soluble in blood, did not cause the changes typical of air emboli.

Three mechanisms have been postulated for the edema formation (which is, however, transient and reversible) seen in a sheep model with venous air embolism

(16): increased capillary permeability, vasoconstriction, and rupture of alveoli. The first mechanism, increased capillary permeability, is evidenced with an increase in lymph flow and the lymph:plasma protein ratio after air embolism. There is ultrastructural evidence of endothelial cell injury and herniation through the basal lamina (14). In addition, there is an increase in hydrostatic pulmonary vascular pressures that favors edema formation. When air bubbles and vasoconstriction mechanically occlude the pulmonary artery (17), there is a corresponding increase in pulmonary arteries and right-side heart pressure. With the absorption of the air emboli, these pressures return to normal. Fluid transudation occurs from the arterial extraalveolar vessels (18).

Air injected into the venous circulation also results in decreased lung compliance, which is, however, short lived and directly related to the absolute amount injected (15, 17). Other factors that may contribute to decreased compliance include alveolar duct constriction, increased airway resistance, and interstitial and alveolar edema. The pulmonary vascular obstruction is of a mechanical nature due to the air bubbles and vasoconstriction. The two locations of this obstruction may then be the right ventricle and the pulmonary vascular bed (13). The lung acts as a filter for the bubbles.

Paradoxically, embolization can occur with massive emboli where the right-side heart pressure is acutely increased and facilitates the shunting of air from the right to the left side through a patent foramen ovale. The air embolus would need to be 30 ml or larger. Air emboli can also enter the arterial circulation through the arteriovenous anastomosis in the lungs; this event can occur with mean pulmonary arterial pressures of more than 29 mm Hg (19).

The second mechanism of pulmonary vascular obstruction is vasoconstriction. Berglund et al. (17) measured pulmonary artery pressure, pulmonary artery flow, pulmonary vascular resistance, left atrial pressure, and aortic pressure in dogs. They showed that unilateral and bilateral air emboli produced similar changes, which would suggest a mechanism other than mechanical obstruction. Pulmonary angiography showed vasoconstriction after unilateral air embolization through corkscrewing, rapid tapering, and delayed emptying of contrast in the pulmonary arterial vessels of the unaffected lung. Pretreatment with α-blockers, vagotomy, atropine, antihistamines, and/or antiserotonin agents did not prevent the vasoconstriction. The follow-up anigiograms, however, showed that the vasoconstriction was a transient effect of a few minutes. As a consequence of the ventilation–perfusion maldistribution, hypoxemia occurred. The major $\dot{V}/Q$ abnormality was shown (20) to be an increase in high $\dot{V}/Q$ areas in the lung and not a shunt with small volumes of air emboli. With larger volumes of air emboli, however, the shunt and physiologic dead space increased proportionately. Pulmonary blood flow obstruction with increased right-side heart and pulmonary vascular pressures and hypoxemia could cause hypotension, impaired coronary flow, and myocardial ischemia.

The third mechanism of air embolism relates primarily to the lungs. If the tension on the alveoli walls reaches a critical level due to intraalveolar gas expansion, the alveoli rupture, allowing entry of air into the interstitial tissue and ruptured blood vessels. Intratracheal pressures of 8 mm Hg (21) or transpulmonic pressures of 60–70 mm Hg (22, 23) have been sufficient to rupture alveolar septa, allowing gas to enter the interstitial space and pass along perivascular sheathes, causing mediastinal emphysema and pneumothorax (24). Air could also enter the pericardium, retroperitoneum, and subcutaneous tissue of the neck. After the pulmonary barotrauma and an intrathoracic pressure drop with breathing, the extraalveolar gas intravasates into torn vessels and then migrates to the left side of the heart and thus to the systemic circulation (25). Scuba diving in water only 4 feet (1.2 m) deep after full inspiration has resulted in intratracheal pressures high enough to rupture alveoli, producing fatal air embolism.

The stiff lungs resulting from increased pulmonary compliance with a nonuniform distribution of lung elasticity may result in the more compliant zones of the lung being subjected to excessive strain, with resultant pulmonary barotrauma. Forced expiration at low lung volumes narrows the airways and acts as a check valve that is exaggerated by immersion in water (26).

In arterial air gas embolism, the major target organ is the brain. The gas emboli lodge in the arteries and arterioles, producing distal ischemia (27) followed by endothelial damage (28–30). Immediate damage to the endothelium is caused by the active bubble surface. Within seconds, the cerebrospinal fluid pressure rises and remains elevated for several minutes to an hour, depending on the volume of air injected (31, 32). The cerebrospinal fluid pressure increase is most likely due to vasodilation and extreme dilatation of open intracranial vessels associated with an increase in intracranial blood volume (33). Neuronal function recedes during a period of reduced local blood flow. A critical-range nutrient blood flow of 12–20 ml/100 ml/min is necessary for nerve survival. Nerve cells can survive in a suspended animation within this range for prolonged periods (ischemic penumbra) (34). The process of progressive shutdown of nutrient flow may involve interaction between blood factors and elements in damaged vascular neurotissue (35). Intravenous pharmacologic agents (prostaglandin-2, heparin, and indomethacin) that produce vasodilation and prevent platelets from aggregating and blocking the coagulation and prostaglandin systems eliminate impairment of reflow after global central nervous system ischemia. This action promotes neuronal recovery after focal ischemia from air embolism (36).

ETIOLOGY OF AIR EMBOLISM AND OCCURRENCE IN CLINICAL PRACTICE

The most serious type of decompression sickness, cerebral air embolism, occurs from diving, whether for pleasure (37–39) or for commercial or naval enterprises. In Florida, Smith (40) described 33 scuba diving deaths over a 3-year period. Forty-two deaths occurred in the Los Angeles area in a 7-year period and 10 occurred in Seattle during a similar period. Greene (41) reviewed the experience with air embolism during submarine escape training from 1954 to 1979 and estimated 91 cases of air embolism with four fatalities in 212,000 ascents.

Cases of massive air embolism after scuba diving accidents continue to be reported and are a major concern of the Diving Alert Network. The Diving Alert Network is attempting to correlate the incidence and symptomatology of scuba air embolism and to indicate the location of hyperbaric facilities for treating air embolism and decompression sickness occurring in divers (42).

Iatrogenic arterial gas embolism is both underrecognized and undertreated. There are a great variety of causes with different degrees of frequency. Stoney et al. (25) surveyed the patient load of 349 cardiac surgeons over a 6-yr period and showed there were 264 deaths from air embolism with disseminated intravascular coagulopathy as a result of bypass cardiac surgery. They recommended that rigorous use of alarm systems and heparin monitoring would reduce the incidence of pump-related accidents. They stressed the underestimation of the frequency of this occurrence since only the most dramatic or worst cases were recognized or remembered and reported. As a total number of accidents, they estimated that there was 1 occurrence/300 procedures, with permanent injury or death occurring in 1/1,000 procedures.

A review of the literature from 1978 to 1988 showed 14 papers related to air embolism during cardiopulmonary bypass and three papers each on air emboli after mitral valve replacement, percutaneous transluminal coronary angioplasty, and cannulation of the ascending aorta as documented causes of air embolism (25, 43–53). During that same period, 20 articles were published on air embolism in the use of central venous catheters, including pulmonary artery catheters; the complications occurred from the insertion of the line, detachment of the intravenous tubing to the venous cannula, sheath malfunctioning, and patient positioning at the time of line insertion (54–61). Neurosurgical procedures have also been associated and recognized with air embolism complications, particularly in the following situations: during surgery performed on the posterior fossa, often with the patient in the seated position (62, 63); during transsphenoidal pituitary procedures (64); after the creation of burr holes (65); after the use of Mayfield skull clamps (66); during epidural catheter insertion (67); through ventriculoarterial shunts (68); after lumbar disk surgery (69); associated with trauma, such as massive head trauma (70), and superior sagittal sinus injury with penetrating craniocerebral trauma (71); after head and neck surgery (72); and after the removal of neck drains (73). Table 23.1 lists other causes of air embolism.

CLINICAL MANIFESTATIONS OF AIR EMBOLISM
Diagnosis

A major problem exists in establishing the diagnosis, which, in general, must be determined by the recovery of air from either the right or left ventricle or by the visualization of air in the coronary or cerebral arteries. Venous air embolism may be recovered from the right atrium. More than 50% of the patients present unconscious or with a history of unconsciousness at some time; the other major presentation is an altered level of consciousness. The neurologic patterns show great variability but, in general, the signs and symptoms may be described as bilateral carotid and vertebral-basilar system dysfunction. Isolated unilateral carotid or brainstem syndromes are less frequent. It is essential to remember that the signs and symptoms may change very rapidly and that there may be sporadic or continued seizure activity. General anesthesia, analgesics, or narcotics can alter the presenting findings, greatly increasing the complexity of diagnosis and evaluation. Apart from the severe neurologic signs, there may well be circulatory collapse, evidence of lung rupture or edema, and a wide range of pain syndromes. The crux of diagnosis is the history of neurologic changes and the circumstances under which these changes developed. (In scuba diving, simple breath holding may produce the symptomatology.)

Confirmation of the diagnosis is always very difficult and one often has to treat on suspicion. One of the methods of confirming the diagnosis is to pass a central catheter into the right ventricle (in the case of a venous embolism) or into the radial or femoral line and to aspirate bubbles in the arterial blood. At surgery, an opening into the aorta or coronary or femoral arteries may release frothy blood, a positive identification of air embolism. Less dramatic evidence of air in the tissues is found in the upper portion of the body where intravascular air bubbles may be seen via superficial incisions or by assessment of the fundal arteries. A venous catheter for monitoring air emboli with a precordial Doppler is used by anesthesiologists in neurosurgical procedures, particularly those related to the base of the skull and posterior fossa.

Table 23.1.
Reported Causes of Air Embolism

Cause	Reference
Positive-pressure ventilation producing pulmonary barotrauma	Kane et al., 1988 (74)
Manual lung inflation	Tracey and Vartian, 1982 (75)
Respiratory distress syndrome and mechanical ventilation	Mahmud, 1979 (76)
Other ventilatory overinflations	Blanco et al., 1979 (77)
	Oppermann et al., 1979 (78)
	Banagle, 1980 (79)
Traumatic invasive procedures on the lungs, such as needle aspiration and biopsy	Aberle et al., 1987 (80)
	Cianci et al., 1987 (81)
	Strange et al., 1987 (82)
	Tolly et al., 1988 (83)
Penetrating lung injury	Meier et al., 1979 (84)
	King et al., 1984 (85)
Induction of artificial pneumothorax	Khalil et al., 1979 (86)
Abdominal surgery, such as peritoneovenous shunts for ascites	Hirst and Saunders, 1981 (87)
	Gui et al., 1986 (88)
Autotransfusion	Bretton et al., 1985 (89)
Liver transplantation and venovenous bypass	Mazzoni et al., 1979 (90)
	Starzl et al., 1978 (91)
	Khoury et al., 1987 (92)
	Delva et al., 1986 (93)
Laparoscopy (accompanied by carbon dioxide embolization)	Parewijck et al., 1979 (94)
	Wadhwa et al., 1978 (95)
	Yacoub et al., 1982 (96)
	Nichols et al., 1981 (97)
Necrotizing enterocolitis	Miller, 1979 (98)
Escherichia coli septicemia	Jones, 1981 (99)
Postpneumatosis cystoides intestinalis	Bonnell and French, 1982 (100)
Hip surgery and hip arthrography	Michel, 1980 (101)
	Anderson, 1983 (102)
	McCauley et al., 1981 (103)
Gynecologic/obstetric procedures and sex practices such as orogenital sex	Fyke et al., 1985 (104)
	Lifschultz et al., 1983 (105)
	Bray et al., 1983 (106)
Uterine surgery (caesarean sections and hysterectomy)	Davies et al., 1980 (107)
	Younker et al., 1986 (108)
	Naulty et al., 1982 (109)
Renal and urethral surgery, including percutaneous nephrolithotomy and laser urethral surgery	Miller et al., 1984 (110)
	Vourc'h et al., 1982 (111)
Transurethral resection	Hofsess, 1984 (112)
Insufflation of the urethra	Vanlinthout et al., 1986 (113)
Hydrogen peroxide wound irrigation	Bassan et al., 1982 (114)
	Bristow et al., 1985 (115)
Kidney dialysis	Baskin and Wozniak, 1975 (116)
	Ward et al., 1971 (117)

Signs and Symptoms

The clinical manifestations of arterial air embolism usually are related to either the coronary or cerebral circulation. A very small volume of air can cause a lethal arterial embolism; a 0.5-ml injection of air into the anterior descending artery, for example, would lead to ventricular fibrillation and death. The arterial air may be distributed to any organ, but the actual location depends on body position. Because air is buoyant in blood, it tends to float upward, thus involving primarily the upper portion of the body. The arterial air traverses systemic capillaries more readily than lung capillaries. The pressure threshold for air passage in an organ capillary is less than the systemic arterial pressure. When air is carried into the right heart, having passed through the systemic capillaries, it is called secondary venous air embolism.

The major clinical symptoms experienced by patients with air embolism depend on which circulation is involved. With cerebral circulation involvement, patients may feel dizzy or peculiar, have a fear of death, or present with blindness or a headache. The most important differentiating factor is its abrupt and sudden onset with rapid progression to overt signs such as convulsions, loss of consciousness, or general or focal seizures. The neurologic deficits include a wide range of symptoms: hemiplegia, paraplegia, monoplegia, hemianopsia, nystagmus, or strabismus. The pupils are generally dilated but may be constricted, and the retinal vessels may show evidence of air. There may be sharply defined areas of tongue pallor (Liebermeister's sign). When the skin is the primary area involved, air embolism presents as a marbling effect; a small incision will release the air.

Blindness may occur and be complete in patients who have not temporarily lost consciousness; it may persist for several days. The pupils are generally noted to be dilated, but occasionally they may be constricted. Cyanosis has often been described, particularly related to the face and neck, but it may also be generalized or very marked, and respiratory disturbances may be present as well. The respiratory rate is most commonly slowed and Cheyne-Stokes breathing may be observed. With peripheral vascular collapse, there may be a thready or imperceptible pulse; a marked fall in blood pressure; and the classic presentation of cold, clammy, pallid skin. On auscultation of the heart, a tumultuous sound is heard but no wheel murmurs, such as is found in pulmonary air embolism. The patient recovering from an acute episode may then present with chest pain referred to the precordial or substernal areas; there may be considerable associated dyspnea. Other signs and symptoms include nausea or vomiting. Symptomatology may persist for hours or days.

The so-called pathopneumonic signs of air embolism include the following:

1. Detection of air in the retinal vessels by ophthalmoscopic examination (9–12). In the acute stages, the actual bubbles may be seen circulating through the vessels as pale, silvery sections in the retinal vessels; however, these bubbles are quite temporary and are best seen immediately after the onset of the accident. Pallor of the retina may be noted for several days after the disappearance of the air bubbles; this condition is associated with diminution or loss of visual acuity.
2. Liebermeister's sign (118). Liebermeister suggested that this sign, which defines the presence of emboli by a sharply delineated area of pallor of the tongue, was due to air bubbles in the lingular vessels or their branches. As the lingual artery is an end artery, there appears to be a small segmental area of anemia of the edge of the tongue to the right of the tip. When the total stem is blocked, the total right half of the tongue

is anemic. The absence of this sign indicates that air embolism is not present. There are no cases in the American literature where this sign has been described; it may, however, be missed in the confusion surrounding the original episode. A single report of this sign in the British literature describes a patient who had two episodes of air embolism: in each situation, he had right hemiparesis and right-side tongue pallor (119). The presence of the right hemiparesis and tongue involvement on the same side is difficult to explain as an air embolic phenomenon, but it may be due to a vasospastic phenomenon associated with the embolism.

3. Marbling of the skin. Marbling is presumed to represent actual air emboli in the skin capillaries, located mainly over the superior portions of the body. Van Allen et al. (120) strongly support this diagnostic sign and note that incisions into the skin over these areas will result in air bubbles bleeding through the wound. Retinographic demonstration of air in the cerebral vessels has been reported (121) but is considered a rarity because the amount of air required to produce this retinographic demonstration is usually fatal. It thus becomes of value in the postmortem situation. In today's world of high technology, the computed tomography (CT) scan can be used to demonstrate air in the cerebral vessels. In my own experience, CT examination has been used on several occasions. In one patient, the CT scan showed a major amount of air in the internal carotid artery system; this unconscious patient never recovered and died with increasing cerebral edema and ultimate inflow obstruction. The patient had received direct input of air into the carotid system while undergoing a carotid artery angiogram to assess the state of an arteriovenous malformation in the brain. In the remaining situations, no air has been visualized on the CT examinations.

Electrocardiogram changes are unlikely to be specific but may add corroborative evidence for cerebral injury. The involvement of the coronary vessels has frequently been demonstrated in both animal models and postmortem studies. As early as 1928, Rukstinat and Le Count (122) were able to demonstrate hemorrhages in the myocardium. Rukstinat (123) used direct injections of air into the coronary arteries to demonstrate a tumultuous heart action with acceleration of rate, leading to bradycardia within 10–20 sec and death in 1–4 min. Injecting air slowly caused only temporary disturbances. Air injection into the left auricle resulted in death from coronary air embolism in 35–70 sec. This work was extended by Moore and Braselton (124). They conclusively demonstrated in cats that the cause of death after air embolism was obstruction of the coronary arteries. Death occurred regardless of the position of the animal. The heart was noted to behave as if the coronary arteries were ligated. The air bubbles in the coronary arteries did not progress along the course of the vessels and there was subsequent progressive heart failure with increased heart rate, weaker contractions, ventricular fibrillation, and, shortly thereafter, death. Despite the presence of air in the coronary arteries, there was no evidence of myocardial infarction because there was insufficient time for the picture of a myocardial infarction to develop. (Arrest is due mainly to conduction problems.) When the patient survives for a longer period of time, the coronary arteries may show no pathologic changes; however, there is evidence of myocardial infarction in the form of focal hemorrhages and flabby cardiac muscle (125). Goldfarb and Bahnson (126) extended this animal experimental work and were able to show that, after embolization, there was consistent impairment of cardiac function and a predisposition to arrhythmias with a decrease in ventricular function, stroke work, and arterial pressure. Lasting myocardial damage was indicated by abnormal electrocardiographic and histologic changes. They showed that air sequestered in the left side of the heart or pulmonary veins became dislodged with position changes, causing damage to the brain or heart—a significant implication for open-heart surgery.

Thus, bubble effects occur with occlusion of vessels and, in addition, a more delayed and diffuse action occurs due to the indirect or surface activity effect of circulating enzymes, which change their configuration and biochemical activity (127). The results of these changes include endothelial edema, platelet thrombi, increased capillary permeability, and the release of biologic mediators such as smooth muscle acting factor. These phenomenon could explain the coagulopathy and bronchospasms in patients with air embolism.

It must be stressed that the late circumstance of gas bubbles physically blocking blood flow is variable and may persist for up to 4 hr. With the vascular blockage, there is cytotoxic cerebral edema due to hypoxia and endothelial damage with platelet thrombi, resulting in a no-reflow phenomenon (14, 128, 129). In the reestablished areas of circulation, there may be abnormal capillary permeability, small hemorrhages, and loss of vascular regulation (130). In reality, autodestruction is now set in place (131), including demyelination in the neuronal deaths. These pathologic changes occurring after air embolism are thought to be more diffuse than those following other kinds of ischemia (132).

Patient outcome is variable; unconscious patients with severe neurologic impairment have made very rapid recoveries, although, in general, the greater the neurologic insult, the longer the recovery. Rather than making a complete recovery, the patient has actually learned to compensate for the neuronal destruction.

PROPHYLAXIS

To prevent bronchial obstruction problems from occurring underwater, individuals with pulmonary cysts, cavitary disease, bronchiectasis, constrictive obstructive lung disease, or acute pulmonary infection are not permitted to dive. Individuals with cyanotic congenital heart disease, asymptomatic septal defects, or pulmonary arteriovenous fistulas should also be excluded from diving because of the dangers of paradoxical air embolism (133).

In the diving world, careful training of divers is essential and breath holding during ascent is to be avoided at all costs. Catastrophe from inadvertent breath holding occurs when a diver panics, as when he/she runs out of breathing gas or experiences some event that affects judgment and caution.

In the medical field, it is essential that particular care be taken during intravenous fluid infusion to ensure that no bubbles occur and that bags are used as containers rather than bottles since the latter allow easy air access. Various protective devices have been developed to guard against arterial air embolism in open-heart surgery and venous air embolism in dialysis. To avoid air embolization during insertion of central venous lines, it is essential that the patient be in a head-down position and on positive end-expiratory pressure ventilation *before* venipunctures are undertaken. The use of Doppler monitoring during neurosurgical or similar procedures in the patient in the upright or head-elevated position is essential to detect cerebral air embolism. The placement of a venous catheter in the superior vena cava or right side of the heart allows one to back-aspirate to determine whether or not air is present in the blood. The routine use of positive end-expiratory pressure in the operating room also reduces the risk of venous air aspiration in surgery. The upright position should be avoided whenever possible. In cardiac bypass surgery, low-level reservoir line alarms should be utilized with all perfusions.

The aspiration of all intracardiac air after cardiac bypass perfusion is difficult; there is a high rate of air embolism when no precautions are undertaken. Nicks (134) reported 40 cases of air embolism with 10 deaths in 340 patients prior to the institution of special precautions. Roe (135) has recommended the use of intravascular carbon dioxide washout to prevent air embolization when air is already present in the aorta. DeLaria et al. (48) placed traction sutures on the leaflets of the valves of the heart to produce incompetence and thus prevent air trapping. Numerous venting techniques are available and include (136–138) multiple aspiration procedures of the superior pulmonary vein, left atrial appendage, left ventricular appendage, and descending aorta with the heart fibrillating.

The extracorporeal circuit is possibly the source of the gas emboli. Small bubbles have been noted during the priming procedure, particularly when it produces no blood (138). The actual formation of bubbles in the liquid is closely allied to the presence or absence of small invisible gas masses called gas nuclei. The gas nuclei attach to the hydrophobic areas or stabilize in surface cracks. Expansion of gas nuclei by multiplication rather than by supersaturation may be the most important factor in bubble formation (139). A bubble trap is particularly helpful in eliminating these small bubbles. A carbon dioxide flush, which is 20 times more soluble than oxygen and 100% more soluble than nitrogen, is the best flushing agent. Finally, a Venturi effect results in a low-pressure phenomenon in the tubing in the pump head, with inadvertent injections of air when the blood sample is taken. It is then essential to use both an arterial Doppler over the cervical vessels and a continuous electroencephalogram print-out.

EMERGENCY AND ADJUNCTIVE THERAPY

The basic approach to air embolism is to give emergency resuscitation with intubation and ventilation and cardiac support as needed. The patient should be placed in the left lateral decubitus position with the feet elevated 30–60° to increase the hydrostatic force and thus dilate both arterial and venous vasculature of the brain, enabling bubbles to pass more freely through the capillaries. The patient should be placed left-side down to prevent air which may be lodged in the right side of the heart from entering the pulmonary outflow tract. The major effects of this Trendelenburg-type position occur within 20–30 min; thereafter, the patient can be placed in the horizontal position. For long-distance transport, air speed is desirable and should be by fixed-winged aircraft; transportation by ground or by low-flying helicopter is advisable for short distances.

When the gas embolism is suspected to have occurred during open-heart surgery, all efforts should be made to clear all gross bubbles in the aorta. The nonhypothermic patient should be cooled and given 100% oxygen. Surgery should be completed under the umbrella of heparinization and/or hypothermia to reduce the amount of neurologic damage from gas embolism (140). Appropriate safety measures with low-level alarms on reservoirs, pump shut-offs, and bubble detectors will all help reduce the risk of air embolism. The open-heart surgery teams should be aware of the location of the local hyperbaric facilities and have a protocol developed for the suspected, presumed, or proven cases of air embolism; the patient should be transferred as soon as possible for hyperbaric oxygen therapy.

Mills and Ochsner (44) recommended retrograde perfusion of the inferior vena cava as soon as the embolization has been recognized. An essential assessment of all post-pump patients should be standard neurologic testing and interviews of the patient's family to determine immediate or delayed return of neurologic function (44). CT of the brain preoperatively and postoperatively can also be used to determine subclinical changes and brain morphology (141).

Steroids are now contraindicated in the treatment of cerebral edema as a consequence of air/gas embolism. Studies by Dick et al. (142) and Dearden et al. (143) demonstrated the noneffectiveness of steroids and the potential for enhancing neurologic oxygen toxicity.

HYPERBARIC OXYGEN THERAPY

The specific recommended therapy for all types of air embolism, both iatrogenic and with decompression diving (115, 116, 144–165), is hyperbaric oxygen therapy. The mechanism of action of hyperbaric oxygen is to compress the gas bubbles and reduce the size of the bubble and thus the mechanical obstructive effect. The addition of oxygen to the breathing mix results in an increased rate of nitrogen bubble breakdown and reabsorption. Hyperbaric oxygen also reduces cerebral edema by lowering the increased intracranial pressure, and the high O_2 level provided reduces the anoxic disruption of the microcirculatory flow. The more quickly the hyperbaric oxygen treatment is given, the better the outcome. The greatest likelihood of the patient returning to normal with complete resolution of the symptomatology occurs when treatment begins immediately or within 2 hr of the incident. The longer the delay between incident and primary treatment, the more difficult it is to resolve the symptomatology. However, delays from 29 to 39 hr still have had successful outcomes (115, 165, 166). The use of early surface oxygen has been recommended as a temporizing measure.

SUMMARY

The diagnosis and treatment of air embolism still remain partly enshrouded in mystery. Because of the highly litigious world that we live in, it would appear to be legally dangerous for the open-heart surgeon or the renal dialysis program to openly admit to their problems with air emboli. Despite the work of Stoney et al. (25), pitifully few patients with postsurgical air embolism are referred for hyperbaric oxygen therapy. This may be due to the low index of suspicion of the event actually occurring, inexperience of the surgeons, or difficulty in making the diagnosis during surgery.

Currently, the major source of referrals to hyperbaric oxygen therapy for air embolism is diving accidents due to rapid, uncontrolled decompression and the resulting barotrauma that produces air embolism. The value of hyperbaric oxygen therapy in the successful treatment and outcome of these cases is well-established through detailed animal research and human experience. The emphasis on early and aggressive treatment includes recompression to a treatment depth ranging from 60 to 165 feet of sea water pressure (3–6 atmospheres absolute [ATA]). Elaborate tables of treatment dive depths and times have been developed which compress the gas bubbles as small as possible and then substitute oxygen for the gas nuclei to help reabsorb the bubbles. The details of the treatment protocols are available at any hyperbaric facility throughout the nation; there are currently more than 240 facilities nationwide (167). A list of these hyperbaric facilities is available through the Hyperbaric Medicine Registry at the Maryland Institute for Emergency Medical Services Systems (Baltimore, MD), and a hyperbaric medicine consultation can be obtained without charge 24 hr a day through the Diving Alert Network located at Duke University (Durham, NC).

The recent work of Leitch et al. (152–155) in the animal raises the question of whether a shallower treatment depth of 60 feet of sea water (2.8 ATA) given immediately after air embolism is as good as the traditionally accepted deep dive of 165 feet of sea water (6 ATA). Confirmation requires further clinical work in patients. However, it again stresses what is known, that is, the sooner the patient is placed in a hyperbaric facility, the better the outcome.

REFERENCES

1. Morgagni J. The seats and causes of diseases. Alexander B, trans., from the Latin. London: 1769 (Cited by Fries CC, Levowitz B, Adler S, Cook AW, Karlson KE, Dennis C. Experimental gas embolism. Ann Surg 1957;145:46.)
2. Bert P. Barometric pressure researches in experimental physiology (1878) [republished]. Bethesda, MD: Undersea Medical Society, 1978:1032.
3. Schlaepfer K. Air embolism following venous diagnostic or therapeutic procedures in diseases of the pleura and lung. Bull Johns Hopkins Hosp 1922;33:321–330.
4. Brandes M. Ein Todesfall durch Embolie nach Injektion von Wismutsalbe in eine Empyemfistel. Muench Med Wochenschr 1912;44:2392–2394. (Cited by Schlaepfer, ref 3.)
5. Brauer L. Die Behandlung der einseitigen Lungenphthisis mit kunstlichem Pneumothorax. Muench Med Wochenschr 1906;7:338–339. (Cited by Schlaepfer, ref 3.)
6. Wever EK. Cerebrale Luftembolie. Beitr Klin Tuberk Spezif Tuberk Forsh 1913;31:159–230.
7. Capps JA. Air embolism versus pleural reflex as a cause of pleural shock. JAMA 1937;109:852–854.
8. Durant TM, Oppenheimer MJ, Webster MR, Long J. Arterial air embolism. Am Heart J 1949;38:481–500.
9. Schattenberg HJ, Ziskind J. Air embolism as complication of artificial pneumothorax. Am J Clin Pathol 1939;9:477–482.
10. Dalgleish PH. Two cases of air embolism. Br Med J 1945;2:256.
11. Wong RT. Air emboli in the retinal arteries: report of a case. Arch Ophthalmol 1941;25:149–150.
12. Reyer GW, Kohl HW. Air embolism complicating thoracic surgery. JAMA 1926;87:1626–1630.
13. Hartveit F, Lystad H, Minken A. Pathology of venous air embolism. Br J Exp Pathol 1968;49:81–86.
14. Warren B, Philip B, Inwood M. The ultrastructural morphology of air embolism: platelet adhesion to the interface and endothelial damage. Br J Exp Pathol 1973;54:163–172.
15. Khan M, Alkalay I, Suetsugu S, et al. Acute changes in lung mechanics following pulmonary emboli of various gases in dogs. J Appl Physiol 1972;33:774–777.
16. Kazuhiro O, Kazuya N, Binder A, et al. Venous air emboli in sheep: reversible increase in lung microvascular permeability. J Appl Physiol 1981;51:887–894.
17. Berglund E, Josephson S, Ovenfors CO. Pulmonary air embolism: physiological aspects. Prog Respir Res 1970;5:259–263.
18. Albert R, Lakshminarayan S, Kirk W, et al. Lung inflation can cause pulmonary edema in zone I of in situ dog lungs. J Appl Physiol 1980;49:815–819.
19. Spencer R. The significance of air embolism during cardiopulmonary bypass. J Thorac Cardiovasc Surg 1965;49:615–634.
20. Hlastala MP, Robertson T, Ross B. Gas exchange abnormalities produced by venous gas emboli. Respir Physiol 1979;36:1–17.
21. Polak B, Adams H. Traumatic air embolism in submarine escape training. US Nav Med Bull 1932;30:165–177.
22. Schaeffer KE, McNulty WP Jr, Carey C, Liewbow AA. Mechanisms in development of interstitial emphysema and air embolism on decompression from depth. J Appl Physiol 1958;13:15–29.
23. Malhotra MC, Wright CAM. Arterial air embolism during decompression and its prevention. Proc R Soc Med (Br) 1960;154:418–427.
24. Macklin MT, Macklin CC. Malignant interstitial emphysema of the lungs and mediastinum as an important occult complication in many respiratory diseases and other conditions: an interpretation of the clinical literature in the light of laboratory experiment. Medicine 1944;23:258–281.
25. Stoney WS, Alford WC Jr, Burrus GR, Glassford DM Jr, Thomas CS Jr. Air embolism and other accidents using pump oxygenators. Ann Thorac Sug 1980;29:336–340.
26. Dayman H. Mechanics of air flow in health and in emphysema. J Clin Invest 1951;30:1175–1190.

27. Waite CL, Mazzone WF, Greenwood ME, Larsen RT. Dysbaric cerebral air embolism. In: Lambertsen CJ, ed. Proceedings of the third symposium on underwater physiology. Baltimore: Williams & Wilkins, 1967:205–215.

28. Broman T, Branemark PI, Johansson B, Steinwall O. Intravital and postmortem studies on air embolism damage of the blood-brain barrier tested with trypan blue. Acta Neurol Scand 1966;42:146–152.

29. Philip R, Inwood MJ, Warren BA. Interactions between gas bubbles and components of the blood: implications in decompression sickness. Aerosp Med 1972;43:946–956.

30. Johansson B. Blood-brain barrier dysfunction in experimental gas embolism. In: Shilling CE, Beckett MW, eds. Proceedings of the sixth symposium on underwater physiology. Bethesda, MD: Federation of American Societies for Experimental Biology, 1978:79–81.

31. Nishimoto K, Wolman M, Spatz M, Klatzo I. Pathophysiologic correlations in the blood-brain barrier damage due to air embolism. Adv Neurol 1978;20:237–244.

32. De La Torre L, Meredith J, Netsky MG. Cerebral air embolism in the dog. Arch Neurol 1962;6:307–316.

33. Fritz H, Hossman KA. Arterial air embolism in the cat brain. Stroke 1979;10:581–589.

34. Astrup J, Symon L, Branston NM, Lassen NA. Cortical evoked potential and extracellular K+ and H+ at critical levels of brain ischemia. Stroke 1977;8:51–57.

35. Hallenbeck JM, Greenbaum LJ Jr, eds. Workshop on arterial air embolism and acute stroke. Bethesda, MD: Undersea Medical Society, 1977.

36. Hallenbeck JM, Leitch DR, Dutka AJ, Greenbaum LJ Jr, McKee AE. PGI$_2$, indomethacin and heparin promote post-ischemic neuronal recovery in dogs. Ann Neurol 1982;12:145–156.

37. Cales RH, Humphreys N, Pilmanis AA, Heilig RW. Cardiac arrest from gas embolism in scuba diving. Ann Emerg Med 1981;10:589–592.

38. Wilmshurst PT, Ellis BG, Jenkins BS. Paradoxical gas embolism in a scuba diver with an atrial septal defect. Br Med J [Clin Res] 1986;293:1277.

39. Ballham A, Allen MJ. Air embolism in a sports diver. Br J Sports Med 1983;17:7–9.

40. Smith FR. Air embolism as a cause of death in scuba diving in the Pacific. Northwest Chest 1967;51:53.

41. Greene KM. Causes of sudden death in submarine escape training casualties. In: Hallenbeck MJ, Greenbaum LJ, eds. Workshop on arterial air embolism and acute stroke. Bethesda, MD: Undersea Medical Society, 1977:8–13.

42. Diving Alert Network. Report on 1987 diving accidents. Durham, NC: Duke University, 1987.

43. Spampinato N, Stassano P, Gagliardi C, Tufano R, Iorio D. Massive air embolism during cardiopulmonary bypass: successful treatment with immediate hypothermia and circulatory support. Ann Thorac Surg 1981;32:602–603.

44. Mills NL, Ochsner JL. Massive air embolism during cardiopulmonary bypass: causes, prevention, and management. J Thorc Cardiovasc Surg 1980;80:708–717.

45. Krebber HJ, Hanrath P, Janzen R, Ritoff M, Rodewald G. Gas emboli during open heart surgery. Thorac Cardiovasc Surg 1982;30:401–404.

46. Kumar AS, Jayalakshmi TS, Kale SC, Saxena BK, Singh V, Paul SJ. Management of massive air embolism during open heart surgery. Int J Cardiol 1985;9:413–416.

47. Ghosh PK, Kaplan O, Barak J, Lubliner J, Vidne BA. Massive arterial air embolism during cardiopulmonary bypass. J Cardiovasc Surg (Torino) 1985;26:248–250.

48. DeLaria GA, Monson DO, Weinberg M Jr. Prevention of air embolism after mitral valve replacement with a porcine heterograft prosthesis. Ann Thorac Surg 1979;27:181–182.

49. Stewart S, Harris JP, Manning JA. Coronary artery air embolism following pulmonary valvotomy for pulmonary atresia: a note of caution. J Thorac Cardiovasc Surg 1983;86:311–313.

50. Tomatis L, Meiroff M, Riahi M, et al. Massive arterial air embolism due to rupture of pulsatile assist device: successful treatment in the hyperbaric chamber. Ann Thorac Surg 1981;32:604–608.

51. Beckman CB, Hurley F, Mammana R, Levitsky S. Risk factors for air embolization during cannulation of the ascending aorta. J Thorac Cardiovasc Surg 1980;80:302–307.

52. Becker RM, Gabbay S, Frater RW. Pulmonary venous-bronchial fistula following left atrial pressure line insertion: iatrogenic cause of air embolism following cardiac surgery. Chest 1982;81:378–380.

53. Bentivoglio LG, Leo LR. Death from coronary air embolism during percutaneous transluminal coronary angioplasty. Cathet Cardiovasc Diagn 1985;11:585–590.

54. Feliciano DV, Mattox KL, Graham JM, Beall AC Jr, Jordan GL Jr. Major complications of percutaneous subclavian vein catheters. Am J Surg 1979;138:869–874.

55. Conahan TJ III. Air embolization during percutaneous Swan–Ganz catheter placement. Anesthesiology 1979;50:360–361.

56. Doblar DD, Hinkle JC, Fay ML, Condon BF. Air embolism associated with pulmonary artery catheter introducer kit. Anesthesiology 1982;56:389–391.

57. Lambert MJ III. Air embolism in central venous catheterization: diagnosis, treatment, and prevention. South Med J 1982;75:1189–1191.

58. Murphy BP, Harford FJ, Cramer FS. Cerebral air embolism resulting from invasive medical procedures: treatment with hyperbaric oxygen. Ann Surg 1985;201:242–245.

59. Kashuk JL, Penn I. Air embolism after central venous catheterization. Surg Gynecol Obstet 1984;159:249–252.

60. Seidelin PH, Stolarek IH, Thompson AM. Central venous catheterization and fatal air embolism. Br J Hosp Med 1987;38:438–439.

61. Cohen MB, Mark JB, Morris RW, Frank E. Introducer sheath malfunction producing insidious air embolism. Anesthesiology 1987;67:573–575.

62. Porter SS, Boyd RC, Albin MS. Venous air embolism in a child undergoing posterior fossa craniotomy: a case report. Can Anaesth Soc J 1984;31:86–90.

63. Cucchiara RF, Bowers B. Air embolism in children undergoing suboccipital craniotomy. Anesthesiology 1982;57:338–339.

64. Newfield P, Albin MS, Chestnut JS, Maroon J. Air embolism during trans-sphenoidal pituitary operations. Neurosurgery 1978;2:39–42.

65. Edelman JD, Wingard DW. Air embolism arising from burr holes. Anesthesiology 1980;53:167–168.

66. De Lange JJ, Baerts WD, Booij LH. Air embolism due to the Mayfield skull clamp. Acta Anaesthesiol Belg 1984;35:237–241.

67. Naulty JS, Ostheimer GW, Datta S, Knapp R, Weiss JB. Incidence of venous air embolism during epidural catheter insertion. Anesthesiology 1982;57:410–412.

68. Nehls DG, Carter LP. Air embolism through a ventriculoatrial shunt during posterior fossa operation: case report. Neurosurgery 1985;16:83–84.

69. Albin MS. Venous air embolism and lumbar disk surgery [Letter]. JAMA 240:1713.

70. Messmer JM. Massive head trauma as a cause of intravascular air. J Forensic Sci 1984;29:418–424.

71. Crone KR, Lee KS, Moody DM, Kelly DL Jr. Superior sagittal sinus air after penetrating craniocerebral trauma. Surg Neurol 1986;25:276–278.

72. Hybels RL. Venous air embolism in head and neck surgery. Laryngoscope 1980;90:946–954.

73. Chang JL, Skolnick K, Bedger R, Schramm V, Bleyaert AL. Postoperative venous air embolism after removal of neck drains. Arch Otolaryngol 1981;107:494–496.

74. Kane G, Hwins B, Grannis FW Jr. Massive air embolism in an adult following positive pressure ventilation. Chest 1988;93:874–876.

75. Tracey JA, Vartian V. Systemic air embolism following manual lung inflation. Can Anaesth Soc J 1982;29:272–274.

76. Mahmud F. Air embolism from mechanical ventilation in respiratory distress syndrome. South Med J 1979;72:783–787.

77. Blanco CE, Rietveld LA, Ruys JH. Systemic air embolism: a possible complication of artificial ventilation. Acta Paediatr Scand 1979;68:925–927.

78. Oppermann HC, Wille L, Obladen M, Richter E. Systemic air embolism in the respiratory distress syndrome of the newborn. Pediatr Radiol 1979;8:139–145.

79. Banagale RC. Massive intracranial air embolism: a complication of mechanical ventilation. Am J Dis Child 1980;134:799–800.

80. Aberle DR, Gamsu G, Golden JA. Fatal systemic arterial air embolism following lung needle aspiration. Radiology 1987;165:351–353.

81. Cianci P, Posin JP, Shimshak RR, Singzon J. Air embolism complicating percutaneous thin needle biopsy of lung. Chest 1987;92:749–751.

82. Strange C, Heffner JE, Collins BS, Brown FM, Sahn SA. Pulmonary hemorrhage and air embolism complicating transbronchial biopsy in pulmonary amyloidosis. Chest 1987;92:364–365.

83. Tolly TL, Feldmeier JE, Czarnecki D. Air embolism complicating percutaneous lung biopsy. AJR 1988;150:555–556.

84. Meier GH, Wood WJ, Symbas PN. Systemic air embolization from penetrating lung injury. Ann Thorac Surg 1979;27:161–168.

85. King MW, Aitchison JM, Nel JP. Fatal air embolism following penetrating lung trauma: an autopsy study. J Trauma 1984;24:753–755.

86. Khalil SN, Madan V, Rigor BM, Fields WS, Unger KM. Systemic air embolism following induction of artificial pneumothorax under anaesthesia, with successful management. Br J Anaesth 1979;51:461–464.

87. Hirst AE, Saunders FC. Fatal air embolism following perforation of the cecum in a patient with peritoneovenous shunt for ascites. Am J Gastroenterol 1981;76:453–455.

88. Gui D, Gianguiliani G, Veneziani A, Giorgi G, Sganga C. Inguinal hernia repair in patients with peritoneovenous shunt: risk of air embolism. Br J Surg 1986;73:122.

89. Bretton P, Reines HD, Sade RM. Air embolization during autotransfusion for abdominal trauma. J Trauma 1985;25:165–166.

90. Mazzoni G, Koep L, Starzl T. Air embolus in liver transplantation. Transplant Proc 1979;11:267–268.

91. Starzl TE, Schneck SA, Mazzoni G, et al. Acute neurological complications after liver transplantation with particular reference to intraoperative cerebral air embolus. Ann Surg 1978;187:236–240.

92. Khoury GF, Mann ME, Porot MJ, Abdul-Rasool IH, Busuttil RW. Air embolism associated with veno-venous bypass during orthotopic liver transplantation. Anesthesiology 1987;67:848–851.

93. Delva E, Sadoul N, Chandon M, Boucherez C, Lienhart A. Air embolism during liver resection: an unusual mechanism of entry from a peristaltic pump. Can Anaesth Soc J 1986;33:488–491.

94. Parewijck W, Thiery M, Timperman J. Serious complications of laparoscopy. Med Sci Law 1979;19:199–201.

95. Wadhwa RK, McKenzie R, Wadhwa SR, Katz DL, Byers JF. Gas embolsim during laparoscopy. Anesthesiology 1978;48:74–76.

96. Yacoub OF, Cardona I Jr, Coveler LA, Dodson MG. Carbon dioxide embolism during laparoscopy. Anesthesiology 1982;57:533–535.

97. Nichols SL, Tompkins BM, Henderson PA. Probable carbon dioxide embolism during laparoscopy: case report. Wis Med J 1981;80:27–29.

98. Miller T. Systemic air embolism in necrotizing enterocolitis [Letter]. AJR 1979;132:322.

99. Jones B. Massive gas embolism in E. coli septicemia. Gastrointest Radiol 1981;6:161–163.

100. Bonnell H, French SW. Fatal air embolus associated with pneumatosis cystoides intestinalis. Am J Forensic Med Pathol 1982;3:69–72.

101. Michel R. Air embolism in hip surgery. Anaesthesia 1980;35:858–862.

102. Anderson KH. Air aspirated from the venous system during total hip replacement. Anaesthesia 1983;38:1175–1178.

103. McCauley RG, Wunderlich BK, Zimbler S. Air embolism as a complication of hip arthrography. Skeletal Radiol 1981;6:11–13.

104. Fyke FE III, Kazmier FJ, Harms RW. Venous air embolism: life-threatening complication of orogenital sex during pregnancy. Am J Med 1985;78:333–336.

105. Lifschultz BD, Donoghue ER. Air embolism during intercourse in pregnancy. J Forensic Sci 1983;28:1021–1022.

106. Bray P, Myers RA, Cowley RA. Orogenital sex as a cause of nonfatal air embolism in pregnancy. Obstet Gynecol 1983;61:653–657.

107. Davies DE, Digwood KI, Hilton JN. Air embolism during caesarean section. Med J Aust 1980;1:644–646.

108. Younker D, Rodriguez V, Kavanagh J. Massive air embolism during cesarean section. Anesthesiology 1986;65:77–79.

109. Naulty JS, Meisel LB, Datta S. Ostheimer GW. Air embolism during radical hysterectomy. Anesthesiology 1982;57:420–422.

110. Miller RA, Kellett MJ, Wickham JE. Air embolism, a new complication of percutaneous nephrolithotomy: what are the implictions? J Urol (Paris) 1984;90:337–339.

111. Vourc'h G, Berretti E, Trichet B, Moncorge C, Camey M. Gas embolism associated with use of lasers for urethral surgery [Letter]. Anesth Analg 1982;61:160.

112. Hofsess DW. Fatal air embolism during transurethral resection. J Urol 1984;131:355.

113. Vanlinthout L, Boghaert A, Thienpont L. Venous air embolism following insufflation of the urethra. Acta Anaethesiol Belg 1986;37:275–279.

114. Bassan MM, Dudai M, Shalev O. Near-fatal systemic oxygen embolism due to wound irrigation with hydrogen peroxide. Postgrad Med J 1982;58:448–450.

115. Bristow A, Batjer H, Chow V, Rosenstein J. Air embolism via a pulmonary artery catheter introducer [Letter]. Anesthesiology 1985;63:340–342.

116. Baskin SE, Wozniak RF. Hyperbaric oxygenation in the treatment of hemodialysis-associated air embolism. N Engl J Med 1975;293:184–185.

117. Ward MK, Shadforth M, Hill AV, Kerr DN. Air embolism during haemodialysis. Br Med J 1971;3:74–78.

118. Liebermeister G. Das Anämische Zungenphanomen, ein wichtiges Frühsymptom der arteriellen Luftembolie. Klin Wochenschr 1929;8:21–23.

119. Smith AW. Case exhibiting Liebermeister's syndrome following on air filling of left pleural cavity. Tubercle 1935;16:454–455.

120. Van Allen CM, Hardina LS, Clark J. Air embolism from the pulmonary vein: clinical and experimental study. Arch Surg 1929;19:567–599.

121. Chase WH. Anatomical and experimental observations on air embolism. Surg Gynecol Obstet 1934;59:569–577.

122. Rukstinat G, Le Count ER. Air in coronary arteries. JAMA 1928;91:1776–1779.

123. Rukstinat G. Experimental air embolism of coronary arteries. JAMA 1931;96:26–28.

124. Moore RM, Braselton CW Jr. Injection of air and carbon dioxide into the pulmonary vein. Ann Surg 1940;112:212–218.

125. Durant TM. The occurrence of coronary air embolism in artifical pneumothorax. Ann Intern Med 1935;8:1625–1632.

126. Goldfarb D, Bahnson HT. Early and late effects on the heart of small amounts of air in the coronary circulation. J Thorac Cardiovasc Surg 1963;46:368–378.

127. Lee WH, Hairston P. Structural effects on blood proteins at the gas bubble interface. Fed Proc 1971;30:1615–1620.

128. Philip RB, Gowdey CW. Platelets as an etiological factor in experimental decompression sickness. J Occup Med 1969;11:257.

129. Smith KH, Stegall PJ, D'Aoust BG. Pathophysiology of decompression sickness. In: International Symposium on man in the sea, 13–15 July 1975, Bethesda, MD: Undersea Medical Society, 1975:V190–205.

130. Waite CL, Mazzone WF, Greenwood ME, Larson RT. Cerebral air embolism. I. Basic studies. Report no. 493. US Nav Submar Med Cent Rep 1966;12:1–14.

131. Hallenbeck JM, Bradley ME. Experimental model for systematic study of impaired microvascular reperfusion. Stroke 1977;8:238–243.

132. Brierley JB. Neuropathological findings in patients dying after open-heart surgery. Thorax 1963;18:291–304.

133. Ponsky JL, Pories WJ. Paradoxical cerebral air embolism. N Engl J Med 1971;284:985.

134. Nicks R. Arterial air embolism. Thorax 1967;22:320–326.

135. Roe BB. Prevention of air embolism with intravascular carbon dioxide washout. J Thorac Cardiovasc Surg 1976;71:628–630.

136. Kurusz M, Shaffer CW, Christmas EW, Tyers GF. Runaway pump head: new cause of gas embolism during cardiopulmonary bypass. J Thorac Cardiovasc Surg 1979;77:792–795.

137. Lemole GM, Pinder GC. A method of preventing air embolus in open-heart surgery. J Thorac Cardiovasc Surg 1976;71:557–558.

138. Marco JD, Barner HB. Aortic venting: comparison of vent effectiveness. J Thorac Cardiovasc Surg 1977;73:287–292.

139. Galletti PM, Brecher GA. Heart-lung bypass principles and techniques of extracorporeal circulation. New York: Grune & Stratton, 1962:230.

140. Peirce EC II. Specific therapy for arterial air embolism. Ann Thorac Surg 1980;29:300–303.

141. Muraoka R, Yokota M, Aoshima M, et al. Subclinical changes in brain morphology following cardiac operations as reflected by computed tomographic scans of the brain. J Thorac Cardiovasc Surg 1981;81:364–369.

142. Dick AR, McCallum ME, Maxwell JA, Nelson R. Effect of dexamethasone on experimental brain edema in cats. J Neurosurg 1976;45:141–147.

143. Dearden NM, Gibson JS, McDowall DG, Gibson RM, Cameron MM. Effect of high-dose dexamethasone on outcome of severe head injury. J Neurosurg 1986;64:81–88.

144. Kindwall EP. Massive surgical air embolism treated with brief recompression to six atmospheres followed by hyperbaric oxygen. Aerosp Med 1973;44:663–666.

145. Takita H, Olszewski W, Schimert G, Lanphier EH. Hyperbaric treatment of cerebral air embolism as a result of open-heart surgery: report of a case. J Thorac Cardiovasc Surg 1968;55:682–685.

146. Hart GB. Treatment of decompression illness and air embolism with hyperbaric oxygen. Aerosp Med 1974;45:1190–1193.

147. Calverley RK, Dodds WA, Trapp WG, Jenkins LC. Hyperbaric treatment of cerebral air embolism: a report of a case following cardiac catheterization. Can Anaesth Soc J 1971;18:665–674.

148. Rapin M, Gordon M, Nouailhat F. Four cases of postabortal neurologic accident treated with hyperbaric oxygenation. In: Brown IW Jr, Cox BG, eds. Proceedings of the third international conference on hyperbaric medicine. Durham, NC: NAS/NRC 1966;1404:455.

149. Bond GF. Arterial gas embolism. In: Davis JC, Hunt TK, eds. Hyperbaric oxygen therapy. Bethesda, MD: Undersea Medical Society, 1977:141.

150. Steward D, Williams WG, Freedom R. Hypothermia in conjunction with hyperbaric oxygenation in the treatment of massive air embolism during cardiopulmonary bypass. Ann Thorac Surg 1977;24:591–593.

151. Bernardt TL, Goldmann RW, Thomas PA, Kindwall EP. Hyperbaric oxygen treatment of cerebral air embolism from orogenital sex suring pregnancy. Crit Care Med 1988;16:729–730.

152. Leitch DR, Greenbaum LJ Jr, Hallenbeck JM. Cerebral arterial air embolism. I. Is there benefit in beginning HBO treatment at 6 bar? Undersea Biomed Res 1984;11:221–235.

153. Leitch DR, Greenbaum LJ Jr, Hallenbeck JM. Cerebral arterial air embolism. II. Effect of pressure and time on cortical evoked potential recovery. Undersea Biomed Res 1984;11:237–248.

154. Leitch DR, Greenbaum LJ Jr, Hallenbeck JM. Cerebral arterial air embolism. III. Cerebral blood flow after decompression from various pressure treatments. Undersea Biomed Res 1984;11:249–263.

155. Leitch DR, Greenbaum LJ Jr, Hallenbeck JM. Cerebral arterial air embolism. IV. Failure to recover with treatment and secondary deterioration. Undersea Biomed Res 1984;11:265–274.

156. Van Genderen L, Waite CL. Evaluation of the rapid recompression–high pressure oxygenation approach to the treatment of traumatic cerebral air embolism. Aerosp Med 1968;39:709–713.

157. US Navy Diving Manual. Change 2, 8-15-22. NAVSHIPS 0994-001-9010, Bureau of Ships, Navy Department, Washington, DC: Government Printing Office, 1973.

158. Leitch DR. Treatment of air decompression illness in the Royal Navy. In: Davis JC, ed. Treatment of serious decompression sickness and arterial air embolism, a workshop. Bethesda, MD: Undersea Medical Society, 1979:11.

159. Spaur WH. US Navy treatment methods. In: Davis JC, ed. Treatment of serious decompression sickness and arterial air embolism, a workshop. Bethesda, MD: Undersea Medical Society, 1979:25.

160. Van Genderen LV, Waite CL. Evaluation of the rapid recompression–high pressure oxygenation approach to the treatment of traumatic cerebral embolism. Report 519. US Naval Submarine Medical Center, Submarine Base, Groton, CT, 1968.

161. Bornmann RC. Experience with minimal recompression. Oxygen breathing: treatment of decompression sickness and air embolism. Memorandum report project SF0110605, task 11513-2. Washington, DC: Navy Experimental Diving Unit, 1967.

162. Ingvar DH, Adolfson J, Lindemark C. Cerebral air embolism during training of submarine personnel in free escape: an electroencephalographic study. Aerosp Med 1973;44:628–635.

163. Berghage TE, Vorosmarti J Jr, Barnard EEP. Background. In: Davis JC, ed. Treatment of serious decompression sickness and arterial air embolism, a workshop. Bethesda, MD: Undersea Medical Society, 1979:xi.

164. Miller JN, Fagraeus L, Bennett PB, Elliott DH, Shields TG, Grinstad J. Nitrogen-oxygen saturation therapy in serious cases of compressed air decompression sickness. Lancet 1978;1:169–171.

165. Murphy BP, Harford FJ, Cramer FS. Cerebral air embolism resulting from invasive medical procedures: treatment with hyperbaric oxygen. Ann Surg 1985;201:242–245.

166. Mader JT, Hulet WH. Delayed hyperbaric treatment of cerebral air embolism: report of a case. Arch Neurol 1979;36:504–505.

167. Myers RAM. Hyperbaric medicine USA 1986. Jpn J Hyperbaric Med 1987;22:1–15.

Index

Page numbers in *italics* denote figures; those followed by "t" denote tables.